Medical Perspectives on Human Trafficking in Adolescents

Kanani E. Titchen • Elizabeth Miller
Editors

Medical Perspectives on Human Trafficking in Adolescents

A Case-Based Guide

Springer

Editors
Kanani E. Titchen
Division of Adolescent and Young Adult Medicine, Department of Pediatrics
University of California San Diego and Rady Children's Hospital
San Diego, CA
USA

Elizabeth Miller
Children's Hospital of Pittsburgh
Pittsburgh, PA
USA

ISBN 978-3-030-43366-6 ISBN 978-3-030-43367-3 (eBook)
https://doi.org/10.1007/978-3-030-43367-3

This Springer imprint is published by the registered company Springer Nature Switzerland AG
The registered company address is: Gewerbestrasse 11, 6330 Cham, Switzerland

Kanani: For my patients, who teach me more than any textbook or standardized test ever could.

Liz: For the young people who have trusted me with their stories over the years and encouraged me to pursue this healing profession.

Foreword

Though the United States Congress passed the Trafficking Victims Protection Action of 2000 nearly 20 years ago, professionals in communities across the United States often misinterpret or altogether fail to recognize the signs of human trafficking and exploitation right here in our midst. Until recently, many professionals engaged in anti-trafficking work viewed adolescent labor and sex trafficking strictly as an international problem, unaware that precisely the same epidemic was rampant in our own communities. Regrettably, the topic of human trafficking is largely absent from the halls of academia, and students routinely graduate from their programs with little to no education in this area. In their regular course of practice, physicians, like my own mother and her colleagues, provided compassionate care in exam rooms and child advocacy centers to their patients experiencing extreme forms of abuse and trauma but failed to understand the precise form of abuse that was taking place: adolescent labor and sex trafficking. This is a far too common problem. The indicators for human trafficking are routinely missed and classified as domestic violence, familial child sexual abuse, intimate partner violence, or another type of abuse or accidental injury. While those elements might be a part of a patient's experience, forced work or the exchanging of sexual acts for something of value is, indeed, human trafficking. Early research tells us that patients experiencing exploitation are likely to seek medical care while under the control of their traffickers, making professional development for healthcare providers not only strategic but critical.

I, too, became educated about human trafficking in the United States well after I graduated from college. Once I understood the exploitation occurring in my own community, providing trafficking-related professional development to community stakeholders became my full-time passion, and, eventually, community mobilization and capacity building became my full-time vocation. One night, I was called by federal law enforcement to the emergency room at a local hospital to assist with a young woman I had been working with who had been brutally beaten. Before the SANE nurse entered the exam room, the federal agent and I gave the staff a quick crash course on human trafficking. That overview for the staff was critical to ensuring that their approach with the patient would be trauma-informed. Meanwhile, the patient was waiting in the exam room wondering whether or not she should simply leave. Though she had disclosed that she had been trafficked against her will, she had experienced stigma in the past and was deeply fearful that she would be judged, or worse, not believed.

How tragic is it that healthcare providers are mostly reactive in their approach to trafficking survivors? And how many survivors arrive at emergency rooms without the benefit of an advocate and law enforcement by their side? Patients experiencing human trafficking routinely seek medical care, and not exclusively at emergency rooms – they also frequent the offices of neurologists, obstetricians and gynecologists, child abuse pediatricians, and other specialists. All of these professionals provide care to patients experiencing exploitation and, therefore, must be equipped to meet the unique needs of that population appropriately.

Community stakeholders, including healthcare providers, benefit from professional development on the topics of human trafficking and exploitation. Medical professionals across the United States are now learning the signs of exploitation, and what to do when they recognize the indicators. This resource is designed to go beyond simply recognizing the signs of trafficking, to providing compassionate care for patients experiencing trafficking.

The authors of this book are physicians who have consistently offered compassionate care to patients experiencing trafficking, and because of their remarkable care, their patients are returning to them. Providing appropriate, compassionate care to survivors of human trafficking is not simply good bedside manner: it is the necessary intervention. This is what it looks like to be truly victim centered.

Healthcare providers play a critical role in bringing about justice for survivors of human trafficking. Other human service providers, prosecutors, law enforcement, and community-based service providers cannot do this work alone. Human trafficking is one of the most egregious human rights violations of our time, but we are not helpless in the face of it. Knowledge is power, and together we can bring about real hope and exact change. We invite you to learn with us and become an effective, strategic ally in the effort to prevent and combat trafficking in persons.

Washington, DC, USA Heather Fischer

Preface

How do we reduce a person's lived experience – a life lived in four dimensions – to a story reported in two dimensions through ink on a page? When reading these lives and while editing these life stories, these thoughts emerge. How would our own lives be reflected in a case study? How much about us – the nuances of our vocal tone, the subtleties of our gestures and expressions, the biting of our wit, the surprise of our dark humor – would be lost?

How can a survivor crack jokes about her torture? Because she is more than *a survivor*. She is a comedienne, a tree hugger, a fire spinner, a mother, an analyst, a soul sister, a runner, a pianist, a legal advocate, a chocolate-lover.

How can a victim wax rhapsodic about the soap he used that time he was scrubbing blood out of his hair? Because he is more than *a victim*. He is a full flesh-and-blood skateboarder, a brother, a disco dancer, a son, a writer, an athlete, an intellectual, a baker.

Within these pages, we have reduced dozens of people full of character and joie de vivre and desperation and angst and passion into the formulaic Case Study. As healthcare workers and trainees, we learn from the Case Study. We take solace in the predictability of the Case Study. The Case Study presents with this condition to that medical setting. On history, they have X and Y and Z, and their vital signs are within normal limits, and their physical exam reveals A and B and C, and follow-up labs and imaging reveal… and our differential diagnosis includes…

But we recognize that behind this charade of medical detachedness and linear thinking lives and breathes and sweats a human being engaged in life – sometimes desperately surviving – and perhaps caught up in the web of human trafficking. Human trafficking *is* a thing. It is a thing right here in our country, in our state, in our town, and maybe even in our neighborhood.

In the case of this textbook, human trafficking is *the* thing. It is why we've opened the pages of this book and scoured its stories for answers. *What* is human trafficking? What is the difference between trafficking in humans and smuggling humans? What is the difference between sex trafficking and "prostitution"? Between labor trafficking and labor exploitation? How do we acknowledge the victimization and the horrific wrongs done to the victim while we also honor the strength, the resilience, and the phoenix rising in the survivor? Where is the line between being trafficked and doing the trafficking? When is that line blurred? What are the signs of human trafficking? What are the signs of human trafficking in the healthcare setting? When should I report human trafficking? When should I refrain from reporting human trafficking? Where is human trafficking occurring? Where – to which medical settings – are these trafficked persons presenting? Who is being trafficked? Who is doing the trafficking? Who is seeing these patients and treating these patients? Who is *not* seeing these patients but unwittingly treating these patients?

Why is human trafficking happening?

As to the *why*, we cannot adequately address human trafficking without also addressing racism, misogyny, homophobia, transphobia, ableism, and poverty. These are the drivers of enslavement, cruelty, and exploitation. They are concepts and realities beyond the scope of this book… or any one book.

No one person can tackle these Goliaths. No one sector of society can defeat them alone. As Ta-Nehisi Coates has said, enslavement is a *system* [1]. The reality is that human trafficking is a system. It is a system from which many of us benefit: within these chapter narratives, we may recognize in *ourselves* the moral failings of those who we condemn or on whom we take pity. It will take all of us – survivors, policy makers, healthcare professionals, legal advocates, law enforcement, social workers, educators, artists, the tech community, business leaders, entrepreneurs, and others – to address oppression and marginalization in our own communities. We will need the community to show us the way.

Enter the Credible Messenger: "The idea that individuals with shared lived experiences are uniquely suited to teach, support, and guide others through similar challenges can be found across ancient faith traditions and indigenous and tribal cultural practices" [2]. Communities – and people – have within them the capacity for transformation. Life experience can be a guiding force for youth on a path leading toward self-destruction, victimization, and conflict with the justice system.

The Credible Messenger approach has been used in confronting gun violence and gang violence in communities in Chicago, from Phoenix to Philadelphia, and from Baltimore to the Bronx. Two of the key elements that define this model are the identification of perpetrators of violence and the transformation of their assumptions about violence, and the redefining of community norms relating to violence through public education and messaging. The program's integrity is built on the community credibility of its Violence Interrupters, who are selected for their own lived experiences with crime and violence. When implemented with high fidelity to the original model developed by physician Gary Slutkin at the University of Illinois at Chicago, results show that gun violence decreases [3].

Building on this model, who are the credible messengers who can help us identify persons at risk for human trafficking and disrupt and prevent human trafficking? And what is the story we need to tell and the message we want to send?

The most obvious answer is that these credible messengers are the survivors of human trafficking who walk among us – survivors who show victims of human trafficking the path to survivorhood, recovery, and resilience. And indeed, these credible messengers are found within and throughout these pages. They are approximated in the chapter case studies. Their insights spill onto the page in Chapter 19. And they are found as co-authors on various other chapters. Some of these survivors have chosen to reveal themselves as survivors. Still others write as their professional personas or contribute anonymously and *choose* not to wear the title of survivor just now.

All of us who encounter and serve victims and survivors of human trafficking – "allies" if you will – serve as credible messengers to our professional communities. We are the authors of this book and are also found within its pages. Likely we are also the readers of this book. We take our own lived experiences to our colleagues: our missed encounters, our botched attempts to help, our cowardice and fear, our confusion and doubt, our courage in speaking up and showing up, our clarity, our joy at seeing patients rise above their circumstances and break the cycle of human trafficking.

Who will serve as credible messengers for the traffickers and exploiters and buyers of humans?

And once we engage these credible messengers, what will the unifying message be? Trauma beats us down, and in cases of complex trauma and trauma bonds, we repeat the same story hoping against hope for a different outcome. But how do we *reframe* the story? How do we tell the story differently? And by doing so, how do we create a different story? How do we see and realize the world that *could* be in spite of the way that it is?

We get different storytellers.

In this book, we hear from many different storytellers. We walk a fine line between exploiting people for their stories and allowing survivors' voices to be heard. At times, we let data lead the narrative while we also acknowledge the need for more data. We *listen* to the stories of complex trauma and survival and resilience, we acknowledge our own blinders and biases, and we *learn*. And one by one, block by block, and town by town, we change the narrative.

San Diego, CA, USA Kanani E. Titchen

References

1. Fresh Air [Internet]. Philadelphia: NPR; 2019. Ta-Nehisi Coates on Magic and Memory and the Underground Railroad; 2019 September 24 [cited 2019 Oct 2]. Available from: https://www.npr.org/templates/transcript/transcript.php?storyId=763477150
2. http://home2.nyc.gov/html/prob/html/messengering/cm_whatis.shtml Accessed Sep 26, 2019.
3. Butts JA, Roman CG, Bostwick L, Porter JR. Cure Violence: a public health model to reduce gun violence. Annu Rev. Public Health. 2015 Mar 18;36:39–53.doi: https://doi.org/10.1146/annurev-publhealth-031914-122,509.

A Brief Guide to Using this Textbook

We are grateful to the many contributors to this textbook who have enabled us to cover an array of topics relevant to care for trafficked persons, specifically adolescents and young adults. The chapters are arranged to be read chronologically and can also be used as "stand-alone" chapters focused on specific topics relevant to trafficking.

A note on privacy: case presentations are sometimes based on one patient or client known to the authors, and sometimes they are an amalgamation of several different patients or clients. In all cases, the identifying details about trafficked persons who serve as case studies through this book have been changed to protect their privacy.

Regarding nomenclature: in some instances, the authors choose to refer to these individuals as *victims* of human trafficking in an effort to acknowledge the great injustice and harm done to them; at other times, authors refer to these individuals as *survivors* in an effort to honor the strength of each person who has emerged from trafficking. The term *victim-survivor* also is used to illustrate the non-linear path to recovery that each may walk.

A note about redundancies: Some of the chapters may repeat key data elements from previous chapters and refer to the same literature. We have opted to keep many of these redundancies, recognizing that many educators who opt to use this textbook may want to select only one or a few chapters to review with their learners or staff.

There is not enough research to guide every aspect of our clinical practice: the research on human trafficking and the clinical response to care for trafficked persons is still in a nascent stage, with few research studies currently informing this response. Thus, several of the chapters also refer to the same studies, especially related to use of certain assessment tools, and this information may appear in slightly different forms across several chapters.

When relevant, we also direct readers to other chapters in this textbook, to encourage cross-referencing. As the field of research on human trafficking grows, we anticipate that there will be a growing body of evidence that will help to further refine and optimize the healthcare response to young people who have been trafficked.

Pittsburgh, PA, USA Elizabeth Miller
San Diego, CA, USA Kanani E. Titchen

Acknowledgments

We are grateful to so many people who contributed to this work. First and foremost, thank you to our patients and clients who share their lives with us daily and to the many survivors who wanted their stories heard; to the hard-working professionals who donated their time and expertise to this project; and to our publishing team Miranda Finch and Anila Vijayan for their guidance and patience.

Kanani: My teammate Lou; my co-editor Liz– truly a guiding light; my mom, journalist Kathy Titchen; Drs. Eliza Chin, Jordan Greenbaum, Hanni Stoklosa, Makini Chisolm-Straker; Holly Austin Gibbs and the team at Dignity Health; the many patients and survivors who continue to teach me so much; Lori Cohen, Esq.; Caroline Davis; Tracy Harold and the crew at SBH in the Bronx; Montefiore's Division of Adolescent Medicine; GEMS, Bronx Rises Against Gun Violence, Sanctuary for Families, HEAL Trafficking, SD HT & CSEC Advisory Council, and my AMWA-PATH family; and the expert, compassionate teams at the Department of Pediatrics and the Division of Adolescent and Young Adult Medicine at UC San Diego/Rady Children's Hospital.

Liz: My spouse Josh; Kanani, extraordinary co-editor and lead on this work; the many advocates and clinicians named above; Cathy Zimmerman, especially for her mentorship in my early years as I was just learning about trafficking; the anti-trafficking coalitions with whom I've worked in Boston, Sacramento, and Pittsburgh; Brad Orsini; Alison Hall; Julie Evans; Jacki Hoover; Brenda Cassidy; Jocelyn Anderson; Shenoa Williams; Deb Shane; the 412 Youth Zone team (Carol Byers, Leslie Luko-Pitetti, Aimee Plowman, Laura Richardson, and many others); and the wonderfully dedicated team in the Division of Adolescent and Young Adult Medicine, UPMC Children's Hospital.

Contents

Contributors

Alessandra Amato, BS Trafficking in Persons Program, Refugee & Immigrant Center, Asian Association of Utah, Salt Lake City, UT, USA

Elizabeth S. Barnert, MD, MPH, MS Department of Pediatrics, David Geffen School of Medicine at UCLA, Los Angeles, CA, USA

Wendy Barnes, AA Human Trafficking Response Program, Dignity Health, Seattle, WA, USA

Uri Belkind, MD, MS, FAAP, AAHIVS Callen-Lorde Community Health Center, New York, NY, USA

Elizabeth A. Berdan, MD Pediatric Surgery, Mary Bridge Children's Hospital and Health Network, Tacoma, WA, USA

Department of Surgery, University of Washington School of Medicine, Tacoma, WA, USA

Kristina L. Borham, MD Department of Obstetrics and Gynecology, Walter Reed National Military Medical Center, Bethesda, MD, USA

Linda Cahill, MD Butler Center for Children and Families, Department of Pediatrics, Children's Hospital at Montefiore Bronx, New York, NY, USA

Amanda C. Castro, MD Department of Behavioral Health Nemours/A.I. Dupont Hospital for Children, Sidney Kimmel Medical College, Wilmington, DE, USA

Christine Cesa, MAICS Office of Victims of Crime (Expert Consultant), Los Angeles, CA, USA

Tonya Chaffee, MD, MPH Department of Pediatrics, University of California, San Francisco, Teen and Young Adult Health Center, Zuckerberg San Francisco General Hospital, San Francisco, CA, USA

Sarah Chaffin, MD Department, Family Medicine, Dignity Health, Sacramento, CA, USA

Ronald Chambers, MD, FAAFP Department, Family Medicine, Dignity Health, Sacramento, CA, USA

Makini Chisolm-Straker, MD, MPH Department of Emergency Medicine Icahn School of Medicine at Mount Sinai, New York, NY, USA

Catherine G. Coughlin, MD Boston Combined Residency Program, Boston Children's Hospital/Boston Medical Center, Boston, MA, USA

Christine Dipaolo, DNP Department of Pediatrics, Division of Adolescent Medicine Nemours/A.I. duPont Hospital for Children, Sidney Kimmel Medical College at Thomas Jefferson University, Wilmington, DE, USA

Julia Einbond, JD Covenant House New Jersey, Newark, NJ, USA

Abigail English, JD Center for Adolescent Health & the Law, Chapel Hill, NC, USA

Amy Gajaria, MD, FRCPC Department of Psychiatry, University of Toronto, Toronto, ON, Canada

Jack Garden, MD Department of Cardiology, Thomas Jefferson University Hospitals, Philadelphia, PA, USA

Micaela Cayton Garrido, JD, MA Legal Aid Society of Metropolitan Family Services, Chicago, IL, USA

Julia Geynisman-Tan, MD Female Pelvic Medicine and Reconstructive Surgery, Department of Obstetrics and Gynecology, Northwestern University, ERASE Trafficking Clinic, Chicago, IL, USA

Patric Gibbons, MD, MSCI Harvard Affiliated Emergency Medicine Residency, Massachusetts General Hospital/Brigham and Women's Hospital, Boston, MA, USA

Kenneth R. Ginsburg, MD, MS Ed, FSAHM Division of Adolescent Medicine The Children's Hospital of Philadelphia, Perelman School of Medicine at the University of Pennsylvania, Philadelphia, PA, USA

Mollie R. Gordon, MD Menninger Department of Psychiatry and Behavioral Sciences Baylor College of Medicine, Houston, TX, USA

Erik Gray, BA Innovations Human Trafficking Collaborative (Programs Director), Olympia, WA, USA

Jordan Greenbaum, MD Institute on Healthcare and Human Trafficking at the Stephanie V. Blank Center for Safe and Healthy Children, Children's Healthcare of Atlanta, Atlanta, GA, USA

International Centre for Missing and Exploited Children, Alexandria, VA, USA

Selina Higgins, LCSW-R Office of Child Trafficking Prevention and Policy, NYC Administration for Children's Services, New York, NY, USA

Sarah Hofer, MPH Aspirus Wausau Hospital, Wausau, WI, USA

Marisa Hultgren, MS San Diego State University, San Diego, CA, USA

Alison Iannarone, LCSW Covenant House New Jersey, Newark, NJ, USA

Brittany A. Jackson, MD Obstetrics and Gynecology, Capital Women's Care-Division 37, Alexandria, VA, USA

Dana Kaplan, MD Department of Pediatrics, Division of Child Abuse and Neglect, Staten Island University Hospital, Northwell Health, Staten Island, NY, USA

Mikaela A. Kelly, BA Department of Pediatrics, David Geffen School of Medicine at UCLA, Los Angeles, CA, USA

Coleen Kivlahan, MD, MSPH Department of Family & Community Medicine University of California, San Francisco, CA, USA

Miriam Langer, MD Department of Pediatrics, Division of Adolescent Medicine Children's Hospital at Montefiore, Bronx, NY, USA

M. Susan Latuga, MD, MSPH Department of Pediatrics, Division of Neonatology, Children's Hospital at Montefiore, Albert Einstein College of Medicine, Bronx, NY, USA

Hayoung Lee, MD Internal Medicine and Pediatrics, Louisiana State University School of Medicine, New Orleans, LA, USA

Shirley Louis, MD Department of Pediatrics, Division of Neonatology, Children's Hospital at Montefiore, Albert Einstein College of Medicine, Bronx, NY, USA

Michelle Lyman, MD, MPH University of North Carolina Hospitals, Chapel Hill, NC, USA

Marti MacGibbon, CADC-II, ACRPS, CAPMS, I-CADC Office for Victims of Crime (Expert Consultant), Sacramento, CA, USA

Kidian Martinez, LCSW Department of Pediatrics, Division of Adolescent Medicine Nemours/A.I. duPont Hospital for Children, Sidney Kimmel Medical College at Thomas Jefferson University, Wilmington, DE, USA

Sofya Maslyanskaya, MD Department of Pediatrics, Children's Hospital at Montefiore, Bronx, NY, USA

Suleman Masood, BS Subject Matter Expert, Falls Church, VA, USA

Aisha Mays, MD Core Faculty, UC Berkeley/UCSF Joint Medical Program UC, Berkeley School of Public Health, Berkeley, CA, USA

Stephanie Mersch, JD Institute to Address Commercial Sexual Exploitation, Villanova, PA, USA

Elizabeth Miller, MD, PhD, FSAHM Division of Adolescent and Young Adult Medicine, UPMC Children's Hospital of Pittsburgh, University of Pittsburgh, Pittsburgh, PA, USA

Robyn R. Miller, MD Department of Pediatrics, Division of Adolescent Medicine Nemours/A.I. duPont Hospital for Children, Sidney Kimmel Medical College at Thomas Jefferson University, Wilmington, DE, USA

Laura T. Murphy, PhD Helena Kennedy Centre for International Justice, Sheffield Hallam University, Sheffield, UK

Nkemakolem Osian, MPH HIV/AIDS Bureau, Division of Community HIV/AIDS Programs, Health Resources and Services Administration, Rockville, MD, USA

Deborah Ottenheimer, MD Women's Holistic Health Initiative, Harlem United/URAM – The Nest Community Health Center, New York, NY, USA

Nat Paul Bolivar, NY, USA

Mary C. Reissinger, PsyD Menninger Department of Psychiatry and Behavioral Sciences Baylor College of Medicine, Houston, TX, USA

Shea Rhodes, Esq. Institute to Address Commercial Sexual Exploitation, Villanova, PA, USA

Stephanie Richard, Esq. Coalition to Abolish Slavery & Trafficking (CAST), Los Angeles, CA, USA

Rachel A. Robitz, MD Department of Psychiatry and Behavioral Sciences University of California, Davis, Sacramento, CA, USA

Corey J. Rood, MD, FAAP Department of Pediatrics, University of California Irvine School of Medicine, Orange, CA, USA

Nadia E. Saldanha, MD Department of Pediatrics, Division of Adolescent Medicine Hofstra Northwell School of Medicine, Cohen Children's Medical Center Queens, New Hyde Park, NY, USA

Sara Schreiber, LMSW SBH Health System, Bronx, NY, USA

Alexandra G. Shumyatsky Department of Cell Biology and Neuroscience, Rutgers University, Piscataway, NJ, USA

Mary Steigerwald, RN, BA, MBA Departments of Women, Children and Psychiatry, Dignity Health, Phoenix, AZ, USA

Hanni Stoklosa, MD, MPH Department of Emergency Medicine Brigham and Women's Hospital, Boston, MA, USA

Heidi Strickler, PhD, LCSW-S, CEDS, CART, CTLS United Healthcare Community & State, Maryland Heights, MO, USA

Miriam L. Tarrash, MD Department of Obstetrics and Gynecology, Northwell Health at Long Island Jewish Medical Center and North Shore University Hospitals, Queens, NY, USA

Kanani E. Titchen, MD Division of Adolescent and Young Adult Medicine, Department of Pediatrics, University of California San Diego and Rady Children's Hospital, San Diego, CA, USA

Sawan Vaden Community Against Sexual Harm (Program Administrator & Survivor Leader), Sacramento, CA, USA

Natalia Vasquez-Canizares, MD Department of Pediatrics, Division of Rheumatology, Children's Hospital at Montefiore, Albert Einstein College of Medicine, Bronx, NY, USA

Jessica Whitney, MSIS San Diego State University, San Diego, CA, USA

Amy Williamson, MD University of Arizona, Dignity Health Medical Group and Phoenix Children's Hospital, Department of Obstetrics and Gynecology and Pediatric and Adolescent Gynecology, Phoenix, AZ, USA

Chapter 1
Human Trafficking: Definitions, Epidemiology, and Shifting Ground

Patric Gibbons, Makini Chisolm-Straker, and Hanni Stoklosa

Human Trafficking Definitions

Albert Einstein said "If I were given one hour to save the planet, I would spend 59 min defining the problem and one minute resolving it." While this is obviously an extreme example, it emphasizes the necessity of defining problems, as these definitions form a foundation on which solutions can be built. Human trafficking is no exception to this concept. How states, agencies, or institutions successfully serve trafficked persons is rooted in clarity around terminology.

Human trafficking encompasses a broad range of abuses of human rights in which individuals are exploited for any number of purposes, most commonly forced labor or commercial sex. The current definitions of trafficking are based on an international consensus that occurred at the turn of the twenty-first century. At that time, a number of countries and stakeholders ratified the "Palermo Protocols," under the umbrella of the United Nations (UN). The Palermo Protocols were part of a larger effort against transnational organized crime, with one protocol titled "The Protocol to Prevent, Suppress, and Punish Trafficking in Persons, Especially Women and Children." As part of this UN protocol, the international definition for human trafficking was created, which defined it as "the recruitment, transportation, transfer,

P. Gibbons
Harvard Affiliated Emergency Medicine Residency, Massachusetts General Hospital/Brigham and Women's Hospital, Boston, MA, USA

M. Chisolm-Straker (✉)
Department of Emergency Medicine Icahn School of Medicine at Mount Sinai, New York, NY, USA

H. Stoklosa
Department of Emergency Medicine Brigham and Women's Hospital, Boston, MA, USA

K. E. Titchen, E. Miller (eds.), *Medical Perspectives on Human Trafficking in Adolescents*, https://doi.org/10.1007/978-3-030-43367-3_1

harboring or receipt of persons, by means of the threat or use of force or other forms of coercion, of abduction, of fraud, of deception, of the abuse of power or of a position of vulnerability or of the giving or receiving of payments or benefits to achieve the consent of a person having control over another person, for the purpose of exploitation" [1]. Importantly, this definition outlined by the Palermo Protocols divides the definition of trafficking into three key elements: the act, the means, and the purpose. The "act" defines what is done, such as recruitment, transportation, or harboring of persons. The means describes how the act is done, whether it be through force, coercion, or deception. Finally, the purpose describes why the act is done, such as for exploitation via commercial sex, forced labor, and/or for harvesting vital organs.

This three-pronged definition for trafficking outlined by the Palermo Protocol was influential in providing a framework for nations around the world to codify their own definitions of human trafficking. The USA adopted a similarly structured definition in its Trafficking Victims Protection Act (TVPA) of 2000, which describes trafficking in persons as "the recruitment, harboring, transportation, provision, or obtaining of a person through the use of force, fraud, or coercion for the purpose of subjection to involuntary servitude, peonage, debt bondage, or slavery" (22 U.S.C § 7102(9)) [2]. Furthermore, the Trafficking Victims Protection Act states that in cases of commercial sex during which the individual is under the age of 18 years, there need not be any element of "force, fraud, or coercion" for the individual to be considered a victim of sex trafficking. This same age caveat does not apply to labor trafficking [3].

While the TVPA provides a definition at the federal level, there remains variability across US states in how they describe either the act, means, or purpose. For example, Vermont law defines sex trafficking as anyone who "benefits financially" from a venture in which an individual is compelled to perform a commercial sex act [4]. In Ohio, for a case to be considered sex trafficking for those aged 16–17 years, the potential trafficker must be considered one in a "position of authority" over the minor, such as a parent, teacher, or coach [5]. Alabama, Mississippi, and Georgia allow businesses and corporations to be prosecuted for trafficking crimes [4]. Variation in state laws affects the legal determination of trafficking, which in turn affects resources available to assist trafficked persons. In this chapter, the US federal definition of trafficking, inclusive of labor and sex trafficking, is used whenever there is reference to "trafficking" or "human trafficking."

Human Trafficking Epidemiology

Limitations of Statistics

Estimates of human trafficking are limited in their accuracy, and researchers continue to struggle in obtaining precise incidence and prevalence statistics. The challenge in quantifying trafficking is multifactorial. Data on trafficking is partly limited due to a lack of standardization of definitions and protocols [6–10]. Techniques used to understand other hidden populations are utilized in the anti-trafficking research space. These include capture-recapture, multiple systems estimation, network sampling, snowball sampling, and respondent-driven sampling [7]. It is important to note that the diversity in methodological approaches contributes to varying estimates of human trafficking. For example, one may review global prevalence estimates, such as those reported by the International Labor Organization (ILO), and perceive that the number of trafficked persons has grown from about 20 to 40 million people in less than 10 years [11, 12]. However, different methodologies were used to obtain these estimates, meaning these estimates are not directly comparable.

Further compounding the inaccuracy of prevalence estimates is a justified reluctance among trafficked persons to seek assistance for fear of reprisal from traffickers; experience of stigma; or fear of law enforcement, including immigration services, and other authoritative institutions [7, 13]. Unification of definitions, increased cooperation among agencies, more public-private partnerships, triangulation of data, and an increased focus on community-level research—to complement macroscale estimates—will facilitate a better understanding of the scope of trafficking [7].

The above examples delineate the challenges in studying trafficked populations as a whole. Studying trafficked adolescent populations specifically reveals even more limitations. First, recognition of an individual's trafficking experience must occur for their experience to be studied. Unfortunately, many first responders lack adequate training to accurately identify adolescents with a trafficking experience, especially survivors of labor trafficking. Moreover, adolescent trafficked individuals may incorrectly be labeled "prostitutes" or "juvenile delinquents" rather than recognized as survivors of trafficking [14]. Trafficked individuals who are adolescents may be placed in foster homes and relocated away from where they were trafficked, making longitudinal data collection difficult. Finally, analysis is often performed on aggregated trafficking datasets that combine adolescents with young and/or adult populations making it difficult to tease apart trends that are unique to adolescents [14]. In the future, the anti-trafficking movement should dedicate specific research, education, and resources to understanding the adolescent demographic.

Vulnerable Populations

Trafficking affects all regions of the USA, with cases reported in all 50 states and the District of Columbia [15]. While research on human trafficking has its limitations, studies have consistently demonstrated that a number of factors at the societal, community, interpersonal, and individual levels are associated with increased risk of being trafficked. Society's demand for more goods at a cheaper cost, without concern for how these goods are produced, has also been a contributing factor [16, 17]. This has been the case on the North American continent since European arrival and in histories of slavery across the globe; human trafficking, though newly defined, is not a new phenomenon here [18–20]. At the individual level, migrant workers, undocumented immigrants, people of color, and those of lower socioeconomic status continue to be at increased risk for experiencing labor and/or sex trafficking [21, 22].

Adolescents are another vulnerable population with a variety of identities and experiences that may increase their risk of being labor and/or sex trafficked. For example, those with a history of child maltreatment are at increased risk for trafficking. Adolescents who are Native American or Alaskan Native, who have been in foster care, are homeless, or those who are lesbian, gay, bisexual, transgender, or queer (LGBTQ) are disproportionately more vulnerable to experiencing trafficking [17, 23–28]. Runaway youth, young people with low self-esteem, or those with minimal social support are at higher risk for trafficking as well [29–31]. Those with cognitive and/or physical disabilities or who have a history of substance use disorders (SUD) also have an increased vulnerability to trafficking [29, 32]. Unsurprisingly, undocumented unaccompanied and separated migrant youth are also vulnerable to trafficking [13, 33]. This vulnerability is multifactorial, including a combination of systemic oppressions and a young person's lack of adult or community support, lack of respected agency, language barrier (for those who are non-English speaking), and living in precarious legal situations [34, 35].

Shifting Ground in Human Trafficking

Human Trafficking Understood Using a Public Health Framework

The ethos of the anti-trafficking movement is evolving. The movement has slowly expanded its conceptualization of trafficking as a criminal justice matter to an issue that requires a broader, more inclusive public health framework [36]. A public health approach requires multi-sectoral responses, and a critical partner in this movement is the health sector. Medical professionals were an integral part of this early transition to understanding trafficking using public health principles. Clinicians are positioned to recognize trafficked persons when they present to healthcare settings, and they provide such patients with essential care and avenues to seek relevant assistance. However, a public health approach goes one major step beyond this, to focus on supporting survivors' healing *and* on trafficking prevention. Conceptualizing labor and sex trafficking within a social-ecological framework provides the structure to develop meaningful and sustainable primary, secondary, and tertiary prevention strategies[1] to protect groups and individuals who are at higher risk for experiencing trafficking [37]. The Centers for Disease Control and Prevention

[1] Adapted from US Department of Health and Human Services: Administration for Children and Families [37]

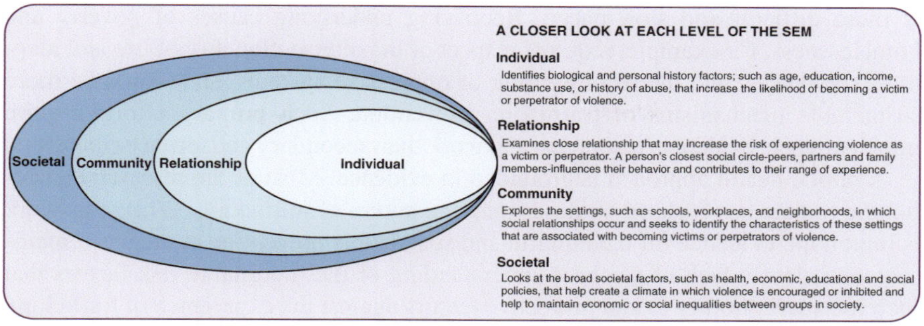

Fig. 1.1 Four-level social-ecological model (SEM) from the CDC. The model identifies risk factors as well as key areas for prevention across a number of levels [38]

(CDC) has applied the social-ecological model (Fig.1.1) to develop prevention practices for other forms of interpersonal violence prevention (e.g., intimate partner violence, youth violence, child maltreatment, etc.). This model suggests intervention across multiple levels for an intersectional anti-trafficking approach; an intersectional framework facilitates more sustainable and meaningful efforts over time than any single strategy or intervention [38].

The social-ecological model can be used to develop meaningful long-term solutions to prevent the trafficking of adolescents and to mitigate the impact of trafficking on adolescents [39]. For example, at the community and individual levels, youth outreach programs, community organizations, and caretakers may focus on populations at high risk for trafficking, such as those with a history of foster care, child maltreatment, or substance use with harm reduction interventions,[2] to mitigate the risk of trafficking [40]. These types of programming represent secondary and tertiary prevention actions. Change at a societal level, leading to primary prevention,

---

Primary prevention stops violence or a problem before it occurs. Strategies focus on strengthening and creating healthy relationships, reducing risks in an individual's environment, rectifying systemic structures that contribute to the problem, and increasing buffers to violence or the problem.

Secondary prevention provides an immediate response to violence or a problem as it happens. This includes basic services and emergency or medical care that address short-term sequelae.

Tertiary prevention practices are long-term responses that occur after violence or a problem occurs, including rehabilitative services (e.g., long-term housing, job training, behavioral counseling, and other supportive services) that seek to prevent or mitigate long-term sequelae and recurrence of the negative experience.

[2] Harm reduction offers people practical means to engage in healthier and/or safer behaviors. Traditionally it has been applied to substance use populations but can be used with those with a trafficking experience too. Harm reduction strategies among trafficked youth can be shared to promote healthy decision-making processes, including how to make risky behaviors less risky (adapted from Hickel and Hallett). For example, for a patient not ready to leave a trafficking situation, regular health appointments for preventive and early intervention healthcare can facilitate continued access to asthma and anti-seizure medications and grow the patient-clinician relationship.

is more difficult and slow-paced. Rectifying underlying causes of poverty and homelessness, for example, requires respect of the intersectionality of life and identity experiences, and the reconfiguring of oppressive systems, and would be more sustainable mechanisms of trafficking prevention. Such primary efforts require more patience, evidence, resources, and work than secondary and tertiary endeavors.

A public health approach is grounded in evidence. Most of the research on trafficking to date has focused on describing the nature of trafficking. While this work is important, evidence for meaningful and sustainable prevention strategies remains scarce as does a lack of a robust understanding of the modifiable risk factors that increase susceptibility to and protective factors against the experience of trafficking [41, 42]. The field also needs more information on how and why others become perpetrators of this kind of interpersonal violence. Future work to expand the evidence base can be accomplished by engaging survivors in design of studies and interventions, enhancing professional collaborations, and standardizing protocols for research and survivor- and community-centered evaluation of best practices.

The importance of the recent anti-trafficking paradigm expansion to a public health framework cannot be overstated. Recognition that prosecution and trafficker imprisonment are insufficient actions to end trafficking has allowed researchers, caretakers, advocates, and policy makers to begin to synthesize a more nuanced and contextualized understanding of human trafficking. The public health framework requires anti-trafficking leaders to consider how racism, inequity, poverty, misogyny, child maltreatment, heteronormativity, xenophobia, and other oppression-based schisms and forms of interpersonal violence are woven into US societal fabric, perpetuating human trafficking. The paradigm expansion has further yielded a movement from a largely reactive response to trafficking into one that is just starting to be proactive. This shift centers on calling attention to root causes of trafficking as well as the human capacity for resilience.

Recognition of Labor Trafficking and the Trafficking of All Genders

The TVPA classified trafficking into labor trafficking or sex trafficking [37]. Since that time, much of the research dedicated to addressing human trafficking has focused on commercial sex and the sex trafficking of women and girls, with a paucity of research dedicated to labor trafficking and the trafficking of other genders (e.g., boys, transgender people, gender nonbinary people) [17, 43].

Labor Trafficking

In particular, child labor trafficking, which includes adolescents, is a frequently neglected and misunderstood form of trafficking. Industries where adolescents are labor trafficked in the USA include domestic servitude, farm work, factory work, janitorial services, health and beauty services, hotel and restaurant (including "fast food") businesses, and illicit drug sales [17, 44, 45]. As previously discussed, reliable estimates for incidence or prevalence rates of adolescent labor trafficking in the USA are unavailable, which hinders the ability to appreciate the true magnitude of the problem [33]. A consistent lack of significant funding for research about labor trafficking poses a barrier. Without research and reporting of labor trafficking, knowledge about people trafficked for labor remains low, leading to a pervasive under-recognition of adolescent labor trafficking by service providers, including health professionals [17, 46–48]. Clinicians may be biased by media portrayals of trafficking, which focus almost entirely on sex trafficking. Practitioners may also find it challenging to tease apart differences between violations of child labor law and human trafficking. Further complicating the issue, child labor laws vary by state and are often based upon age, school attendance, and labor sector criteria; clinicians are not trained to be experts here. Labor trafficking, in contrast to labor law violations, is based on the presence of force, fraud, or coercion, but clinicians are not yet systematically trained on this either [14, 49, 50]. Furthermore, labor trafficked adolescents may not be aware of their rights or even that a situation is exploitative. They may be compelled to work in illicit or legal industries and fear reporting their exploitation due to reasonable concerns for arrest or deportation. Additionally, datasets often aggregate labor trafficking with sex trafficking, and labor trafficking-specific initiatives tend to focus primarily on adults [14, 17].

Boys and TGNB Adolescents

Research on trafficking of boys and transgender and gender nonbinary (TGNB) adolescents is both limited and inconsistent throughout the current literature. For example, some studies and reports demonstrate mostly girls experiencing labor trafficking, while others show mostly boys are affected by labor trafficking. This apparent discrepancy could be due to regional variation in trafficking trends or may be a product of study design reflecting a bias against the recognition of boys as experiencing sex trafficking or trafficking at all [49, 51]. A systemic lack of awareness of trafficking of boys yields a deficiency of services for these survivors [52]. Furthermore, research about trafficking of boys is often aggregated with adults, making it difficult to isolate factors specific to this younger population that might increase vulnerability [17]. Very few studies have specifically examined TGNB adolescent trafficking experiences, but existing data indicate that being TGNB may be a risk factor for being trafficked [see Chap. 11] [29].

The under-recognition of labor trafficking and trafficking overall impacting those other than cis-girls[3] has hindered the creation of relevant evidence-based approaches to trafficking prevention efforts, the development of trafficking response

[3] Use of the term "cis" before a gender denotes the person's present gender identity is the same as the gender that was assigned to them at birth.

programs, and methodologically rigorous estimates. Since 2010, significant strides have been made in educating social workers, law enforcement, and healthcare professionals on trafficking recognition, but again these efforts have focused mostly on sex trafficking. This has allowed for an increase (albeit inconsistent) in the recognition of girls and women with sex trafficking experience and in their connections to resources [53]. Since 2010, an increased number of initiatives have used research for evidence-based policy change [54]. Moving forward, a comprehensive anti-trafficking approach that includes labor trafficking and survivors of all genders is essential.

Recognition and Inclusion of Survivor Leadership

The majority of researchers and policy makers are not survivors of trafficking. This bears repeating: The majority of researchers and policy makers are *not* survivors of trafficking. Therefore, prevailing literature (including this chapter), policies, and interventions frequently lack the needed perspectives of survivors [55]. If the voices of survivors continue to be marginalized by scholars, researchers, and policy makers, anti-trafficking efforts *will* fail. Minh Dang, co-founder of Survivor Alliance, eloquently wrote, "For non-survivors, their knowledge is limited through the lived experience of studying slavery from the outside looking in. For survivors of slavery, their knowledge is limited by the experience of being on the inside, looking out" [55]. A trafficking survivor may live under threats of death or physical harm and may experience powerful psychological coercion. Should non-survivors presume to know the complexity of the cognitive and emotional transformations of this experience? Can programmers effectively design interventions without understanding these experiences? Lived experience is an expertise this movement cannot do without. Nonacademic survivors are often engaged by the academic field to "share experiences" and use their stories to raise awareness [56]. These perspectives are important, but only inviting survivors to tell their trafficking story minimizes survivors' ability to contribute to the anti-trafficking movement, encourages voyeurism, and enables non-survivors to occupy space that is not theirs to occupy. Survivors should not be outside looking in. Actors in the anti-trafficking movement must recognize survivors' ability to meaningfully teach, effect anti-trafficking policy change, develop social service programming, and engage in research with non-survivor colleagues [55]. This is not the fight of non-survivors; nor can it be the fight of survivors, alone. In the brilliant words of Lilla Watson, "If you have come here to help me, you are wasting your time. But if you have come because your liberation is bound up with mine, then let us work *together* [emphasis added]."

Survivor leadership remains scarce in the academic arena, and trafficked young people are especially ignored [3]. Trafficked youth are often considered to be lacking the necessary self-determination of adults. Those caring for adolescent survivors often default to acting in the child's "best interest" without meaningfully and respectfully engaging the child [3]. The "best interest" principle, while well-intentioned, neglects the capacity of the minor to participate in the decision-making process [3, 57]. Adolescents may be vulnerable, but they are not helpless [58]. Practitioners, caretakers, and policy makers must respect the incredible survival skills and the resilience of these young people; adults must encourage the self-efficacy of young people as the foundation of their paths to recovery and (re)integration into mainstream society.

Actions to increase survivor contribution to academic research include budgeting for survivor participation in study design, implementation, analysis, and interpretation, as well as subject participation, and hiring survivor leaders to teach non-survivors how to substantively incorporate survivors into research or policy ventures [55]. Non-survivors should also be aware of how their own assumptions and lived experiences influence data collection and interpretation. They must ask themselves, and survivors, how research projects can be constructed so that projects are founded on the voices of survivors [55]. The culture of academic research must shift to engage with survivors as peer scholars. By expanding the number of survivor scholars, a more complete understanding of trafficking will be unearthed.

In summary, definitions of trafficking in the USA, which were shaped by international colleagues, guide the current framework of anti-trafficking efforts today. While more is understood about the scope and nature of trafficking today than when trafficking was defined in 2000, labor trafficked and non-female adolescent populations remain marginalized in research and the general anti-trafficking response in the USA. Using a public health approach to actively engage adolescent health professionals, coupled with meaningful partnerships with survivors, will be critical in genuinely turning the tide of trafficking and exploitation of adolescents in this country.

References

1. United Nations Convention against Transnational Organized Crime and the protocols thereto. Palermo, Italy: United Nations Office on Drugs and Crime; 2000.
2. The United States Department of Justice. Human trafficking [Internet]. 2019 [cited 2019 Jan 4]. Available from: https://www.justice.gov/humantrafficking.
3. Goździak EM. Forced victims or willing migrants? Contesting assumptions about child trafficking. In: Seeberg ML, Goździak EM, editors. Contested childhoods: growing up in migrancy. Cham: Springer; 2016. p. 23–41.
4. National Conference of State Legislators. Human trafficking state laws [Internet]. 2019 [cited 2019 Jan 5]. Available from: http://www.ncsl.org/research/civil-and-criminal-justice/human-trafficking-laws.aspx.
5. Ohio Human Trafficking Task Force. Overview of state and federal trafficking laws [Internet]. 2019 [cited 2019 Jan 5]. Available from: http://humantrafficking.ohio.gov/links/Anti-Trafficking-Laws.pdf.
6. Farrell A, Pfeffer R. Policing human trafficking: cultural blinders and organizational barriers. Ann Am Acad Pol Soc Sci. 2014;653:46–64.
7. Brunner J. Inaccurate numbers, inadequate policies: enhancing data to evaluate the prevalence of human trafficking in ASEAN. East-West Center; 2015.

8. Farrell A, McDevitt J, Fahy S. Where are all the victims? Understanding the determinants of official identification of human trafficking incidents. Criminol Public Policy. 2010;9:201–33.
9. Newton PJ, Mulcahy TM, Martin SE. Finding victims of human trafficking. Bethesda, MD: University of Chicago, National Opinion Research Center; 2008.
10. Wilson DG, Walsh WF, Kleuber S. Trafficking in human beings: training and services among US law enforcement agencies. Police Pract Res. 2006;7:149–60.
11. Global estimates of modern slavery: Forced labour and forced marriage. Geneva, Switzerland: International Labour Organization; 2017.
12. ILO global estimate of forced labour: Results and methodology. Geneva, Switzerland: International Labour Organization; 2012.
13. Child labor trafficking. Washington, D.C.: Office of Juvenile Justice and Delinquency Prevention; 2016.
14. Kaufka WK. Child labor trafficking in the United States: a hidden crime. SI. 2017;5:59.
15. 2015 NHTRC annual report: National Human Trafficking Hotline [Internet]. 2016 [cited 2019 Sep 25]. Available from: https://humantraffickinghotline.org/resources/2015-nhtrc-annual-report.
16. Chon KY, Khorana S. Moving forward: next steps in preventing and disrupting human trafficking. In: Chisolm-Straker M, Stoklosa H, editors. Human trafficking is a public health issue: a paradigm expansion in the United States. Cham: Springer International Publishing; 2017. p. 415–41.
17. Greenbaum J, Bodrick N, Committee on Child Abuse and Neglect, Section on International Child Health. Global human trafficking and child victimization. Pediatrics. 2017;140.
18. Zinn H. A people's history of the United States: 1492-present. Routledge; 2015.
19. Reséndez A. The other slavery: the uncovered story of Indian enslavement in America. New York: Houghton Mifflin Harcourt; 2016.
20. Warren W. New England bound: slavery and colonization in early America. New York: Liverwright Publishing Corporation; 2016.
21. Banks D, Kyckelhahn T. Characteristics of suspected human trafficking incidents, 2008–2010. US Department of Justice, Office of Justice Programs, Bureau of Justice Statistics: Washington, D.C; 2011.
22. The Joint Commission. Quick Safety 42: Identifying human trafficking victims [Internet]. 2018 [cited 2019 Mar 27]. Available from: https://www.jointcommission.org/issues/article.aspx?Article=Dtpt66QSsiI%2fHRkIecKTZPAbn6jexdUPHflBjJ%2fD8Qc%3d#.
23. Pember MA. Mapping the market for sex: New report details Minneapolis sex trade [Internet]. 2014 [cited 2019 Mar 27]. Available from: https://newsmaven.io/indiancountrytoday/archive/mapping-the-market-for-sex-new-report-details-minneapolis-sex-trade-H0pAGc00cE-qXKjqZ2j-deQ/.
24. Sweet V. Trafficking in native communities [Internet]. National Council of Juvenile and Family Court Judges Newsletter. 2015 [cited 2019 Mar 27]. Available from: https://www.ncjfcj.org/resource-library/publications/synergy-vol-18-no-1.
25. Estes R. The commercial sexual exploitation of children' ' in the U.S., Canada and Mexico. Philadelphia, PA: University of Pennsylvania, School of Social Work, Center for the Study of Youth Policy; 2001.
26. Tyler KA, Hoyt DR, Whitbeck LB, Cauce AM. The impact of childhood sexual abuse on later sexual victimization among runaway youth. J Research Adolescence. 2001;11:151–76.
27. Whitbeck LB, Chen X, Hoyt DR, Tyler KA, Johnson KD. Mental disorder, subsistence strategies, and victimization among gay, lesbian, and bisexual homeless and runaway adolescents. J Sex Res. 2004;41:329–42.
28. Ahrens KR, Katon W, McCarty C, Richardson LP, Courtney ME. Association between childhood sexual abuse and transactional sex in youth aging out of foster care. Child Abuse Negl. 2012;36:75–80.
29. Chisolm-Straker M, Sze J, Einbond J, White J, Stoklosa H. A supportive adult may be the difference in homeless youth not being trafficked. Child Youth Serv Rev. 2018;91:115–20.

30. Guidance to states and services on addressing human trafficking of children and youth in the United States. Washington, D.C.: U.S. Department of Health and Human Services, Administration for Children, Youth and Families; 2013.
31. Clawson HJ, Dutch N, Solomon A, Grace LG. Human trafficking into and within the United States: a review of the literature. Office of the Assistant Secretary for Planning and Evaluation, U.S. Department of Health and Human Services: Washington, D.C; 2009.
32. Middleton JS, Gattis MN, Frey LM, Roe-Sepowitz D. Youth experiences survey (YES): exploring the scope and complexity of sex trafficking in a sample of youth experiencing homelessness. J Soc Serv Res. 2018;44:141–57.
33. United Nations. International migration report. New York, NY: United Nations; 2017.
34. Chester H, Lummert N, Mullooly A. Child victims of human trafficking: Outcomes and service adaptation within the U.S. Unaccompanied Refugee Minor programs [Internet]. 2015 [cited 2019 Sep 24]. Available from: http://www.socialserviceworkforce.org/resources/child-victims-human-trafficking-outcomes-and-service-adaptation-within-us-unaccompanied.
35. Zhang SX. Looking for a hidden population: trafficking of migrant laborers in San Diego County. San Diego, CA: San Diego State University; 2012.
36. Chisolm-Straker M, Stoklosa H, editors. Human trafficking is a public health issue: a paradigm expansion in the United States. Cham: Springer International Publishing; 2017.
37. Information memorandum definitions and principles to inform human trafficking prevention. U.S. Department of Health and Human Services Administration for Children and Families, Office on Trafficking in Persons; 2019.
38. The social-ecological model: A framework for prevention [Internet]. Centers for Disease Control and Prevention. 2015 [cited 2019 Sep 25]. Available from: https://www.cdc.gov/violenceprevention/publichealthissue/social-ecologicalmodel.html.
39. Macias-Konstantopoulos W. Human trafficking: the role of medicine in interrupting the cycle of abuse and violence. Ann Intern Med. 2016;165:582–8.
40. Hickle K, Hallett S. Mitigating harm: considering harm reduction principles in work with sexually exploited young people. Child Soc. 2016;30:302–13.
41. Kiss L, Zimmerman C. Human trafficking and labor exploitation: toward identifying, implementing, and evaluating effective responses. PLoS Med. 2019;16:e1002740.
42. Rothman EF, Stoklosa H, Baldwin SB, Chisolm-Straker M, Kato Price R, Atkinson HG, et al. Public health research priorities to address US human trafficking. Am J Public Health. 2017;107:1045–7.
43. Oram S, Stöckl H, Busza J, Howard LM, Zimmerman C. Prevalence and risk of violence and the physical, mental, and sexual health problems associated with human trafficking: systematic review. PLoS Med. 2012;9:e1001224.
44. Chisolm-Straker M, Sze J, Einbond J, White J, Stoklosa H. Screening for human trafficking among homeless young adults. Child Youth Serv Rev. 2019;98:72–9.
45. National Human Trafficking Hotline. Labor trafficking [Internet]. 2019 [cited 2019 Apr 1]. Available from: https://humantraffickinghotline.org/type-trafficking/labor-trafficking.
46. Making progress against child labour: Global estimates and trends 2000-2012. Geneva, Switzerland: International Labour Organization. p. 2013.
47. National Research Council. Confronting commercial sexual exploitation' ' and sex trafficking of minors in the United States. 2013.
48. Stransky M, Finkelhor D. How many juveniles are involved in prostitution in the U.S.? Durham, NH: Crimes Against Children Research Center, University of New Hampshire; 2008.
49. Owens C, Dank M, Breaux J, Bañuelos I, Farrell A, Pfeffer R, et al. Understanding the organization, operation, and victimization process of labor trafficking in the United States. Washington, D.C: Urban Institute; 2014.
50. Atkinson HG, Curnin KJ, Hanson NC. U.S. state laws addressing human trafficking: education of and mandatory reporting by health care providers and other professionals. Journal of Human Trafficking. 2016;2:111–38.

51. Turner-Moss E, Zimmerman C, Howard LM, Oram S. Labour exploitation and health: a case series of men and women seeking post-trafficking services. J Immigr Minor Health. 2014;16:473–80.
52. Friedman S, Willis B. And boys too: An ECPAT-USA discussion paper about the lack of recognition of the commercial sexual exploitation of boys in the United States. Brooklyn, NY: End Child Prostitution and Trafficking (ECPAT-USA); 2013.
53. Brennan D. Life interrupted: trafficking into forced labor in the United States: Duke University Press; 2014.
54. Miller CL, Lyman M. Research informing advocacy: an anti-human trafficking tool. In: Chisolm-Straker M, Stoklosa H, editors. Human trafficking is a public health issue: a paradigm expansion in the United States. Cham: Springer; 2017. p. 293–307.
55. Dang M. Epistemology of survival: a working paper. University of Nottingham, Rights Lab; 2019.
56. Dang M. Survivors are Speaking. Are we Listening? The Global Slavery Index [Internet]. 2019 [cited 2019 Apr 12]. Available from: https://www.globalslaveryindex.org/resources/essays/survivors-are-speaking-are-we-listening.
57. Connor B. In loco Aequitatis: the dangers of "Safe Harbor" Laws for youth in the sex trades. Stanf J Civ Rights Civ Liberties. 2016:12.
58. Iman J, Fullwood C, Paz N, Daphne W, Hassan S. "Girls do what they have to do to survive: illuminating methods used by girls in the sex trade and street economy to fight back and heal: a participatory research study of resilience and resistance." Young Women's Empowerment Project; 2009.

Chapter 2
Adolescent Medicine: Physical and Neurocognitive Development

Elizabeth Miller and Kenneth R. Ginsburg

Physical and Physiologic Changes

The emergence of secondary sexual characteristics is the most obvious aspect of pubertal development. Youth develop at highly variable rates. There is a wide range of what is normal in terms of age that physical changes start to happen (such as onset of menses) and at what pace. Pubertal changes that are still within the normal range can start as early as 8 years of age among females and as late as 14 years among males. Youth who experience physical maturity earlier than most of their peers or who develop later than their peers each have their unique struggles. A young person who has developed secondary sexual characteristics early (such as breast development) may be especially vulnerable to sexual abuse and trafficking, as these children appear older while they are cognitively and emotionally still young.

Chronic medical conditions, deprivation, and maltreatment all impact typical pubertal development. As discussed in subsequent chapters, disordered eating, substance use, and malnutrition can all contribute to changes in the hypothalamic-pituitary-gonad axis, which can result in weight loss and secondary amenorrhea. Onset of pubertal changes and slow growth can also be associated with such chronic stressors. However, there is also a growing body of research on the impact of childhood abuse (specifically sexual abuse) on early menarche [1, 2]. The neuroendocrine pathways for this finding remain unclear. This may be one additional mechanism for how exposure to childhood sexual abuse (commonly seen among

E. Miller (✉)
Division of Adolescent and Young Adult Medicine, UPMC Children's Hospital of Pittsburgh, University of Pittsburgh, Pittsburgh, PA, USA

K. R. Ginsburg
Division of Adolescent Medicine The Children's Hospital of Philadelphia, Perelman School of Medicine at the University of Pennsylvania, Philadelphia, PA, USA

K. E. Titchen, E. Miller (eds.), *Medical Perspectives on Human Trafficking in Adolescents*, https://doi.org/10.1007/978-3-030-43367-3_2

youth who have been trafficked) may increase likelihood of early pubertal maturation, thus further increasing vulnerability to sexual violence (including exploitation) in adolescence.

Cognitive, Emotional, and Identity Development

A review of the many theories from the last century about adolescent development is beyond the scope of this chapter. Readers may find texts related to adolescence and adolescent health, typical development, and strategies to foster resilience helpful [3, 4]. Similar to physical development, cognitive and emotional development also occur at a highly individualized and varied pace.

Several key points are relevant for the care of youth who have been trafficked:

1. Certain developmental characteristics may increase vulnerability for trafficking. Youth who face challenging circumstances such as homelessness or needing to provide care for younger siblings may be forced to develop more quickly than their peers of similar age. These "adultified" youth may perceive that they are older and more mature than their actual age (and this may be reinforced by adult caregivers in their lives), and thus they may be susceptible to traffickers who use comments about the young person's "maturity" and "no one else understands you" as strategies to seduce young people [5]. Healthcare professionals should consistently keep a developmental framework in mind as they interact with youth, as a young person may display tremendous insight for certain situations and severe emotional immaturity in other contexts.
2. Intellectual impairment is a significant risk factor for being trafficked. Reasons for such intellectual impairment are myriad including genetics, exposure to substances in utero, poverty and limited access to educational opportunities in early childhood, exposure to maltreatment and lack of stimulation, and traumatic brain injury [5]. Traffickers will specifically seek out youth with intellectual impairment as an easy target to control [6]. As intellectual impairment can also manifest with externalizing behaviors such as inattention, hyperactivity, aggression, and emotional outbursts, such impairment often can be misdiagnosed as a mental health problem. While there is a growing recognition of intellectual disabilities among youth who are caught in the juvenile justice or child welfare systems, there is still significant advocacy needed to ensure that youth who have had exposures to adversities (including trafficking) should have a more thorough neuropsychiatric evaluation as part of treatment.
3. Identity development is a particularly salient task during adolescence. Trying to figure out who one is and who one wants to become is critical to the transition into adulthood. Young people can seem to have settled on a fixed identity one moment ("I'm going to be a model") and then drastically change their mind the next ("I hate models"). For young people living in unstable situations (such as experiencing homelessness) that increase their likelihood for trafficking, the

usual task of trying out different identities may feel unsafe and scary. Some youth may adopt more "fixed" identities than they are ready to assume, due to the environment feeling unsafe for more explorations [7]. Experiences of homelessness, racism, and other forms of discrimination can profoundly influence identity development, leading to harmful internalizing of negative stereotypes [8].

The Developing Adolescent Brain

Some of the most exciting developments in adolescent health research in recent years have emerged from modern imaging techniques that allow much more detailed perspectives on how adolescents' brains are changing over time and responding to different stimuli. While a comprehensive review is well beyond the scope of this chapter, there are some key points to underscore from this research:

- Historically, we have assumed (too simplistically) that adolescents do not have developed frontal lobes and therefore have poor impulse control. More recent research has identified that by the time puberty occurs, adolescents do have a brain structure similar to adults [9]. Adolescence is a time for pruning and fine-tuning these networks, but the key ingredients are already there.
- The ability to exert cognitive control continues to improve as adolescents transition to adulthood [9]. The brain is working on fine-tuning and integrating the various components needed for cognitive control throughout adolescence and well into young adulthood (into the mid- to late-20s) – these include inhibitory control (being able to inhibit an impulse to do something), performance monitoring (being able to reflect on a behavior as it is happening), and working memory (being able to hold information about what is going on in one's surroundings temporarily for processing and to guide decision-making).
- Unique changes in brain structure as maturation occurs support interactions between various parts of the brain (specifically the dopaminergic and GABAergic systems) which helps the whole brain network to synchronize better and to be able to fine-tune "signal-to-noise" ratio (the ability to focus on what's important).
- Over time, the specialization and strengthening of connectivity in networks supports the transition to adult levels of cognitive control [10].
- Adolescent developmental neuroscience is finding that this dynamic period from early puberty to young adulthood is an "adaptive period" during which time high levels of experience seeking are necessary to help encourage brain systems to "learn" and to improve cognitive control [11]. Specifically, adolescent brains are particularly "turned on" to rewards (increased sensation seeking and reward seeking behaviors as well as goal-directed activity). This increase in dopamine sensitivity appears to support early adolescents to try new things, explore the world, and take risks – all necessary from a developmental perspective.
- While there are differences by developmental stages, across middle and later adolescence and into adulthood, the number of dopamine receptors decreases

and is distributed away from the reward and behavior pathways. This means over time there is greater cognitive control over the reward seeking behaviors. Given this difference in pace of development between two processes – reactivity and regulation – healthcare professionals can keep in mind that youth in early- and mid-adolescence especially may need more physical space and strategies to calm themselves to regain control over some of the impulsivity [12]. These are skills that can be learned.

- Environmental contexts and social experiences such as nutrition, exercise, trauma, poverty, discrimination, and education are all associated with changes in the structure and function of the brain and how white and gray matters are organized. *These findings, however, never should imply that adolescents who have experienced trauma have "damaged" brains.*
- The limbic system, the part of the brain that generates emotions and arousal, has been particularly well-developed in the context of chronic or toxic stress [13]. The amygdala within the limbic system processes emotional responses (such as fear, anxiety, anger, and aggression). When trauma and violence (especially chronic adversities) have necessitated constantly needing to be hypervigilant about new dangers, the amygdala may be particularly dominant and "fire" its signals readily.
- Understanding how stress activates different parts of the brain is key to understanding behavior and a person's ability to self-regulate and make wise decisions in stressful moments. For youth who have grown up with chronic adversity, their level of sensitivity to threats may be acutely high, and they may perceive new interactions that are not true dangers as threats. Those perceived threats produce the same biological response. In a youth whose stress load is high, connections with the "thinking brain" are disconnected, leading to emotional, cognitive, social, and prosocial dysregulation.
- When a young person does not have their basic needs met or, worse, experiences the world as an unpredictable and dangerous place, their brain may be wired to remain hypervigilant and reactive to perceived threats (however significant or not) and will take longer to calm down. *And they can settle in the context of safe, supportive relationships that help them develop skills necessary for self-regulation.*
- Safety is a critical ingredient for being able to integrate learning from the environment. Calm, safe communication promotes self-regulation in a young person. Maintaining a consistent safe space for interaction assures the "fired-up" amygdala (the emotional processing part of the brain) that there is no danger and allows for more wise decision-making and planning.
- The pace of development varies tremendously from child to child and is deeply influenced by the interactions and environments in which they have developed. By recognizing that the brain is continuing to fine-tune and refine itself over time into young adulthood, advocates for trafficked youth may be better equipped to build programs that are safe, supportive, and nurturing while providing enough scaffolding for youth to make their own decisions about safety and life goals.

While understanding the brain science is critical for informing best practices in supporting young people, health professionals should remain vigilant about how the emerging research on the adolescent brain may be misinterpreted or misused. Adolescents are not "unfinished" or incomplete. In particular, adolescents who have experienced trauma (as described in subsequent chapters) may certainly have behavioral challenges from emotion regulation, poor attachment, hypervigilance, and self-harm. Simply because the brain science shows changes in the adolescent brain in the context of abuse, this does not mean that the brain cannot heal or continue to develop. In fact, the latest developmental neuroscience underscores that adolescence is a time of tremendous growth and potential, of incredible neuroplasticity. This is a time when healthy environments are beneficial and critical for brain development – safe schools, good nutrition, sufficient sleep, absence of substances, and so forth. This research then can support advocacy for creating more safe environments for adolescents and young adults. Health professionals can model having high expectations for all youth and advocate to ensure resources are available to meet and exceed those expectations.

Among our roles in guiding youth toward adulthood is to have them learn to self-regulate and gain self-control. This is vital for every young person's developmental path. As youth who have hard lives have also been wired for hypervigilance, their tendency to scan their environment for safety, or lack thereof, can make them more volatile and less focused. As health professionals and advocates for youth, we must strive to create safe environments combined with sustained relationships which will enable them to reveal their best selves.

Developmental Considerations and the Clinical Encounter

Assessing the developmental stage of a young person who may be trafficked or at risk for trafficking is both challenging and critical. Healthcare professionals need to remember that young people may have significant difficulty disclosing what is going on, may not recognize the current situation as abnormal, and have limited ability to describe specific symptoms as well as their medical history. Asking young people to only share what they feel comfortable sharing, using easy-to-understand language and asking for verbal feedback to ensure comprehension, and use of visual cues (including drawings) to explain a clinical problem that needs treatment and why (such as pelvic inflammatory disease) are among the strategies healthcare professionals can use to offer youth-centered, developmentally relevant care.

Developmental Considerations with Child Abuse Reporting Requirements

Healthcare professionals' requirements for involving child protective services and law enforcement in situations of abuse of minors including trafficking vary across states, territories, and tribes. This means that healthcare professionals need to know who they can reach out to in their region for guidance. This includes building formal partnerships with victim service advocates who are able to support youth while simultaneously navigating complex social service and judicial systems.

Healthcare professionals should have a low threshold for notifying authorities regarding concerns about trafficking so that a "paper trail" is created for a young person living in vulnerable social circumstances with the goal of increasing access to supportive services and safety. This needs to be balanced with building a trusting relationship with that young person and strengthening the therapeutic alliance. The child welfare and juvenile justice systems are often imperfect and under-resourced with staff who may not have had adequate training in youth development much less trafficking. This means that healthcare professionals should (whenever possible) invite a young person to complete a call to child protective services and/or law enforcement together, so that the young person has an opportunity to discuss ways to increase their options for safety.

Healthcare professionals must also explain "reporting" in easy-to-understand terms for their patients who are minors as young people will often assume they are being "reported" because they have done something wrong. Healthcare professionals should consider phrasing that is nonjudgmental such as "Sometimes the situations that young people are experiencing are more than even a professional adult like me can manage alone, and I am required to pull in other experts to help keep young people safe." Most importantly, offering options and choices throughout the health encounter will allow a clinician to engage the young person as an active partner in their healthcare visit, build rapport, and give the clinician a better understanding of where this young person is developmentally (See Chap. 18 for more discussion of mandatory reporting requirements and medicolegal aspects of trafficking).

In summary, the dynamic physiologic changes of adolescence combined with rapid emotional, cognitive, and social development during adolescence mean that differences in where a young person is developmentally will influence their understanding and insights about what is happening to them and their willingness to engage in treatment and services. Healthcare professionals will benefit from remembering that adolescents develop at different paces and that exposures to adversities influence adolescents differently. While the developing adolescent brain may be particularly vulnerable to trauma and exposure to substances, the plasticity of the adolescent brain and resiliency of young people offer immense opportunity to support young people to envision a different and more hopeful future for themselves.

References

1. Boynton-Jarrett R, Wright RJ, Putnam FW, Lividoti Hibert E, Michels KB, Forman MR, et al. Childhood abuse and age at menarche. J Adolesc Health. 2013;52:241–7.
2. Henrichs KL, McCauley HL, Miller E, Styne DM, Saito N, Breslau J. Early menarche and childhood adversities in a nationally representative sample. Int J Pediatr Endocrinol. 2014;2014:14.

3. Reaching Teens Strength-Based Communication Strategies To Build Resilience and Support Healthy Adolescent Development. Edited by Kenneth R. Ginsburg and Sara B. Kinsman. 2014. American Academy of Pediatrics.
4. Neinstein LS, Katzman DK, Callahan T, Gordon CM, Joffe A, Rickert V, editors. Neinstein's adolescent and young adult health care: a practical guide (Adolescent health care a practical guide). 6th ed: LWW; 2016.
5. National Research Council. Confronting commercial sexual exploitation and sex trafficking of minors in the United States. 2013.
6. Trafficking of Persons with Disabilities in the United States. The Human Trafficking Legal Center.
7. Chapter 12 - Interventions for Identity Issues [Internet]. [cited 2019 Sep 25]. Available from: https://keck.usc.edu/adolescent-trauma-training-center/treatment-guide/chapter-12-interventions-for-identity-issues/.
8. Trent M, Dooley DG, Dougé J, Section on Adolescent Health, Council on Community Pediatrics, Committee on Adolescence. The impact of racism on child and adolescent health. Pediatrics. 2019;144:e20191765.
9. Luna B, Marek S, Larsen B, Tervo-Clemmens B, Chahal R. An integrative model of the maturation of cognitive control. Annu Rev Neurosci. 2015;38:151–70.
10. Larsen B, Luna B. Adolescence as a neurobiological critical period for the development of higher-order cognition. Neurosci Biobehav Rev. 2018;94:179–95.
11. Murty VP, Calabro F, Luna B. The role of experience in adolescent cognitive development: integration of executive, memory, and mesolimbic systems. Neurosci Biobehav Rev. 2016;70:46–58.
12. Romer D. Adolescent risk taking, impulsivity, and brain development: implications for prevention. Dev Psychobiol. 2010;52:263–76.
13. Herman JP, Ostrander MM, Mueller NK, Figueiredo H. Limbic system mechanisms of stress regulation: hypothalamo-pituitary-adrenocortical axis. Prog Neuro-Psychopharmacol Biol Psychiatry. 2005;29:1201–13.

Chapter 3
Human Rights and Human Trafficking of Adolescents: Legal and Clinical Perspectives

Abigail English and Coleen Kivlahan

Introduction

When young people are victimized by human trafficking—for labor or for sex—their human rights are violated in profound ways. The health effects of trafficking are serious and often result in long-term consequences which are human rights violations in themselves. Some trafficked adolescents are subjected to mistreatment so severe that it amounts to torture. Thus, the role of healthcare professionals in addressing the human trafficking of adolescents and young adults is a critical one. Healthcare professionals can work to identify youth engaged in human trafficking, provide trauma-informed care for survivors, and act as advocates to support the human rights of young people through prevention and treatment. The purpose of this chapter is to illuminate the ways in which young people's human rights are violated when they are trafficked, explain the legal protections that exist for their human rights, and describe the key role healthcare professionals can play as clinicians and as advocates in responding to human trafficking of youth.

There is no fixed age-based definition of the term "adolescent" in law, medicine, or public health. In law, the critical distinction is between "minors"—who are generally under the age of 18—and adults, who are age 18 or older. In medicine and public health, the age ranges vary among governmental entities and nongovernmental organizations (NGOs). The World Health Organization (WHO), for example, defines "adolescents" as individuals in the 10–19-year age group, "youth" as ages

A. English
Center for Adolescent Health & the Law, Chapel Hill, NC, USA

C. Kivlahan (✉)
Department of Family & Community Medicine University of California, San Francisco, CA, USA

K. E. Titchen, E. Miller (eds.), *Medical Perspectives on Human Trafficking in Adolescents*, https://doi.org/10.1007/978-3-030-43367-3_3

15–24 years, and "young people" as the age range 10–24 years [1]. In this chapter, discussion related to adolescents who are legally minors will indicate that; otherwise the terms are used interchangeably without reference to a fixed age range.

Adolescents are at risk of human trafficking anywhere in the world, including the USA [2]. Certain situations heighten that risk. Young people who are migrants, refugees, or in conflict zones are at especially high risk [3, 4]. This has been documented repeatedly and recently as adolescents have fled from Syria, Afghanistan, Africa, Central America, and elsewhere, seeking safety in their own regions or distant countries, and often being victimized by traffickers "en route" or when they arrive [3, 5, 6]. But young people who never leave their home communities can also be at risk. All of these youth may suffer serious violations of their human rights.

Many of the human rights protections that exist in international treaties and conventions and in national and local laws are relevant to the health and safety of adolescent trafficking survivors and those at risk. However, these protections frequently are not enforced. Healthcare professionals can help make human rights protections real for adolescents by providing trauma-informed clinical care and by acting as advocates for their safety and treatment.

Human Rights of Adolescents

Important and long-standing articulations of the human rights of adolescents are contained in the Universal Declaration of Human Rights, 1948, and the United Nations Convention on the Rights of the Child, 1989 [7, 8]. Although the USA signed but did not ratify the Convention on the Rights of the Child (CRC), both the Declaration of Human Rights and the CRC are viewed as setting well-established and widely accepted standards.

The Universal Declaration of Human Rights specifies several rights that are particularly relevant in the context of human trafficking:

- Life, liberty, security of person (Article 3)
- Freedom from slavery or servitude (Article 4)
- Freedom from torture, cruel, inhuman, or degrading treatment or punishment (Article 5)
- Freedom of movement (Article 13)
- Freedom of expression (Article 19)
- Health, well-being, and medical care (Article 25) [7]

When a young person is trafficked either for sex or for labor, virtually all of these rights are violated.

The CRC similarly articulates rights of great significance for trafficked youth:

- Life (Article 6)
- Freedom from violence (Article 19)

- Highest attainable standard of health, treatment of illness, and rehabilitation of health (Article 24)
- Protection from economic exploitation (Article 32)
- Protection from sexual abuse and sexual exploitation (Article 34)
- Protection against abduction, sale, or trafficking (Article 35)
- Freedom from torture, cruel, inhuman, or degrading treatment or punishment and protection against unlawful deprivation of liberty (Article 36) [8]

Again, when adolescents who are minors under age 18 are trafficked, these CRC rights are violated in almost every case.

Legal Protections in International Law

The rights articulated in the Universal Declaration of Human Rights most relevant to human trafficking have been elaborated over the past seven decades in numerous conventions adopted under the auspices of various international entities. Three important international groups that have issued anti-trafficking conventions and other agreements designed to provide legal protection for human rights are the United Nations, the International Labor Organization, and the Council of Europe.

The UN Convention on the Rights of the Child has two relevant protocols: the Optional Protocol on Sale of Children, Child Prostitution, and Child Pornography and the Optional Protocol on the Involvement of Children in Armed Conflict [9, 10]. Other important UN conventions are the Convention on Transnational Crime, which includes the Protocol to Prevent, Suppress, and Punish Trafficking in Persons, Especially Women and Children (the "Palermo Protocol") [11], and the UN Convention Against Torture [12]. The International Labor Organization has adopted the Convention on Forced Labor, the Convention on the Worst Forms of Child Labor, and the Minimum Age Convention [13–15]. The Council of Europe adopted a Convention on Action Against Trafficking in Human Beings and the Convention on Protection of Children Against Sexual Exploitation and Sexual Abuse [16, 17]. Each of these contains important protections for young people.

The Palermo Protocol defines human trafficking (or "trafficking in persons") as:

> the recruitment, transportation, transfer, harbouring or receipt of persons, by means of the threat or use of force or other forms of coercion, of abduction, of fraud, of deception, of the abuse of power or of a position of vulnerability or of the giving or receiving of payments or benefits to achieve the consent of a person having control over another person, for the purpose of exploitation. Exploitation shall include, at a minimum, the exploitation of the prostitution of others or other forms of sexual exploitation, forced labour or services, slavery or practices similar to slavery, servitude or the removal of organs[.] [11]

For the past two decades, this definition has been the standard for laws enacted in countries and in state or local jurisdictions around the world.

Legal Protections in US Laws

In the same year that the Palermo anti-trafficking protocol was adopted, the US Congress enacted the Trafficking Victims Protection Act of 2000 (TVPA) [18], which has since been reauthorized multiple times. The TVPA includes a definition of "severe forms of trafficking" that closely parallels the Palermo Protocol definition but excludes trafficking in human organs [19]. Notably, the consent of a victim is irrelevant for victims of any age; force, fraud, or coercion is not required for children, including adolescent minors, to be considered a victim of sex trafficking.

All US states and the District of Columbia have enacted anti-trafficking laws [20]. Many of these laws focus on the criminal justice aspects of human trafficking, emphasizing prosecution of traffickers more than the prevention of trafficking or the protection of trafficking victims and survivors. This emphasis is beginning to shift as recognition grows of the public health dimensions of human trafficking and the key role of healthcare professionals [21]. To understand fully the legal aspects of human trafficking, it is essential to consider the laws that directly address trafficking and the many other state laws that affect adolescents. Laws in all of the following domains are highly relevant: prostitution; juvenile delinquency; status offenses and runaway and homeless youth; criminalization of sex with a minor; child abuse reporting; healthcare; child welfare and foster care; education, housing, and employment; and "Safe Harbor" laws [20].

A growing number of states are enacting laws—referred to as "Safe Harbor" laws—that are designed to do two things: stop treating children and adolescents who are victims of commercial sexual exploitation and trafficking as perpetrators of crimes such as prostitution; and provide trafficking victims and survivors with comprehensive and appropriate services to meet their needs [22, 23]. Typical provisions of Safe Harbor laws include defining child and adolescent victims as abused and neglected, granting them immunity from prosecution for prostitution and related offenses, and diverting them from juvenile delinquency to child protection proceedings. These laws are a significant improvement in the treatment of children and adolescents who are victimized by traffickers, but limitations remain. Some of the Safe Harbor laws do not extend protection up to age 18 but end it at a younger age; some are limited to first-time offenders; and few protect young adults or victims of labor trafficking. As the Safe Harbor laws redirect trafficked youth to the child welfare and foster care systems, the demands on those systems increase, and the challenges they face in responding are revealed.

The Safe Harbor laws generally do not protect adolescents or young adults past age 18, but other mechanisms are being developed that would provide alternatives to criminal prosecution and punishment for individuals who are arrested for offenses such as prostitution or drug-related offenses but also have been victimized by human trafficking. For example, several states have established specialized "human trafficking" courts to address the needs of human trafficking survivors [24]. Although these courts are not universally viewed as the best way to offer protection from criminal prosecution to trafficking survivors who have been arrested, some alternative method is needed to meet their needs without criminalizing them [25].

Adolescents on the Move

In addition to the many adolescents and young adults throughout the USA who are at risk for or are being trafficked in their home communities, children and adolescents who are "on the move" [4] throughout the world are at especially heightened risk: These include young people fleeing war zones and other areas characterized by severe violence. The circumstances and treatment of unaccompanied immigrant youth dramatically demonstrate the impact of human rights violations of youth in the USA.

Tens of thousands of unaccompanied minors arrive in the USA each year, mostly across the southern border. Historically, these youth were confined in adult detention facilities and suffered profound deprivations. In 1985 a lawsuit was filed on their behalf, challenging their detention in restrictive adult settings, the conditions of the confinement, and the lack of education and healthcare services. The litigation resulted in a landmark settlement in 1997—the "*Flores* Settlement Agreement" [26]—that subsequently has undergone a protracted implementation process to secure for unaccompanied minors the services they are entitled to in the least restrictive and most family-like setting. Ultimately, court orders resulted in generally limiting their detention in secure facilities to no more than 20 days. Responsibility for unaccompanied minors was transferred from law enforcement agencies (Homeland Security and Customs and Border Patrol) to child welfare agencies (Department of Health and Human Services and Office of Refugee Resettlement). Regulatory efforts to undermine many of the key protections contained in the *Flores* Settlement Agreement [27] have been resoundingly rejected in federal court [28]. Nevertheless, abuses and human rights violations have persisted.

Examples of these human rights violations and their profound implications for the physical and mental health of the affected adolescents can be seen in the treatment of unaccompanied minors held in detention. Advocacy organizations conducted visits to detention facilities and "shelters" for these youth in 2018 and found:

> At a detention center in Homestead, Florida, a group of immigrant teens are packed into cold rooms that can hold 70 to 250 kids, given a substandard education and detained for more than six months, according to interviews done by five legal and child psychology experts [29].

Detention of unaccompanied minors in other facilities led—as a follow-up to the *Flores* litigation—to the filing of a new lawsuit (*Lucas R. v. Azar*) [30] in which:

> Five immigrant children challenged the government for unlawfully detaining them in jail-like conditions for prolonged periods, drugging them with powerful psychotropic medication without consent, arbitrarily denying release to their family, and denying access to legal counsel [31].

Tragically, many of these youth had already suffered brutality at the hands of human traffickers before and during their journeys to the USA, only to be subjected to further violations of their human rights. These harms underscore the absolute necessity for healthcare professionals to be involved not only by providing comprehensive and trauma-sensitive clinical care but also by acting as vocal advocates for human rights protections.

The Role of Healthcare Professionals

Health and human rights are inextricably linked by the principle that all people have the right to the highest attainable standards of health and well-being. Clinicians are uniquely placed to use their education, experience, expertise, and positions to identify, treat, and document violations of human rights and to advocate for and educate peers, patients, organizations, and communities for the protection of human rights.

Identifying Trafficking Survivors in Healthcare Settings

While the total number of trafficking survivors in the world is unknown, estimates are in the millions. Women and children predominate: in a 2018 UN study, up to half of the survivors were women and one third were children, with girls accounting for 23% and boys 7% [2]. While data on male trafficking survivors are scarce, research suggests that women are trafficked primarily for sexual purposes and men trafficked primarily for forced labor [2].

Survivors of trafficking are often victims of physical, sexual, and psychological abuse, and healthcare clinicians are likely to see exploited men, women, children, and adolescents in multiple care settings [32, 33]. Worldwide, young male and female survivors of labor or sex trafficking are found to have suffered severe health consequences [34, 35].

A 2014 study involving focus groups with 107 US survivors of sex trafficking ranging in age from 14 to 60 suggests that almost 88% of trafficking survivors had accessed healthcare services and 63% were seen at the hospital/emergency department at some point [36]. Survivors also report using urgent care, primary care clinics, teen clinics, school clinics, shelters, specialty clinics, community health centers, and dental clinic settings and present with acute and chronic medical conditions, infections, injuries, substance use disorders, and mental health challenges. Health systems have a responsibility to accurately identify survivors, treat their medical conditions, and work to mitigate the negative impacts of trafficking [36].

Trained clinicians can identify signs of trafficking, provide care, and intervene to help prevent further health problems [20, 37]. In order to identify adolescents at risk for exploitation during clinical interactions, it is necessary to understand the development of the adolescent brain (see Chap. 2 on physical and neurocognitive development); be familiar with specific social, medical, and environmental risks; and have a high clinical index of suspicion.

There are a number of markers for identifying children and adolescents at risk for commercial sexual exploitation and trafficking. Some of the most important individual clues in healthcare settings include signs such as being controlled by another person, bruises or other physical injuries, fear of authorities, and lack of personal identification documents. Pattern recognition supplements a high index of suspicion. Co-occurrence of the following should prompt concern: the adolescent's ambiguity about their exact address, another person speaking for the patient, evidence of hypervigilance, submission, fear, anxiety, avoidance of eye contact, numerous inconsistencies in their history, and leaving without being seen or against medical advice [38, 39]. Additionally, specific indicators for labor trafficking include working during school hours, owing debts, living away from home or with an employer, not having control of their own money, and being unable to safely quit jobs [40].

Risk Factors: Adolescent Development

Limited life experiences, a rapidly developing brain driven by reward and limited ability to control impulses, difficulty in thinking critically about alternative options or decisions, challenges in analyzing risks and benefits, and limited options for control of their lives are elements of normal adolescent development. Simultaneously, adolescents are learning about their own sexuality and puberty. Studies suggest that two processes of brain maturation may predispose to impulsivity in adolescents: early nucleus accumbens maturation (which plays a significant role in reward, aversion, and motivation) and increased dopaminergic innervation in the prefrontal cortex with an increased reward sensitivity (which is implicated in complex decision-making) [41–43]. Children who are chronically exposed to trauma and danger are very sensitive to perceived threats, showing amygdala activation on brain imaging [44]. The hippocampus is also impacted by prior trauma and affects contextual learning and memory. Without context and history, it is easy to understand why adolescents respond to many situations as if they were in danger. Children who are highly reactive to threats develop overactive alarm systems and can react with unwarranted aggression. Many trafficking survivors are traumatized during early childhood and while they are being trafficked. They lack trust in law enforcement, adults in authority, and even family or caregivers [45, 46].

Other Significant Risk Factors

For some young people, trafficking victimization commences at a young age, although data are limited according to National Human Trafficking Hotline reports [46]. In addition to risks associated with brain development, these children are more likely to have a history of abuse and neglect, incest, rape, educational disruption, running away, and early sexual experiences [20] (see Table 3.1 for a summary of individual, family, and community risk factors for human trafficking). Sexual abuse,

Table 3.1 Summary of individual, family, and community risks [20, 60]

Individual	Family	Community
Behavioral, mental health, and substance use problems	History of sexual or physical abuse or neglect	Association with gangs; drug sales
Immigration status	Runaway and homeless youth, throw-away youth	Neighborhoods with high crime rates, adult prostitution, or poverty
LGBTQ youth	Families with other dysfunction such as domestic violence, substance misuse, criminality, illness/death of parent, maternal trauma	Areas with transient male populations (military bases, truck stops, convention centers)
History of juvenile justice or child protective services involvement	Immigration status	Countries with political or social upheaval or police/political corruption
Developmental and learning challenges; school attendance	Poverty and homelessness	Societal attitudes of gender bias and discrimination, sexualization of girls, and glorification of the pimp culture

early initiation of sexual activity, and overall childhood adversity exposure are risk factors for sex trafficking of children. Boys and girls share several risks for involvement in commercial sexual exploitation of children (CSEC) and sex trafficking, including a history of child maltreatment, family violence, foster care, and other out-of-home residential placement [20]. A disturbing report in 2017 estimates that one of seven runaway children who were reported to the National Center for Missing and Exploited Children was likely to be a sex trafficking victim, and 88% had been in the custody of social services or foster care [47].

While child victims were most commonly trafficked for sex (45%), they were also trafficked for labor (34%) and for domestic servitude (11%) [48]. The intersectionality of risks for these children is especially striking. Abused and neglected children, and those in foster care, are more likely to run away which increases their risk of exploitation for sex and labor. Children with prior trauma may develop strong bonds with their traffickers, replicating their behavior with an abusive parent. In a study of adolescents in a residential setting for treatment of trauma after CSEC, 40% reported medical treatment for child abuse, 58% had a childhood history of significant neglect, and 54% described long-standing emotional abuse. More than 85% reported at least one episode of sexual abuse as a child, with most events occurring between the ages of 6 and 12 years. A quarter of these children also witnessed acts of violence, and another 22% were witnesses to serious intentional injuries. Finally, 90% of these adolescents reported that they were engaged in trafficking or exploitation prior to age 16. While most adolescents in this cohort were physically healthy, they exhibited a high prevalence of oppositional behavior, depression, conduct disorder, anger, and anxiety, and almost half had significant substance use [45]. Research demonstrates links between "precocious transitions," such as early sexual activity, teenage pregnancy, early cohabitation, and early marriage with negative long-term emotional, behavioral, and physical health outcomes. Early physical maturation has also been associated with greater health risks in adolescence [20, 49]. Females sexually abused as children reported twice as many subsequent rapes or sexual assaults, 1.6 times as many episodes of physical abuse, and almost 4 times as many events of self-inflicted harm than did the comparison group, making child sexual abuse a significant risk factor for trafficking [49].

LGBTQ youth are at special risk for exploitation. Up to 40% of homeless youth identify as LGBTQ. Almost half of these youth run away due to rejection from their families and are 7 times more likely to experience acts of sexual violence and 3–7 times more likely to engage in survival sex to meet basic needs. They experience greater discrimination, violence, and economic instability. As they face life on the streets, they find ways to meet their basic needs, including engaging in sex for money and food, and may become targets for trafficking [20, 50]. [See Chap. 11 for more on LGBTQIA+ youth and human trafficking.]

Intergenerational Trauma

Literature suggests that there is an increased likelihood of impairment in some aspects of parenting and subsequent risk of sexual victimization of children of mothers who experienced early sexual abuse. Specifically, there is evidence that mothers who experienced child sexual abuse had greater difficulty setting boundaries with children, at times being overly permissive and at others using harsh discipline [51, 52]. For female sex workers and prostitutes, the prevalence data suggests that about 70–90% of them are mothers with dependent children [53, 54]. These women report high levels of stress, somatization, depression, fatigue, frustration, sleep, smoking and alcohol problems, and more frequent and serious PTSD symptoms, making parenting very challenging [55]. Little is known about sex workers as parents [56]. Qualitative research finds that many women who enter sex work continue to support their families [57] and that stigma is ubiquitous [58] leading to severing of social ties with family and friends and avoidance of health and social services resulting in reduced ability to parent. Sex working mothers report anxiety when they work because of fear that their children will discover their occupation, as well as worries about their children being hurt, no longer loving or respecting them, or becoming involved in trafficking [59].

Healthcare Settings and Trafficking

Survivors of human trafficking present to healthcare settings in a variety of ways (see Table 3.2). A helpful categorization of common presentations includes acute illness (UTI, STIs, asthma), injuries (ecchymoses, burns, lacerations, fractures,

Table 3.2 Summary of indicators of human trafficking in clinical settings [61, 62]

Indicators common to sex and labor trafficking
Homelessness, couch surfing, multiple addresses
Evidence of controlling or dominating relationships as though they are forced or coerced
Inability to produce their own identification and legal documents
Poor school attendance
Excessive anxiety and fear in the healthcare setting
Little or no contact with family or loved ones
Experienced threats made against them or their family members
Distrust of authorities, including clinicians because of fear of reporting, arrest, or retribution
Unexplained or unusual scars, tattoos or other types of branding that the adolescent is reluctant to explain
Indicators specific to sex trafficking
Discrepancies between behavior and reported age
Multiple or frequent pregnancies
Large number of sexual partners
Relationships with older men
Use of specific words referring to a boyfriend as "Daddy" or other controlling words
Dressed in inappropriate clothing
Multiple or frequent STIs
Evidence of genital trauma

electrocution), chronic illness (dental caries, diabetes, malnourishment), pregnancy, and mental health and substance-related conditions (depression, anxiety, suicide gestures, and PTSD). Most survivors have a limited history of past medical care and many lack health insurance [32].

In the clinical setting, it is essential to consider both the safety of the adolescent and the clinical staff [63]. Steps to increase safety include checking to see if the trafficker is still in the facility or has left, assessing the survivor's perceived level of safety, assessing real or perceived threats of injury or harm, and acting on opportunities to help the adolescent feel safer during the visit. Other strategies include separation of the adolescent from his/her escort and placing their belongings in a safe space while reducing contact with mobile phones, GPS, or tracking devices.

Once safety is assured, the clinician should introduce themselves to the adolescent in a comfortable environment, providing the adolescent physical and emotional space to express their needs for the visit. Successful clinicians use a warm, empathic listening approach that is attentive, observant, and nonjudgmental. Clinicians should express their role clearly and describe available services and why they care about the survivor's situation. The goal of the introduction should be to understand the survivor's needs and answer their questions early on in the visit to build trust [62]. The first minutes of the visit are crucial to understanding the survivor's needs, since for most adolescents, the likelihood of repeat visits or following through on longer-term interventions is usually limited.

Adolescent survivors may suffer from daily, long-standing threats, intimidation, deception, unpredictability, isolation, and forced dependency, often resulting in complex trauma [20]. Complex trauma is the sustained exposure to chronic and severe traumatic events and is characterized by high levels of depression, dissociation, borderline personality disorder, self-harm, and suicidal ideation [20, 63]. The clinician is likely to see withdrawn, aggressive, or hostile behavior in the healthcare setting, suggesting the need for a trauma-informed approach to care. Being aware of the impact of trauma on the survivor allows clinicians to prioritize the patient's sense of safety, control, and trust [64]. Seeing manipulative, fearful, confused, angry, and defensive behavior through a trauma-informed lens reduces the likelihood of premature judgment and frustration on the part of clinicians. In addition, it should be expected that survivors will not be honest until trust has been built [36]. Asking the adolescent about their needs first, followed by open questions about their living or working conditions, is helpful prior to directly inquiring about physical or sexual abuse. Clinicians should use the language of the patient to avoid judgmental or triggering words and conduct evaluations in the patient's native language with a medical interpreter [20]. Avoid using words such as sex trafficking or prostitution since many survivors do not identify themselves in that way.

The Medical and Social History

After assuring safety and reviewing conditional confidentiality (including mandatory reporting requirements), a clear introduction and an assessment of acute needs are next, followed by a medical history including relevant past medical, family, and social history using open-ended questions [61]. When the survivor presents with a traumatic injury, the clinician should obtain details of the history of the injury. Offering information and resources (such as hotline numbers) about healthy and unhealthy relationships and trafficking universally to adolescents (when they are alone) can also signal that the healthcare setting is a safe setting to discuss such experiences. While disclosure is not the goal (resource provision and reducing isolation are), certain open-ended questions may help to initiate a conversation about trafficking (see Table 3.3).

The Physical Examination

A comprehensive physical examination includes an assessment of overall health status, documentation and treatment of acute physical injuries and illnesses, and provision of appropriate referrals [39, 62, 63]. The clinician should first care for any immediate needs, including treatment of acute physical trauma, sexually transmitted infections, diagnosis of pregnancy, assessing for suicidal ideation, septic abortion, and untreated serious chronic health problems [37]. Unreported conditions should be considered such as head injury, anogenital injury, pelvic inflammatory disease, HIV, and urinary tract infections. The adolescent's chronic illnesses may be

Table 3.3 Suggested open-ended questions to identify human trafficking. Adapted from [65]

Tell me about a time when you felt threatened, intimidated, or pressured to do something that you didn't want to or felt uncomfortable doing
Describe your fears about trying to leave, to escape this person/situation, or what might happen if you didn't do what you were told to do
Explain where your legal papers and identification (passport, visa, driver's license) are located or how they were lost or taken
Tell me about a time you felt pressured to engage in any sexual acts against your will or for favors or money
Describe the times that anyone took photos/videos of you and what they used them for
Describe any times you were forced to work or engage in sex with family, friends, clients, or business associates (online websites, escort services, street prostitution, informal arrangement, brothel, massage business or strip club)
Tell me about your work and your boss and any times you felt forced to do something you did not want to do
Describe any times that someone tricked you or made you sign something you did not understand
Explain any times when someone you worked for refused to pay you or kept all or most of the money you made
Tell me about times you were physically beaten, slapped, hit, kicked, punched, burned, or harmed in any way by someone
Describe times you were unable to leave a place you worked, or talk to people you wanted to talk to, even when you weren't working, because the person you worked for threatened or controlled you

poorly controlled and cause acute symptoms such as dental pain and caries, asthma, traumatic brain injury, gastrointestinal conditions such as irritable bowel syndrome, and chronic pain and fatigue. Mental health problems—such as complications of substance abuse, post-traumatic stress disorder, major depression, anxiety, and complex trauma—should also be assessed during the medical visit (Table 3.4 lists steps of the physical exam).

When survivors are brought into an examination room, some experience traumatic stress as they face being undressed, being placed into a small exam room with closed doors, touched on private parts of their bodies, exposed to gels and lubricants for exams or invasive procedures, and lying on exam tables. The exam room environment—with doctors, interpreters, and social workers directing the adolescent's behavior—can create power dynamics similar to their trafficking lives. Emotion regulation is a challenge for many trauma survivors. In the examination room, this presents as anxiety, minimization, dissociation, unwillingness to undress, extraordinary fear, and concern about being judged and shamed. Slow movements on the part of the clinician with continuous reassurance are helpful. Seeking consent for each part of the examination and providing an ongoing narrative for the patient about the next steps in the evaluation are essential. The physical examination should begin with body parts which have reportedly not been injured or hurt and slowly move toward areas most likely to trigger re-traumatization. The patient should be given the option to stop the examination or take a break at any point if they grow uncomfortable.

Table 3.4 Steps of the physical examination [20]

1. Obtaining informed consent for the examination
2. Assessing and treating acute and serious chronic conditions, as discussed above
3. Assessing overall health, nutritional status, signs of drug use
4. Performing a head to toe physical examination
5. Documenting acute/healed injuries, genital and extragenital physical abuse
6. Testing for pregnancy, STIs, sexual abuse
7. Testing for alcohol and drugs
8. Providing referrals and treatment

When treating sex trafficking survivors, there may be dual goals for clinicians. The medical examination and care are always the first priority, with the goal of diagnosing and treating medical conditions. In addition, forensic evaluation may be indicated. This evaluation should follow or be done simultaneously with the medical examination and is meant to document injuries and medical findings for law enforcement, child protection services, or judicial proceedings.

Assuring appropriate referrals are the final step in the medical interaction. All adolescents deserve a trusted medical home for treatment of STIs, immunizations, family planning options, trauma-focused behavioral health services, obstetrics management, and substance use assessment and treatment. Supportive community referrals include housing assistance, mentorship programs, interpreter services, immigration assistance, legal services, mental health and addiction services, and educational and vocational training [33]. Establishing a medical home and identifying appropriate referrals for young trafficking survivors can be challenging but is an important goal.

Forensic Medical Documentation

Forensic documentation, if performed, follows the provision of urgent medical care and treatment. A distinct informed consent/assent of the survivor/guardian is sought, and the forensic evaluation is performed by a clinician trained in the documentation of intentional injury, torture, and sexual abuse. Forensic documentation is not appropriate for all trafficking survivors. The decision to perform a forensic medical examination should be based on the detailed history and physical examination, severity of injuries, the survivor's interest in cooperating with law enforcement, allegations of sexual assault, and—in child victims—of violence by a caregiver. Medical forensic documentation of intentional injuries can support legal action, protection, and rehabilitation of the survivor and may positively impact the lives of others [64]. Clinicians trained in forensic documentation can often simultaneously perform both the physical and forensic examinations, which include additional steps (Table 3.5).

Table 3.5 Steps of the medical forensic examination

Detailed forensic interview of all alleged events
Document skin signs of physical abuse such as scars, bites, strangulation, tattoos, branding, as well as internal injuries
Perform a genital examination, using a sexual assault evidence kit and chain of custody as indicated
Use body diagrams and photographs to document all injuries, acute and healed
Document behavioral observations
Diagnostic testing as appropriate (X-rays for rib fractures, etc.)
Referrals as indicated

Trafficking survivors are often exposed to physical and sexual abuse from a number of perpetrators over time; there is rarely a single perpetrator during a single event, and the survivor's clinical presentation is rarely within 72 h of the abuse. Survivors are frequently exposed to prolonged confinement and torture, including food and water deprivation, and have extensive trauma histories. Thus, the purposes of forensic evaluations in trafficking survivors are to document patterns of injury and abuse which may lead to identification of traffickers, to identify the survivor's risk based on the extent of injuries, to identify other youth at risk of exploitation in the community, and to support law enforcement in ongoing investigations. When the forensic examination is complete, the medicolegal documentation and all related evidence is released to the appropriate authority and is generally not part of the medical record [66].

Health Impact of Human Trafficking

In addition to the developmental impact of trafficking, adolescents experience a number of short-term health effects when they are exploited. These may include addiction, emotional exhaustion, depersonalization, fear, anxiety, acute pain, and impaired judgment leading to excessive risk taking and even death. Long-term effects include depression, suicidal ideation, post-traumatic stress disorder (PTSD) with continuous arousal and hypervigilance, untreated STIs, sexual dysfunction, chronic pain, infertility, and difficulty establishing/maintaining healthy relationships [33].

The long-term consequences for sexually exploited adolescents can be predicted by the impact on adult men and women involved in commercial sex work. Adult survivors report having physical health problems such as chronic joint pain, chest pain, genital symptoms, and HIV [67]. Women who were sexually abused as children experience more negative health outcomes in adulthood, such as cardiac and gastrointestinal problems, chronic pain, headache, eating disorders, and somatic symptoms [68]. In men, childhood sexual abuse has been associated with cardiovascular problems [69]. Sexual dysfunction and gynecologic problems have been reported among women with a history of sexual abuse, including chronic pelvic pain, dyspareunia, sexually transmitted infections, reproductive health problems, premature births, and the sequelae of genital injuries [20, 70]. Adolescent survivors of sex trafficking are at risk of facing similar future health challenges.

Psychological sequelae are profound. Adolescents and young adults with a history of childhood sexual abuse were three times more likely to become depressed or suicidal than unexposed populations [71]. Studies of adult women survivors of childhood sexual abuse show increased rates of PTSD, depression, anxiety, and substance abuse; higher rates of promiscuity; and later involvement in commercial sex work. Childhood sexual abuse also has been shown to be associated with earlier initiation of injection drug use among intravenous drug users [72]. Survivors show extremely high rates of fear and anxiety, disrupted relationships with others, addiction and substance abuse, and self-destructive behaviors, including suicidality [73, 74]. [See Chap. 9 for more about the intersection of psychology, psychiatry, and human trafficking.]

Clinician Training

Significant gaps exist in health professional education and awareness of human trafficking. In one study of providers in urban, suburban, and rural health facilities, 63% reported no previous training on identification of sex trafficking survivors. Those who received training were significantly more likely to report having encountered a survivor in their practice and felt more confident in their ability to identify survivors [75].

National organizations have issued policy statements calling upon healthcare professionals to receive training on human trafficking [38, 63, 75, 76] (see Chap. 20 on education of health professionals). Acquisition of skills, as well as cross-training in performing forensic evaluations, can occur through educational programs focused on forensic documentation for child abuse, sexual violence, domestic violence, and torture/asylum forensic examinations. Development and dissemination of national consensus guidelines for forensic medical examinations in adolescent trafficking survivors is needed.

Reporting

If clinicians suspect that a survivor is in immediate danger, notifying law enforcement may be the best option though risks should be weighed carefully along with legal and ethical confidentiality requirements. The clinician should record as much information about the situation as possible, being careful not to put staff or the survivor at further risk. Whenever possible, a report to child protective services or law enforcement (depending on the situation) should be made together with the young person so that they can provide additional detail, understand that the report is being made on their behalf for their safety (not because they have done something wrong), and have a better understanding of next steps. If there is no immediate danger, clinicians may provide hotline numbers for anti-trafficking service providers, giving this information directly to the survivor only when he/she is alone (such as the National Human Trafficking Resource Center 1–888–373-7888).

Every state requires the reporting of child abuse and neglect, as they are required to do under the federal Child Abuse Prevention and Treatment Act (CAPTA) [77, 78]. Although definitions vary among states, every state includes some forms of sexual abuse and sexual exploitation in their child abuse laws [20, 77]. In all states, abuse and neglect by a parent or person responsible for the child must be reported; in a large majority of states, abuse by third parties is also reportable [77]. The explicit inclusion of human trafficking in mandatory child abuse reporting laws is evolving: states are increasingly amending their child abuse reporting mandates to cover sex trafficking, and some include labor trafficking as well [79]. In the states where reports of child abuse or neglect are generally required only when they result from the action of parents or persons responsible for the child, the requirement to report trafficking often extends to third-party perpetrators.

Reporting to law enforcement or social services has risks and benefits for both the clinician and the patient [80]. Mandatory reporting laws such as those for child abuse and interpersonal violence (IPV) are designed for victim protection and to connect victims to protective services, so that the risks of reporting are usually offset by the availability of robust services. For trafficking survivors, reporting by clinicians could deter survivors from trusting health systems, sharing sensitive information, and even seeking healthcare and treatment due to fear of injury from their traffickers, prosecution by court systems, or deportation [20, 80]. When immediately available protection and services are in place, survivors are more likely to seek care, accept referrals, and trust that reporting their abuse will result in benefit [80].

Opportunities

Doctors often face ethical dilemmas during their training and in practice. Learning about human rights advocacy augments doctors' natural desire to serve their patients' needs. Human rights training is likely to increase awareness of our patients' unique needs and support the provision of equitable care for diverse patients; recognition of ethical dilemmas; and advocacy for action by political, institutional, and economic systems to protect the well-being of patients.

Healthcare professionals who care for children, adolescents, and young adults must be trained to identify and treat potential trafficking survivors. Trained clinicians can learn how to identify survivors using short screening tools [81], meet survivors' acute medical needs, document cases for court when indicated, and practice trauma-informed care.

Clinicians can also:

- Partner with lawyers, law enforcement, and community service providers to improve community safety, reduce professional isolation, gain new insight into community strategies, and encourage systemic solutions to this complex problem.
- Exercise advocacy by using clinical skills in the provision of medical forensic evaluations for torture and abuse survivors, by supporting efforts to reduce demand for paid sexual contact, by improving the prosecution of traffickers, and by educating the public and law enforcement about the special health needs of survivors.
- Advocate for better research and more robust technology such as the creation of a national legal database for human trafficking cases across jurisdictions [62, 82].

As occurred with the evolution of the fields of child abuse and neglect, domestic violence, and documentation of torture, the partnership between attorneys and health professionals can advance the identification, treatment, and prevention of human trafficking in adolescents and further the protection of their human rights.

Conclusion

Adolescent survivors of trafficking often have experienced severe violations of their human rights with profound adverse consequences for their health. Implementing legal protections of their human rights requires partnership between legal, advocacy, and healthcare organizations. Health professionals who care for trafficking survivors can partner with lawyers and other advocates to make protection of human rights a reality for adolescents. Clinical care and advocacy for adolescent trafficking victims and survivors can be more effective when informed by a human rights perspective and supported by human rights protections.

References

1. World Health Organization. Adolescent health and development. Available from: http://www.searo.who.int/entity/child_adolescent/topics/adolescent_health/en/.
2. United Nations Office on Drugs and Crime. Global report on trafficking in persons; 2018. [cited 2019 October 4]. Available from: https://www.unodc.org/documents/data-and-analysis/glotip/2018/GLOTiP_2018_BOOK_web_small.pdf.
3. United Nations Office on Drugs and Crime. Trafficking in persons in the context of armed Conflict; 2018. [cited 2019 October 4]. Available from: https://www.unodc.org/documents/data-and-analysis/glotip/2018/GloTIP2018_BOOKLET_2_Conflict.pdf.
4. Bhabha J, Bohne C, Digidiki V, Donger E, Frounfelker R, Glenn J, et al. Children on the move: an urgent human rights and child protection priority. Boston: Harvard FXB Center for Health

and Human Rights; 2016. [cited 2019 October 4]. Available from: https://cdn1.sph.harvard.edu/wp-content/uploads/sites/2464/2017/12/Oak-report2016.pdf.
5. Hiskey JT, Córdova A, Orcés D, Malone MF. Understanding the Central American refugee crisis: why they are fleeing and how U.S. policies are used to deter them; 2016 Feb. [cited 2019 October 4]. Available from: https://www.americanimmigrationcouncil.org/sites/default/files/research/understanding_the_central_american_refugee_crisis.pdf.
6. Center for Gender and Refugee Studies. Childhood and migration in Central and North America: Causes, policies, practices and challenges; 2015 Feb. [cited 2019 October 4]. Available from: https://cgrs.uchastings.edu/sites/default/files/Childhood_Migration_HumanRights_English_1.pdf.
7. United Nations. Universal Declaration of Human Rights; 1949. [cited 2019 October 4]. Available from: https://www.un.org/en/universal-declaration-human-rights/.
8. United Nations. Convention on the Rights of the Child; 1989. [cited 2019 October 4]. Available from: https://www.ohchr.org/EN/ProfessionalInterest/Pages/CRC.aspx.
9. United Nations Office of High Commissioner on Human Rights. Optional Protocol to the Convention on the Rights of the Child on the sale of children, child prostitution and child pornography; 2000. [cited 2019 October 4]. Available from: https://www.ohchr.org/EN/ProfessionalInterest/Pages/OPSCCRC.aspx.
10. United Nations Office of High Commissioner on Human Rights. Optional Protocol to the Convention on the Rights of the Child on the involvement of children in armed conflict; 2000. [cited 2019 October 4]. Available from: https://www.ohchr.org/en/professionalinterest/pages/opaccrc.aspx.
11. United Nations Convention Against Transnational Organized Crime and the Protocols Thereto. [cited 2019 October 4]. Available from: https://www.unodc.org/documents/middleeastandnorthafrica/organised-crime/UNITED_NATIONS_CONVENTION_AGAINST_TRANSNATIONAL_ORGANIZED_CRIME_AND_THE_PROTOCOLS_THERETO.pdf.
12. United Nations Convention against Torture and Other Cruel, Inhuman or Degrading Treatment or Punishment; 1984. [cited 2019 October 4]. Available from: https://www.ohchr.org/en/professionalinterest/pages/cat.aspx.
13. International Labour Organization, Convention Concerning Forced or Compulsory Labour (No. 29); 1930. [cited 2019 October 4]. Available from: https://www.ilo.org/dyn/normlex/en/f?p=NORMLEXPUB:12100:0::NO::P12100_ILO_CODE:C029.
14. International Labour Organization. Convention concerning the Prohibition and Immediate Action for the Elimination of the Worst Forms of Child Labour (No. 182); 1999. [cited 2019 October 4]. Available from: https://www.ilo.org/dyn/normlex/en/f?p=NORMLEXPUB:12100:0::NO::P12100_ILO_CODE:C182.
15. International Labour Organization. Convention concerning Minimum Age for Admission to Employment (No. 138); 1973. [cited 2019 October 4]. Available from: https://www.ilo.org/dyn/normlex/en/f?p=NORMLEXPUB:12100:0::NO::P12100_ILO_CODE:C138.
16. Council of Europe, Convention on Action against Trafficking in Human Beings, CETS 197, May 16, 2005, Article 10(4)(a). [cited 2019 October 4]. Available from http://www.refworld.org/docid/43fded544.html.
17. Council of Europe. Convention on the Protection of Children against Sexual Exploitation and Sexual Abuse. 2007. [cited 2019 October 4]. Available from: https://rm.coe.int/1680084822.
18. Trafficking Victims Protection Act. U.S.C. 22. Sect. 7101 – 7114.
19. Trafficking Victims Protection Act. U.S.C. 22. Sect. 7102(11).
20. IOM (Institute of Medicine) and NRC (National Research Council). Confronting commercial sexual exploitation and sex trafficking of minors in the United States. Washington, DC: The National Academies Press; 2013.
21. Lachapelle Henry AM, Grodin MA. Human trafficking: a health and human rights agenda. Ann Intern Med. 2018;168(9):674–5. https://doi.org/10.7326/M18-0357.
22. Polaris. Human trafficking issue brief: safe harbor. 2015. [cited 2019 October 4]. https://polarisproject.org/wp-content/uploads/2019/09/2015-Safe-Harbor-Issue-Brief.pdf.
23. ECPAT USA. Steps to safety: a guide to drafting safe harbor legislation to protect sex-trafficked children; 2015. [cited 2019 October 4]. Available from: https://static1.squarespace.

com/static/594970e91b631b3571be12e2/t/5977af9a2e69cffa18f34c54/1501015971553/ECPAT-USA_StepsToSafety.pdf.
24. U.S. Department of Justice, Office for Victims of Crimes. Human trafficking task force e-guide: human trafficking courts. Available from: https://www.ovcttac.gov/taskforceguide/eguide/6-the-role-of-courts/64-innovative-court-responses/human-trafficking-courts/.
25. Kendis B. Human trafficking and prostitution courts: problem solving or problematic? Case Western Reserve L. Rev. 2019;69(3):805–41.
26. Stipulated Settlement Agreement, Flores, et al. v. Reno, et al., Case No. CV 85-4544 (C.D. Cal., Jan. 1, 1997).
27. Apprehension, Processing, Care, and Custody of Alien Minors and Unaccompanied Alien Children, 84 Fed. Reg. 44,392–44,535 (Aug. 23, 2019).
28. Jenny L. Flores, et al. v. William P. Barr, et al. Order of Judge Dolly M. Gee, Case No. 2:85-cv-04544-DMG-AGR, U.S. District Court, Central District of California (September 27, 2019). Available from: https://youthlaw.org/wp-content/uploads/2019/06/9.27-Flores-Order.pdf.
29. Chapin A. Florida detention center expands, packing in migrant children 'like sardines'. HuffPost; 2019 Feb 12. [cited 2019 October 4]. Available from: https://www.huffpost.com/entry/florida-detention-center-immigrant-children_n_5c5e1a64e4b0910c63f071e1.
30. Lucas R. et al. v. Alex Azar et al. Complaint for Injunctive Relief, Declaratory Relief, and Nominal Damages, Case No. 2:18-CV-05741, U.S. District Court, Central District of California (June 29, 2018).
31. National Center for Youth Law, Lucas R. v. Azar. [cited 2019 October 4]. Available from: https://youthlaw.org/wp-content/uploads/1997/05/Flores-Supplemental-Complaint-June-2018.pdf.
32. Greenbaum J, Crawford-Jakubiak J. Child sex trafficking and commercial sexual exploitation: health care needs of victims. Pediatr. 2015;135(3):566–74.
33. Barnert E, Iqbal Z, Bruce J, et al. Commercial sexual exploitation and sex trafficking of children and adolescents: a narrative review. Acad Pediatr. 2017;17(8):825–9.
34. Kiss L, Yun K, Pocock N, Zimmerman C. Exploitation, violence, and suicide risk among child and adolescent survivors of human trafficking in the greater Mekong subregion. JAMA Pediatr. 2015;169(9):e152278. https://doi.org/10.1001/jamapediatrics.2015.2278.
35. Oram S, Abas M, Bick D, Boyle A, French R, Jakobowitz S, et al. Human trafficking and health: a survey of male and female survivors in England. Am J Public Health. 2016;106:1073–8. https://doi.org/10.2105/AJPH.2016.303095.
36. Lederer LJ, Wetzel CA. The health consequences of sex trafficking and their implications for identifying victims in healthcare facilities. Ann Health Law. 2014;23:61–91.
37. Dovydaitis T. Human trafficking: the role of the health care provider. Midwifery Womens Health. 2010;55(5):462–7.
38. National Human Trafficking Resource Center, Polaris Project. Identifying victims of human trafficking: potential indicators and red flags; 2014. [cited 2019 October 4]. Available from: https://traffickingresourcecenter.org/sites/default/files/What%20to%20Look%20for%20during%20a%20Medical%20Exam%20-%20FINAL%20-%202-16-16.docx.pdf.
39. National Human Trafficking Resource Center, Polaris Project. identifying victims of human trafficking: what to look for during a medical exam/consultation; 2016. [cited 2019 October 4]. Available from: https://www.traffickingresourcecenter.org/sites/default/files/What%20to%20Look%20for%20During%20a%20Medical%20Exam.pdf.
40. Littrell J. Human trafficking in America's schools: risk factors and indicators. Washington, DC: U.S. Department of Education; 2015. [cited 2019 October 4]. Available from: https://safesupportivelearning.ed.gov/human-trafficking-americas-schools/risk-factors-and-indicators.
41. Arain M, Haque M, Johal L, et al. Maturation of the adolescent brain. Neuropsychiatr Dis Treat. 2013;9:449–61.
42. Romer D. Adolescent risk taking, impulsivity, and brain development: implications for prevention. Dev Psychobiol. 2010;52:263–76.

43. Datta D, Arnsten A. Loss of prefrontal cortical higher cognition with uncontrollable stress: molecular mechanisms, changes with age, and relevance to treatment. Brain Sci. 2019;9(5):113–28. https://doi.org/10.3390/brainsci9050113.
44. Lambert HK, Sheridan M, Sambrook KA, et al. Hippocampal contribution to context encoding across development is disrupted following early-life adversity. J Neuropsychiatry. 2017;37(7):1925–34.
45. Landers M, McGrath K, Johnson M, et al. Baseline characteristics of dependent youth who have been commercially sexually exploited: findings from a specialized treatment program. J Child Sex Abus. 2017;26(6):692–709.
46. 2017 Trafficking Hotline statistics/Polaris. [cited 2019 October 4]. Available from: https://polarisproject.org/resources/u-s-national-human-trafficking-hotline-statistics/2017nhthstats-1-pdf/.
47. National Center for Missing and Exploited Children. "Child sex trafficking." [cited 2019 October 4]. Available from: http://www.missingkids.org/footer/media/keyfacts.
48. Cockbain E, Olver K. Child trafficking: characteristics, complexities, and challenges. In: Child abuse and neglect: forensic issues in evidence, impact and management: Elsevier Inc; 2019. p. 95–116.
49. Noll JG, Horowitz LA, Bonanno GA, et al. Revictimization and self-harm in females who experienced childhood sexual abuse: results from a prospective study. J Interpers Violence. 2003;18(12):1452–71.
50. Schmitt, V. Sex trafficking and LGBTQ youth. Polaris; 2016. [cited 2019 October 4]. Available from: https://polarisproject.org/resources/sex-trafficking-and-lgbtq-youth.
51. DiLillo D, Dameshek A. Parenting characteristics of women reporting a history of childhood sexual abuse. Child Maltreat. 2003;8(4):319–33.
52. Schuetze P, Das ER. The relationship between sexual abuse during childhood and parenting outcomes: modeling direct and indirect pathways. Child Abuse Negl. 2005;29:645–59.
53. Elmore-Meegan M, Conroy RM, Agala CB. Sex workers in Kenya, numbers of clients and associated risks: an exploratory survey. Reprod Health Matters. 2004;12(23):50–7.
54. Feldblum PJ, Nasution M, Hoke TH, et al. Pregnancy among sex workers participating in a condom intervention trial highlights the need for dual protection. Contraception. 2007;76(2):105–10.
55. Young-Eun J, Song JM, Chong J, et al. Symptoms of posttraumatic stress disorder and mental health in women who escaped prostitution and helping activists in shelters. Yonsei Med J. 2008;49(3):372–82.
56. Beard J, Biemba G, Brooks MI, et al. Children of female sex workers and drug users: a review of vulnerability, resilience and family-centered models of care. J Int AIDS Soc. 2010;13(Suppl 2):S6.
57. Basu A, Dutta MJ. 'We are mothers first': localocentric articulation of sex worker identity as a key in HIV/AIDS communication. Women Health. 2011;51(2):106–23.
58. McClelland GT, Newell R. A qualitative study of the experiences of mothers involved in street-based prostitution and problematic substance use. J Res in Nurs. 2008;13(5):437–47.
59. Sloss CM, Harper GW. When street sex workers are mothers. Arch Sex Behav. 2004;33(4):329–41.
60. Pilnik. L. Responding to youth homelessness: a key strategy for preventing human trafficking. Washington, DC: The National Network for Youth; 2018. [cited 2019 October 4]. Available from: https://www.nn4youth.org/wp-content/uploads/NN4Y-2018-white-paper-human-trafficking-FINAL-0918.pdf.
61. National Human Trafficking Resource Center, Polaris Project; 2011. Comprehensive human trafficking assessment. [cited 2019 October 4]. Available from: https://traffickingresourcecenter.org/sites/default/files/Comprehensive%20Trafficking%20Assessment.pdf.
62. U.S. Department of Health and Human Services Administration for Children, Youth and Families (ACYF). Guidance to states and services on addressing human trafficking of children

and youth in the United States. 2013. 1-16. [cited 2019 October 4]. Available from: https://www.acf.hhs.gov/sites/default/files/cb/acyf_human_trafficking_guidance.pdf.
63. National Human Trafficking Resource Center, Polaris Project, 2016. Medical assessment tool. [cited 2019 October 4]. Available from: https://www.traffickingresourcecenter.org/sites/default/files/Assessment%20Tool%20-%20Medical%20Professionals.pdf.
64. Obertova Z, Cattaneo C. Child trafficking and the European migration crisis: the role of forensic practitioners. Forensic Sci Int. 2018;282:46–59.
65. Mostajabian S, Santa Maria D, Wiemann C, et al. Identifying Sexual and Labor Exploitation among Sheltered Youth Experiencing Homelessness: a comparison of screening methods. Int. J Environ Res Public Health. 2019;16(3):363–78.
66. Alempijevic D, Jecmenica D, Pavlekic S, et al. Forensic medical examination of victims of trafficking in human beings. Torture. 2017;17(2):117–21.
67. Farley M, Barkan H. Prostitution, violence, and posttraumatic stress disorder. Women Health. 1998;27(3):37–49.
68. Bonomi A, Anderson ML, Rivara FP. Health care utilization and costs associated with childhood abuse. J Gen Int Med. 2008;23(3):294–9.
69. Fuller-Thomson E, Bejan R, Hunter JT, et al. The link between childhood sexual abuse and myocardial infarction in a population-based study. Child Abuse Negl. 2012;36(9):656–65.
70. McClain NM, Garrity SE. Sex trafficking and the exploitation of adolescents. J Obstet Gynecol Neonatal Nurs. 2011;40(2):243–52.
71. Brown GR, Anderson B. Psychiatric morbidity in adult inpatients with childhood histories of sexual and physical abuse. Am J Psychiatry. 1991;148(1):55–61.
72. Trickett PK, Noll JG, Putnam FW. The impact of sexual abuse on female development: lessons from a multigenerational, longitudinal research study. Dev Psychopathol. 2011;23(2):453–76.
73. Willis B, Levy B. Child prostitution: global health burden, research needs, and interventions. Lancet. 2002;359:1417–22.
74. Diaz A, Simantov E, Rickert VI. Effect of abuse on health: results of a national survey. Arch Pediatr Adolesc Med. 2002;156(8):811–7.
75. Beck ME, Lineer MM, Melzer-Lange M, et al. Medical providers' understanding of sex trafficking and their experience with at-risk patients. Pediatr. 2015;155(4).
76. Ahn R, Alpert EJ, Purcell G, et al. Human trafficking: review of educational resources for health professionals. Am J Prev Med. 2013;44:283–9.
77. U.S. Department of Health & Human Services, Administration for Children & Families. Child welfare information gateway. Available from: https://www.childwelfare.gov/topics/systemwide/laws-policies/state/.
78. 42 U.S.C. § 5106a(b)(2)(B).
79. Todres J. Can mandatory reporting laws help child survivors of human trafficking? Wis L Rev Forward. 2016:69–78.
80. English A. Mandatory reporting of human trafficking: potential benefits and risks of harm. AMA Journal of Ethics. 2017;19(1):54–62.
81. Greenbaum VJ, Dodd M, McCracken C. A short screening tool to identify victims of child sex trafficking in the health care setting. Pediatr Emerg Care. 2018;34(1):33–7.
82. Sadwick R. 8 Tech Innovations that would counter sex trafficking. Forbes; 2016 May 24. [cited 2019 October 4]. Available from: https://www.forbes.com/sites/rebeccasadwick/2016/05/24/counter-trafficking/#6d5d526f677d.

Chapter 4
Medical Perspectives on Human Trafficking in Adolescent Sex Trafficking: A Review

Aisha Mays

Introduction

The United States Federal Trafficking Victims Protection Act (TVPA) of 2000 defines both sex and labor trafficking as severe forms of human trafficking and was the first comprehensive US law designed to protect affected individuals by providing protection, prosecution, and prevention efforts [1]. This chapter focuses on sex trafficking of adolescents. For an in-depth review of labor trafficking in adolescents, please see Chap. 5, Labor Trafficking: A Review.

Sex trafficking is defined as the human trafficking of an individual for the purposes of a commercial sex act by means of force, fraud, or coercion, whereby a commercial sex act is defined as any sex act in which anything of value is given to or received by any person [2]. Commercial sex acts may include but are not limited to sexual intercourse, sex tourism, mail-order-bride trade, early marriage, pornography, stripping, performing in sexual venues, and children and adolescents engaging in "survival sex" for life necessities [3, 4]. Adults, adolescents, or children can be affected by sex trafficking, and trafficking can exist irrespective of transit across domestic or international borders [5].

If an individual being sex trafficked is a minor (<18 years of age), this is defined as commercial sexual exploitation of children (CSEC). CSEC is the engagement in any sexual act in exchange for anything of value, *irrespective* of force, fraud, or coercion [2, 6–8]. This means that force, fraud, or coercion does not have to exist or be proven to consider transactional sexual acts with minors as CSEC. CSEC is an umbrella term which includes international, domestic, and transnational minor sex trafficking. Exploited adolescents can be trafficked across national borders, within

A. Mays (✉)
Core Faculty, UC Berkeley/UCSF Joint Medical Program UC, Berkeley School of Public Health, Berkeley, CA, USA

K. E. Titchen, E. Miller (eds.), *Medical Perspectives on Human Trafficking in Adolescents*, https://doi.org/10.1007/978-3-030-43367-3_4

a country, a state, or a single neighborhood [9]. Other names for CSEC include child sex trafficking, commercial sexual exploitation of youth (CSEY) [9], or youth affected by commercial sexual exploitation (YACSE). For the purposes of this chapter, we will refer to the act of commercial sexual exploitation of children and youth as "CSEC" and the population of commercially sexually exploited youth (including minors and young adults) as "CSEC youth." Where studies involve a subset of this population, we will indicate this.

The commercial sexual exploitation of minors who are US citizens or US legal residents *and* who are exploited within the USA is defined as domestic minor sex trafficking (DMST) [2, 10, 11]. The acronyms CSEC and DMST are often used interchangeably. While the TVPA originally focused on minors trafficked into the USA from other countries, in recent years through ratifications [12], the law has recognized that in addition to youth who are foreign born, US-born adolescents are also affected by sexual exploitation [9] and these two groups often have similar experiences and needs [4]. Moreover, for the first time in 2018, the United Nations Office of Drugs and Crimes (UNODC) Annual Report on Trafficking Persons found that the majority of trafficked individuals are exploited in their country of origin [13].

In line with these federal definitions, any minor engaging in commercial sex, even if they are not working with a third party, is considered to be a commercially sexually exploited individual [14], and anyone engaging with or providing a minor for a commercial sex act is considered a third party (trafficker). Overall, CSEC is considered child abuse [15–17]. Legally, CSEC is considered a severe form of human trafficking [2, 18], and there has been increasing legislation to support youth who are affected [19, 20] (such as an increasing number of states enacting "safe harbor laws") [21, 22] and to prosecute both traffickers and solicitors [23].

Although the legal definition of CSEC specifically pertains to minors affected by sex trafficking, it is well known among the anti-CSEC community and human trafficking scholars that vulnerability to and experience of the grave consequences of sexual exploitation does not end at age 18, but equally affects young adults [24]. This assertion was supported in the 2013 Institute of Medicine (IOM) review of CSEC, which notes, "If a 17-year-old being sold for sex is a victim of commercial sexual exploitation or sex trafficking, is he or she no longer a victim on the day that he or she turns 18" [4]? It is important to include transitional age youth ages 16–24, especially those aging out of foster care, in discussions about and in advocating for commercially sexually exploited youth [25]. This chapter focuses on the sex trafficking and commercial sexual exploitation of adolescents, both minors and transitional age youth (see also Chap. 8 for more details on youth in foster care).

The prevalence of CSEC in the USA is difficult to quantify due to the complex and concealed nature of human trafficking [14, 26] and the lack of universal data collection systems [27]. Although accurate prevalence data is not available, human trafficking experts, researchers, and advocates agree that national estimates are likely to be underestimates of the extent of the problem [4]. A 2013 study of homeless youth (a demographic at disproportionately high risk for exploitation) who were receiving services at a large metropolitan youth shelter found that 15% of the youth were involved in trafficking with an additional 8% engaging in sex in exchange for something of value (also called "survival sex" or "transactional sex") [28]. Efforts to address CSEC should include collaboration between researchers, human trafficking organizations, interdisciplinary professionals, and governmental organizations to more accurately quantify the scope of this problem [11].

Risk Factors

Risk factors that leave youth vulnerable to exploitation (whether for sex or labor) are multifactorial with most societal, community, and relationship risk factors leading to the individual risk factors.

The CDC's social ecological model (see section "Human Trafficking Understood Using a Public Health Framework" in Chap. 1) as a framework for human sex and labor trafficking illustrates the interconnectedness of risk factors and protective factors and the influence that human trafficking has on society, and this model can help to highlight systemic risk factors that lead to individual risk and vulnerabilities. Societal risk factors for CSEC include lack of awareness and education about CSEC, limited prevention strategies and focus on CSEC youth strengths/resilience factors [11], and gender inequities including the sexualization of girls and victimization due to sexual orientation [29, 30]. Community risk factors include community normalization, housing displacement, and community disenfranchisement (including poverty and violence) [30]. Living in poverty creates multiple risk factors for CSEC. In a qualitative study of Bay Area CSEC youth, Jones et al. found that over half of their participants had to leave their homes due to financial insecurity and soon were exploited in the form of "survival sex" (or transactional sex) in exchange for food and shelter [31]. Relationship risk factors include having a family member or close peer who is involved in exploitation, as well as exposure to family violence which may lead to family instability and a young person's decreased sense of safety [4, 32, 33]. Individual risk factors are most often cited in the literature and include youth's personal history of sexual abuse [34, 35], involvement in the foster care system [36], involvement in the juvenile justice system, identification as LGBTQ [29], and experiences of homelessness [36] and housing instability [4]. Additionally, youth with cognitive or emotional disabilities may be more vulnerable as they may be easier for a trafficker to control [14]. Overall, youth who are socially isolated and economically or emotionally vulnerable are at greater risk of exploitation [14].

It is important to consider why youth with particular social vulnerabilities or identity status are more vulnerable to CSEC. Future research and youth interventions must address the societal, community, and relationship factors that leave particular populations of youth more vulnerable to exploitation.

Health Outcomes for CSEC Youth

CSEC youth suffer from severe physical and mental health consequences of exploitation. Numerous studies of CSEC health outcomes show that CSEC youth are disproportionately impacted by sexually transmitted infections (STIs) and HIV, pelvic inflammatory disease(PID), pregnancy, substance use, depression, anxiety, posttraumatic stress disorder, and suicide [8, 37–40]. Additional studies also indicate that due to physical and sexual assault, CSEC youth also suffer from excessive injuries, including lacerations, burns, traumatic brain injuries, anogenital trauma, peritonitis, and bladder and urethral injuries [11, 41–43].

These health outcomes result in both short- and long-term health consequences, disability, and poor functioning among CSEC youth [11, 44, 45]. Although data are based on limited empirical evidence, advocates note that once youth have experienced exploitation, life expectancy may be substantially reduced, and a 2018 review of sex trafficking on health highlighted an exponential increase in morbidity due to communicable diseases, poor reproductive health, and violence [46, 47].

CSEC and Disparities

Extreme socioeconomic and structural inequities, including the intersections of poverty, gender inequality, and racism, directly drive the heightened rates of adolescent sex trafficking [12, 48–50]. These structural barriers limit young people's access to resources, including housing and employment opportunities, and contribute to negative health outcomes [4, 51]. As a result of these inequities, in the USA, youth of color, particularly Black and Latino youth [52–55], are disproportionately affected, with Black youth representing 50–80% and Latino youth representing 25% [52, 56–60] of the CSEC population [61]. In addition to structural inequities, societal hyper-sexualization (the disproportionate, extreme imposition of sexuality on a person and/or valuing a person only as an object of sexual desire) [62] of black [63–66] and brown youth [67, 68] continue to perpetuate their vulnerability to commercial sexual exploitation [69, 70]. In a 2013 study of African American girls vulnerable to CSEC with high exposure to popular media, Kruger et al. described the influence of societal hyper-sexualization upon African American girls in qualitative interviews where girls defined their sexuality as a commodity, describing that to maintain male interest, they needed to wear tight clothing and even perform sexual acts at peer social events. Future CSEC prevention efforts should incorporate addressing racism and the hyper-sexualization of black and brown and female youth as among the drivers of this epidemic [69].

Call for a Public Health Approach

The commercial sexual exploitation of youth is layered in its impact on societies, communities, and individuals; complex in the traumatic and multigenerational health effects on individuals; and multifactorial in its influence on social disparities, individual safety, and community values [30, 33, 71]. The CDC socioecological (Chap. 1 – Fig. 1.1) [72] model illustrates how societal, community, relationship, and individual factors can make youth vulnerable to CSEC and recommends that optimal prevention efforts address risk across these levels. A strong public health approach – one that emphasizes multidisciplinary collaboration, community relationships, and global education – is needed to comprehensively address the multiple dimensions of this issue [30, 44]. A public health approach to confronting CSEC calls for interdisciplinary collaboration between systems that interact with YACSE such as healthcare, education, child welfare, juvenile justice, and youth serving community-based organizations [4]. In 2018, using the CDC social ecological model, Greenbaum and colleagues presented multilevel strategies to address human trafficking as a holistic public health approach to address this systemic issue [30]. They explored how healthcare providers have diverse skills and strong influence which can support CSEC prevention at all socioecological levels and recommended that providers harness their positionality, not only to care for CSEC youth and families in a clinical setting (individual and relationship levels) but also to collaborate with multidisciplinary stakeholders (community level) and to participate in advocacy efforts (societal level) [30].

The following case illustrates how the medical community interacts with and in turn can provide support for an adolescent experiencing CSEC.

Case Presentation

Alanna is an 18-year-old cisgender female who comes to the same-day clinic at your community health center asking to see a doctor. During triage, the nurse asks Alanna why she'd like to be seen, and Alanna looks over at the young male who is with her and answers, "I think I need an STD test?" As the nurse escorts Alanna from the waiting room to the exam room, the young man follows along with Alanna. The nurse explains to them that under clinic policy all patients are seen alone for their medical visit. Alanna responds hurriedly, "Oh, it's ok, he's my boyfriend." The nurse informs them that it is still clinic policy to see patients alone. Alanna's boyfriend says that he is coming with her, especially because she said that it's ok. The nurse, resignedly, rooms Alanna and her boyfriend. Once in the exam room, the nurse asks why Alanna wants to be tested for sexually transmitted infections (STIs), and Alanna giggles, looks over at her boyfriend, and says, "There's *stuff* coming out of my vagina." The nurse asks her how long she has been having these symptoms. Alanna, looking at her boyfriend, answers "Um...I don't know." The nurse leaves the room and gives report to you as the same-day physician in clinic, letting you know that the patient is ready and that there seems to be something "weird" going on.

The Role of the Medical Community

The medical community can play a vital role in supporting adolescents affected by commercial sexual exploitation as it is a natural, safe, and confidential environment where individuals can access comprehensive care [73]. Studies have shown that trafficked individuals have multiple encounters with the healthcare community while being exploited [73–75] with estimates that between 50 and 80% of human trafficked individuals have seen a healthcare professional within the past 6 months [51]. Similarly, youth affected by sex trafficking have been found to frequently seek medical care [8, 39, 40, 61]. A New York City study of CSEC youth found that 82% of CSEC youth had also seen a healthcare professional in the past 6 months for varied reasons, including a general checkup, STI or HIV testing, or because they were pregnant [61]. Additionally, YACSE have been found to present for medical care in a variety of settings including emergency rooms, primary care clinics, family planning clinics, medical clinics co-located in community-based organizations, and school-based health centers [43, 76]. Because we know that CSEC youth seek healthcare across diverse healthcare settings, it is important that all healthcare professionals are aware of commercial sexual exploitation of youth and the common signs that may indicate that an adolescent is being affected.

In 2014, the Institute of Medicine declared in their report on CSEC and healthcare that each interaction with a medical professional is an opportunity for positive intervention and that health professionals must be prepared to identify and support youth affected by sex trafficking [4].

Below are commonly reported signs that may present in the clinical setting which can indicate that an adolescent may be affected by sex trafficking.

Signs that a Patient May Be Experiencing Sex Trafficking

Youth affected by sex trafficking may present with a common constellation of signs and symptoms as a result of being subject to exploitation. It is important for healthcare professionals to be aware of these common indicators as CSEC youth often do not self-identify as being exploited and/or may not disclose their exploitation to any member of the medical team [10, 11]. These common indicators are compiled from research data investigating CSEC risk factors along with clinical experiences from experts in the field and should serve as a guide to identifying signs of CSEC. These lists of common indicators are not representative of all CSEC youth's clinical presentations or experiences, and it is important to remember that some youth do not present with any of these signs: every youth has a unique set of experiences and circumstances. Additionally, it is important to recognize that one individual clinical sign, evaluated in isolation, may indicate a level of vulnerability for an adolescent but may not indicate that the youth is being commercially sexually exploited. It is important not to single out or stereotype youth based on individual clinical signs or social vulnerabilities. That said, youth who are affected by sex trafficking will often present with several common clinical indicators [11] See Table 4.1.

Part 2: Case Continued

When you enter the exam room, it seems as if Alanna and her boyfriend have been arguing. Alanna looks upset and her eyes are tearful. You introduce yourself to Alanna and her boyfriend and review with them the clinic policy of seeing all patients alone. Alanna's boyfriend looks annoyed, gets up, and leaves the room. You

Table 4.1 Initial clinical presentation – potential indicators [4, 8, 38, 77]

Presentation Signs of compromised relationships, internalized trauma, and lack of physical stability	Medical history Signs of inconsistent, extreme, or poor access to medical care	Social history Signs of social disconnection, isolation, abuse, or maltreatment	Physical exam Signs of physical control, harm, and involvement in dangerous behaviors
Appears younger than stated age	Repeat emergency room visits	Frequent missed appointments	Tattoos with name, sexually explicit
Physical signs not consistent with history	Repeat visits for emergency contraception	Lack of personal identification	Withdrawn or hypervigilant
Domineering older adult who speaks for the youth	Repeat visits for physical injuries	Lost to follow up	Attachment to cell phone (or two cell phones)
Delayed presentation for medical care	History of multiple pregnancies/ abortions	History of involvement with child protective services	Physical signs of inflicted injury
Withdrawn, submissive, or aggressive	History of multiple STIs	Chronic truancy	Large amounts of cash, expensive clothing
Significantly older partner		History of sexual abuse	Signs of injection drug use
Adult with youth pays for visit with cash		History of running away from home	

ask Alanna to tell you more about the symptoms that brought her in. Alanna says that she doesn't know, but there's just stuff coming out of her vagina. You ask her if she's had symptoms like this before and she responds, "I don't know." You ask her if she's been tested for STIs in the past, and looking irritated, she responds "Umm. I don't know." Alanna then looks at you and asks if she can just get tested; she doesn't want to answer any more questions. Her boyfriend said she should get tested so that's what she wants to do.

Trauma Bonding

Trauma bonding, also known as Stockholm syndrome or traumatic coercive bonding, refers to the powerful emotional attachment created between abused individuals and their abusers as a result of a complex and often confusing combination of "loving" and violent interactions, coercive control, and severe power imbalances [78–80]. Through this dynamic, the abused individual begins to sympathize with and care for and even protect the abuser [17]. The abused individual gradually loses their sense of self, adopts the worldview of the abuser, and often takes responsibility for the abuse [80].

Youth experiencing CSEC often develop trauma bonds with the trafficker as a coping response to the extreme stress of CSEC in an attempt to feel a sense of safety and reduce suffering [80]. Trauma bonds between CSEC youth and the trafficker are further strengthened and complicated as the youth often relies on the trafficker for protection from the violence of solicitors ("buyers" or "customers") [61]. Along with the distorted emotional connections CSEC youth experience, trauma bonds also hamper the adolescent's psychological and neurophysiological development [76, 80, 81], thereby making it difficult for the youth to recognize their exploitation [17, 76, 82]. An adolescent who has developed trauma bonds with a trafficker may try to protect the trafficker, may disengage from anyone who speaks negatively of the trafficker, and may refuse to leave the trafficker. Trauma bonding with traffickers is one of the strongest forces that keeps youth in the cycle of exploitation [45, 83]. Signs of trauma bonding between CSEC youth and traffickers include:

- CSEC youth exhibits positive feelings toward the trafficker.
- Trafficker exhibits positive feelings toward the CSEC youth.
- CSEC youth may protect or defend the trafficker.
- CSEC unable to engage in behaviors that may assist their detachment from the trafficker.
- CSEC youth may have negative feelings toward family, friends, and authority figures trying to support them to leave the trafficker.

In the beginning of the patient scenario, we see Alanna repeatedly looking at her boyfriend before answering any questions. Further, she advocates for him to remain in the exam room, even after the nurse asks him to leave. We also see the boyfriend using Alanna's advocacy to justify his remaining in the exam room. These types of behaviors may indicate trauma bonding between the adolescent and the trafficker.

Recently, some scholars have begun to coin another term to describe the traumatic attachments between CSEC youth and traffickers: traumatic coercive bonding [80]. Traumatic coercive bonding is specifically used to describe the CSEC relationship, as this captures the intentional ways in which traffickers will encourage the young person to become "attached" to them which allows for even deeper and more insidious control. Traumatic coercive boding used to describe CSEC youth attachments differs from the more widely known Stockholm syndrome where the abuser and abused individual develop bidirectional attachments [80, 84]. Traumatic coercive bonding is a relatively new theory that merits further empirical research and exploration.

Importance of Seeing Patients Alone

A core value of adolescent medicine is to provide a private environment for youth to discuss their health with the clinician. Both the US Society for Adolescent Health and Medicine and the American Academy of Pediatrics support confidential care for adolescents [80, 85, 86]. Providing privacy during the clinical encounter is of vital importance when caring for CSEC youth or youth who are at-risk for CSEC [8]. Any person accompanying an adolescent to a medical visit could be a trafficker, irrespective of their relationship to the adolescent; therefore, it should be standard policy that all adolescent patients have time alone with the clinician.

Posting a privacy statement in the medical waiting areas and in all of the exam rooms is one way to reinforce the privacy policy to all individuals in the medical environment. A sample privacy policy that could be posted in the clinical areas might read, "Our Policy on Patient Privacy: In order to ensure the privacy of patients, it is our policy that all patients are seen alone with the medical provider."

Building Rapport

Most importantly, clinicians must support and sustain connection with CSEC and at-risk youth by building genuine rapport with the adolescent. Building sincere connection, without judgment, supports CSEC youth empowerment and self-efficacy [43, 87, 88] and supports their engagement with their own healthcare [43, 76].

A qualitative study of CSEC youth reported that a major barrier to their accessing medical care and trusting healthcare staff was feeling judged by the clinician and feeling that the clinician was not invested in getting to know them [43].

Healthcare professionals should use nonjudgmental approaches that are both empowering and strength-based to build rapport and to create therapeutic relationships with CSEC youth [43].

For example, clinicians should use the strength-based HEEADSSS psychosocial assessment (SHEEADSSS) to begin to build rapport with youth affected by sexual exploitation. Drawing on the adolescent's strengths [89] with the SHEEADSSS will give the provider a deeper understanding of the context of the adolescent's life, demonstrate the medical provider's desire to understand the holistic needs of CSEC youth, and foster an authentic relationship between the clinician and the young person seeking care. Table 4.2 outlines the SHEEADSSS assessment.

The SHEEADSSS is only an initial psychosocial assessment of the adolescent, a way to begin to build rapport with CSEC youth. Often clinicians will not be able to ask all of the SHEEADSSS questions in the initial medical encounter with CSEC youth; nor is it necessary. Instead, the clinician should plan to build on the SHEEADSSS assessment in future visits with the adolescent.

Of note, the SHEEADSSS is an assessment tool and not a screening or diagnostic tool. If the SHEEADSSS assessment raises concerns for health issues (e.g., depression or substance dependency), the clinician should use the appropriate adolescent screening or diagnostic tool. (see Chaps. 9 and 13 for more detailed information on psychiatric disorders and substance use, respectively. See Chap. 11, Table 11.1, for the similar SSHADESS assessment tool).

Table 4.2 Strengths-based psychosocial assessment

Strengths-based HEEADSSS assessment – SHEEADSSS [89, 90]	
STRENGTHS	What do you do really well? What are some of your talents?
HOME	Whom do you live with? How are things going where you live?
EDUCATION	Tell me about school. What do you like about school? What don't you like?
EATING	What healthy things do you like to eat? How easy is it for you to find healthy food to eat?
ACTIVITIES	What do you do for fun? Who do you hang out with? How do you feel when you're with them?
DRUGS	How much would you say you smoke, if any? What about alcohol? Or any other drugs?
SEX	Have you ever had sex? What feels good about having sex? What about any times when someone has made you do sexual things when you didn't want to?
SUICIDE/ DEPRESSION	What do you do when you feel sad? Who's a safe adult you can talk to about how you're feeling?
SAFETY	What do you do to feel safe?

The Medical Interview

The medical interview with CSEC youth can sometimes be challenging as youth can present to the medical environment with varied dispositions ranging from cheerful to distressed. The CSEC youth may have recently experienced trauma or an assault and may be scared or angry; the youth may be depressed, belligerent, or somnolent from chronic traumatic stress; or they may be anxious and worried about potentially encountering the police in the clinical environment [8, 39, 43, 76]. It is important for the clinician to be aware of and sensitive to these types of presentations and to create a compassionate and open environment where the adolescent feels comfortable speaking openly and honestly. During the medical interview, it is most important to establish rapport and build trust with the adolescent patient as opposed to collecting data or interrogating them [77]. The World Health Organization has published guidelines for conducting the medical interview with individuals affected by sex trafficking that emphasize ensuring patient safety, avoiding retraumatization when discussing sensitive issues, and trauma-informed practices [91].

Limits of Confidentiality

Clinicians must ensure privacy and confidentiality when caring for CSEC youth. A challenge to ensuring confidentiality with minor CSEC youth is that, in some cases, the information discussed falls outside of the limits of confidentiality and mandate reporting to authorities, such as child protective services and law enforcement. It is therefore essential to discuss with the adolescent the limits of confidentiality *at the beginning of the medical interview* in the event that some of the information discussed requires you to break the confidentiality agreement with the CSEC youth (see also Chap. 18 for further discussion of balancing a young person's safety and autonomy and processes for reporting to authorities).

Below is a sample script on how to introduce conditional confidentiality with your adolescent patients.

> Everything that we discuss here is private. This means that by law I am not allowed to discuss with anyone outside of your medical team what we talk about today, unless you give me permission to do so. However, if you tell me that you are going to hurt yourself, hurt someone else, or if someone is hurting you, then in those cases, I will need to tell someone and get help.

There are differences in the limits of confidentiality between minor adolescents and TAY which are discussed in detail in Chap. 18, Medicolegal Aspects and Mandatory Reporting. Please refer to Table 3.3 in Chap. 3 for a list of sample open-ended questions.

Of particular importance for CSEC youth and those at-risk for sex trafficking is to inform the patient that they are not required to answer any questions that they are asked and that at all times they are in control of the medical interview [11]. Explicitly explaining to CSEC youth that they have this autonomy is critical, as CSEC youth are living in conditions where their control and autonomy is constantly compromised and manipulated [11].

Trauma-Informed Care

One of the hallmarks of providing medical care to CSEC youth or adolescents at-risk for sex trafficking is to apply trauma-informed principles to your clinical practice. All individuals, regardless of their experience of sexual exploitation, have experienced some form of trauma in their lives, so trauma-informed principles, also known as trauma-informed care, should be applied to all patient interactions [92] and, in particular, to the care of CSEC youth, as they have been subjected to severe, complex trauma [3, 76, 87, 93].

Trauma-informed principles recognize the signs of trauma, understand the impact of past and present trauma on an individual's life and coping, and incorporate this understanding into practices to support an individual's empowerment and avoid retraumatization [93, 94]. Trauma-informed care employs these principles as a strength-based approach to maximize the patient's accessibility, safety, agency, and trust in the healthcare environment [95].

Trauma-informed care will help the clinician to understand that traumatic stress may manifest in the medical encounter in the form of a patient's withdrawn affect, belligerence, or guardedness [11, 76, 94]. These principles will help the clinician to avoid being defensive and to instead focus on the patient's healing (For more on trauma-informed care and complex trauma, see Chap. 9, The Psychiatric Patient).

The goal of trauma-informed care with CSEC youth (adapted from Alpert et al.) [96]:

1. Avoid retraumatization.
2. Highlight youth's strengths and resilience.
3. Promote healing and recovery.
4. Support the development of healthy short- and long-term coping mechanisms.

Many patients, regardless of their experience of sexual exploitation, have had some form of trauma in their lives that may present during the medical encounter. CSEC youth or adolescents with other social vulnerabilities should not be treated differently or stereotyped as needing "trauma-informed care" more than other patients. *Trauma-informed care and principles should be applied to all medical encounters with all patients.*

Part 3: Case Continued
You tell Alanna that you're happy that she came in for testing and explain to her that you would like to perform a pelvic exam to assess the vaginal discharge and send it for testing. Alanna says that it's often irritated "down there," but she knew that you'd want to look, so she agrees. You bring your medical assistant into the room as chaperone for the exam, and upon speculum examination you notice mucopurulent discharge in the vaginal vault. You collect a sample of the discharge and ask Alanna if it's ok to place two fingers inside her vagina to feel if her cervix is painful or irritated. She looks at you with a worried gaze and says "OK." You let her know that if at any time she feels uncomfortable or has pain, she can stop the exam. She replies, "good, OK." She does not have cervical motion or adnexal tenderness on exam. Microscopic wet mount examination reveals more than 10 white blood cells per high-powered field.

The Physical Exam with CSEC Youth

Performing a physical exam with youth who are affected by sexual exploitation may be frightening, as the adolescent may feel a loss of control or may be triggered by any portion of the physical exam [11]. Because of the coercive, exploitative, and purposefully disempowering nature of human trafficking, routine and customary procedures inherent to ordinary medical practice – such as asking a patient to undress for an exam, performing a gynecological exam, or even engaging in mundane activities such as checking a blood pressure – may be anxiety-provoking or perceived as threatening [83] (see Table 4.3).

It is vital that the clinician apply trauma-informed principles by asking the youth's permission to perform the physical exam and by explaining why specific physical exam maneuvers are important [11, 97]. It is equally key to inform the patient that they can refuse any portion of the physical exam at any time, while also explaining plainly how this could limit accurate diagnosis and treatment.

The physical exam should focus on a thorough assessment of the patient's presenting complaints along with evaluating any additional physical findings the

Table 4.3 Traumatic experiences and the physical exam

CSEC traumatic experiences	Traumatic experiences that could be associated with the physical exam
Forced sexual acts	Being asked to undress for physical exam
Violent interactions with traffickers, solicitors, or others	Performing a gynecological exam
Trauma bonding with trafficker	Drawing blood or taking blood pressure

Adapted from Physicians for Reproductive Health, Adolescent Reproductive Sexual Health Education Program. Commercial Sexual Exploitation of Children (CSEC): Addressing the Healthcare Provider's Role in Identifying the Health Needs and Providing Support for Commercially Sexually Exploited Children [96]

patient may have [11]. The patient should be kept informed of any incidental physical findings. Frequent check-ins with the adolescent throughout the exam may alleviate anxiety and strengthen trust. If the patient requires a sexual assault exam or any other form of extensive physical exam, it is imperative that you have a collaborative, trauma-informed medical team (including a sexual assault examiner, mental health provider, social worker, and medical provider) introduced to the patient [98]. Before any type of extensive exam is undertaken, it is imperative that the clinician first have a discussion with the CSEC youth about why the exam is important [97].

(See Chap. 3, Table 3.4, for a summary of the steps for the physical exam with traumatized patients. For a more detailed discussion on sexual assault and the trauma-informed gynecologic exam, please refer to Chap. 16, Table 16.1).

Laboratory Testing and Medication Administration

The extent of laboratory testing and medication administration will differ based on the clinical site where you are caring for a CSEC adolescent. In some situations, the clinician will be caring for a CSEC youth or at-risk youth in an acute setting, while for others, care may be provided in a primary care clinical care setting.

For the acute care setting where CSEC youth may have been involved in a recent traumatic encounter, it is recommended to provide standard laboratory testing and medications listed in Table 4.4. When testing for STIs, it is important to test all possible sites of infection, including genital, anorectal, and pharyngeal (see section "Forensic Medical Documentation" in Chap. 3 and corresponding Table 3.5 for a summary of the forensic exam and documentation).

Many CSEC youth receive ongoing clinical and primary care outside of an acute or emergency situation. Providing ongoing nonjudgmental, compassionate, primary medical care to CSEC youth is important for affirming their agency and proactivity in caring for their health and for supporting long-term positive health outcomes [43, 77, 87].

The laboratory testing and medication delivery for CSEC youth in the ongoing clinical care setting will look similar to other youth being assessed for similar health conditions, as noted in Table 4.5.

Table 4.4 CSEC youth receiving acute or emergency care

CSEC acute/emergency care	
Laboratory testing	Medications
STIs: CT, GC, *Trichomonas*, Hep B sAg, Hep C Ab, syphilis (RPR), HIV Ag/Ab	Presumptive treatments for GC, CT, *Trichomonas*
Transaminases (ALT, AST)	Postexposure prophylaxis (PEP)[a]
Creatinine	
Pregnancy	Emergency contraception

[11, 44]
[a]If the adolescent is amenable to adherence

Table 4.5 CSEC youth receiving ongoing clinical or primary care

CSEC primary care	
Laboratory testing	Medications
STIs: CT, GC, *Trichomonas*, Hep A, Hep B sAg, Hep C Ab, syphilis (RPR), HIV Ag/Ab	Condoms[a]
Transaminases (ALT, AST)	Pre-exposure prophylaxis (PrEP)[b]
Creatinine	Chronic primary care and mental health medications/refills
Pregnancy	Contraception[a]

[99]
[a]If the adolescent desires
[b]If the adolescent is amenable to adherence

Part 4: Case Wrap-Up

You discuss with Alanna the results of her pelvic exam, informing her that you will send the vaginal discharge to the lab to test for gonorrhea and chlamydia. You also let her know that it is important to treat her today for an infection of her cervix because you saw a high number of "infection" cells on microscopic examination. Alanna looks fearful and starts to cry. She says that she knew that she was going to "catch something." You ask Alanna what she means by this, and she replies "I don't want to talk about it." You inform Alanna that you would like to give her a one-time dose of azithromycin and a shot of ceftriaxone in clinic today to treat the infection and that it's important that she does not have sex for 1 week. Alanna looks up at you startled and says, "What about having sex?" You repeat that she should not have sex for 1 week. Fearfully, Alanna looks at you and asks, "Can you write that in the instructions?" You also ask her if she would like assistance with notifying and treating any sexual partners. She replies, "I'll take care of it."

The Medical Provider Role in Assessment and Identification

Healthcare professionals are essential frontline responders and allies in supporting youth who are affected by or at-risk of CSEC [73]. For any healthcare professional, regardless of training background, it may feel overwhelming to consider how to provide compassionate, high-quality care to CSEC youth that addresses their complex needs.

Quality comprehensive care for CSEC youth requires that clinicians work with a multidisciplinary team which includes nurses, medical assistants and support staff, mental health professionals, social workers, and community-based partners (such as CSEC service advocates and legal experts) with expertise in adolescent sex trafficking and experience in providing compassionate, trauma-sensitive care [76, 100].

The clinician should keep in mind two overall goals to best utilize the clinical environment to support the holistic needs of CSEC youth: universal assessment and identification [83].

Primary Goal: Universal Assessment

The primary goal in caring for CSEC youth or youth at-risk for CSEC is the assessment to provide support, resources, and safety, NOT screening for identification or definitive disclosure of CSEC. It may take CSEC youth many visits to disclose their exploitation or they may never choose to disclose. Focusing solely on screening for disclosure is neither patient-centered nor trauma-informed, and screening practices in a vacuum without a clear system for connecting youth to supports and services should be avoided.

The clinician should NOT withhold supportive resources for individuals affected by or at-risk for CSEC while awaiting a disclosure. Instead, the clinician can and should provide universal education and resources for all youth.

Universal CSEC assessment of all youth presenting to the clinical environment can be achieved by utilizing the SHEEADSSS assessment, validated CSEC assessment tools (presented below), referencing common clinical indicators (see clinical indicator section above), and building rapport with the patient.

As part of universal CSEC assessments of all youth, clinicians should have a supportive conversation with adolescents about healthy and unhealthy relationships. Normalizing these conversations helps the adolescent to acquire a healthy understanding of how intimate relationships affect their lives. A 2019 review of best practices in intimate partner violence and healthcare recommended the CUES approach (Table 4.6) to facilitate healthy relationship discussion with adolescents [101]. For further information on trauma-informed responses, see Chap. 21, Fig. 21.1, to learn about the PEARR tool.

The clinician and healthcare team should remember that youth have the right to decline support for any resources offered. The clinician's role is to inform the patient of available resources, to support their autonomy and health, and to welcome the adolescent to accept the support on their terms and when they are ready.

While disclosure is not required for mandated reporting and a report can be made based on suspicion of CSEC, abuse, and/or concern about safety, engagement of the young person in any reporting processes is strongly recommended (see Chap. 18 for more information on mandated reporting).

Table 4.6 CUES universal education approach to addressing trauma and violence [101]

CUES: A Universal Education Approach to Addressing Trauma and Violence Including Human Trafficking[a]
C: Confidentiality = safety
Always see patients alone
Discuss limits of confidentiality, including local reporting requirements
UE: Universal education + empowerment
Normalize discussion by reminding patients that everyone receives information about importance of healthy relationships and impact of unhealthy ones
Include resources and information about human trafficking including hotline number
Encourage helping others by offering two educational cards+ "in case you ever need this for yourself or so you can help someone you know"
Offer information to all patients regardless of disclosure ("if safe to take with you"); may follow this brief education with direct inquiry: "Is any of this part of your story?"
S: Support for disclosures
Though disclosure is not the goal, be prepared if a patient discloses to provide warm referrals to local and/or national advocacy hotlines/services
Provide harm reduction strategies – such as offering contraceptive method that partner cannot interfere with; offer use of phone in clinic to call an advocate; create a care plan that takes social context such as housing instability or other circumstances into consideration
Develop a plan for follow-up
Document referrals in patient's chart to help facilitate follow-up

[a]Adapted from CUES: Addressing Domestic and Sexual Violence in Health Settings. Futures Without Violence and modified with permission from Futures Without Violence and Dr. Elizabeth Miller. +Palm size educational cards available at futureswithoutviolence.org/?s=safety+card#chev589

Secondary Goal: Identification

Identification – adolescent disclosure or classification of CSEC or CSEC risk based on screening – in the medical setting should be the clinician's secondary goal in caring for CSEC youth or youth at-risk for CSEC. Numerous factors may inhibit youth from disclosing their exploitation including fear of their trafficker and lack of identifying with their own exploitation [102–104]. In the clinical setting, CSEC youth may be identified through various means including CSEC or human trafficking-specific assessment tools, self-disclosure, or community informants. Definitive CSEC youth identification or disclosure may allow the clinician to more confidently file a mandated report (if required), connect the youth to more specific sex trafficking resources, or provide more detailed information to the CSEC youth regarding supportive services to which they are entitled (i.e., victims of crime support) [4, 105]. Definitive CSEC identification may also be useful to support initiating or ongoing legal cases against traffickers or solicitors by adding to the body of evidence against these offenders.

It bears repeating that the clinician should remember that all of the clinical support for CSEC youth and youth at-risk for CSEC can and should be provided with or without disclosure, so it is important the medical provider not wait for definitive identification to provide support.

Assessment Tools

Asking validated questions related to trafficking in the medical environment is acceptable as part of a full CSEC assessment provided that the clinical setting is equipped to provide supportive on-site resources for the youth (social work, mental health, security services) and the clinical team is aware of and able to make referrals to community-based organizations working with CSEC, especially ones that can provide emergency housing with connection to longer-term housing resources. This interdisciplinary wraparound support is vital if screening for CSEC is occurring. If wraparound support services are not available, they should be developed *before* screening is implemented to ensure that the clinical site is prepared in the event of an identification or disclosure. If the clinical site does not have the appropriate resources on-site or by referral, then screening for CSEC or other forms of human trafficking is not recommended.

For resources about how to identify resources in your area and to create a comprehensive CSEC and human trafficking support response protocol in your healthcare setting, please see the Polaris Project Resources Referral Directory [106] and HEAL Trafficking: Human Trafficking Medical Protocol Toolkit [107].

Human trafficking experts and researchers across the USA have created trauma-informed screening CSEC tools [102, 104, 108], and several have been validated for screening accuracy [102, 109, 110]. In 2018, multisite study by Greenbaum et al. in emergency departments, child advocacy centers, and teen clinics evaluated the efficacy of a CSEC screening tool in the healthcare setting: this shows promising results as a screening and prevention tool, yet lacks ideal specificity to distinguish CSEC youth from youth who have experienced other forms of sexual violence [109].

To date there is no evidence that increased identification improves patient health [111]. Existing validated tools [102, 109] show promising results for the development of universal, standard-of-care CSEC evaluations for all adolescents, through integrating CSEC screening tools with patient assessments. Additional research is needed to improve the validity of medical CSEC screening tools to be used as identification measures, to evaluate the effectiveness of these tools in connecting adolescents to supports and services, and to gauge the effects of identification and treatment on physical and mental health outcomes for this population.

Table 4.7 highlights suggested questions for directly exploring potential sex trafficking or CSEC at a healthcare site with an established multidisciplinary response and protocol.

Table 4.7 Sample questions for CSEC identification [8]

Sample questions for CSEC identification
1. Has anyone ever asked you to have sex in exchange for something you wanted or needed (money, food, shelter, or other items)?
2. Has anyone ever asked you to have sex with another person?
3. Has anyone ever taken sexual pictures of you or posted such pictures on the Internet?

Patient Follow-Up and Ongoing Care

A special role for clinicians caring for young people is the ability to regularly interact and form long-term, trusting relationships with adolescents. This unique position should be marshalled to engage and support CSEC youth and youth at-risk for CSEC and to provide consistent ongoing and collaborative medical care with a focus on encouraging routine follow-up [25].

To provide comprehensive clinical care, the clinician does not need to inquire about all potentially sensitive issues (e.g., nature of relationships, sexual practices) during the first clinical encounter, as the youth may feel uncomfortable with or offended by discussing personal topics from an unfamiliar person [43].

Instead, a key to caring for reluctant or guarded CSEC youth is to schedule frequent follow-up visits to continue to build rapport and establish trust. Gradual yet intentional steps in relationship building can be the most important element in promoting overall positive health interactions with CSEC youth [43] (see Table 4.8).

Importance of Clinic-Wide Education and Clinical Protocols to Respond to Sex Trafficking in the Medical Setting

The IOM (now the National Academy of Medicine, NAM) in 2013 called for increased training among a wide audience including members of the medical community to prevent, identify, and respond to CSEC. Further recommendations by the Institute/Academy call for collaboration across the medical, educational, and law enforcement sectors to increase awareness among the public – including among youth and patients who are minors – and to engage in collaborative prevention, connection to community resources, and research of CSEC [4].

Despite these recommendations, healthcare professionals' understanding of how to support CSEC in the clinical setting remains low, with 60% to 80% of healthcare professionals acknowledging limited training in or knowledge or awareness of how to respond CSEC youth [112–115]. To increase awareness among the medical community, it is important that clinical systems provide human trafficking trainings for the entire healthcare team and develop tailored human trafficking response protocols [116] to use in their clinical setting that address patient

Table 4.8 Guiding principles for providing medical care to CSEC youth [43]

Guiding principles for providing medical care to CSEC youth
1. Utilize trauma-informed approach for all patients
2. Partner with community agencies outside the health sector to provide wraparound services for youth
3. Utilize healthcare tools designed to care for CSEC patients
4. Collaborate and seek support from colleagues within the health sector who have been engaged in anti-trafficking work

assessment, safety, and support for individuals affected by or at-risk of human trafficking. To this end and at the time of this writing, some states through public health laws are beginning to require that all staff in healthcare settings receive training in recognizing and assisting patients who are victims of either sex or labor trafficking (or both) [117–119].

A 2016 systematic review of healthcare protocols to identify and treat individuals affected by human trafficking found that only 50% of protocols recommended that providers have initial training on human trafficking as part of protocol implementation [116].

To best respond to human trafficking in the clinical environment, trafficking response protocols should consist of a collaborative, multidisciplinary team of clinicians, mental health providers, social workers, and human trafficking community-based agencies to provide wraparound evaluation and ongoing support for affected and at-risk individuals [116].

HEAL Trafficking: Human Trafficking Medical Protocol Toolkit and the Asian Health Services, Oakland, California, Clinic-Based CSEC protocol [104, 107] are two examples of clinical site human trafficking protocols that can be tailored to the medical community in which you serve.

Conclusion

Sex trafficking of youth is a largely underrecognized problem in the USA. Healthcare professionals are on the front lines and are positioned to provide assessment and support for youth who are affected by or at-risk for commercial sexual exploitation. Healthcare professionals need to understand the socioecological factors that leave youth vulnerable to exploitation, recognize the common clinical signs that may indicate that an adolescent is being exploited, and be proficient in applying trauma-informed principles when working with CSEC and at-risk youth.

References

1. National Human Trafficking Hotline. Federal Law [Internet]. [cited 2019 May 17]. Available from: https://humantraffickinghotline.org/what-human-trafficking/federal-law.
2. Trafficking Victims Protection Act of 2000. 22 U.S. Code §§ 7102(4), (9), and (10). Sect. No. 106–386, 114. Oct 8, 2000.
3. Barnert E, Iqbal Z, Bruce J, Anoshiravani A, Kolhatkar G, Greenbaum J. Commercial sexual exploitation and sex trafficking of children and adolescents: a narrative review. Acad Pediatr. 2017;17:825–9.
4. Institute of Medicine (U.S.) Committee on the Commercial Sexual Exploitation and Sex Trafficking of Minors in the United States., Clayton EW, Krugman RD, Simon P, Institute of Medicine (U.S.), National Research Council (U.S.). Confronting commercial sexual exploitation and sex trafficking of minors in the United States. Washington, D.C.: National Academies Press; 2013.

5. United States Department of State. Trafficking in persons report. 2013 Jun.
6. United States Department of Justice. Federal Strategic Action Plan on Services for Victims of Human Trafficking in the United States 2013-2017. 2013.
7. McCoy M. Measurements of vulnerability to domestic minor sex trafficking: a systematic review. J Hum Traffick. 2017;5:1–12.
8. Greenbaum J, Crawford-Jakubiak JE. Committee on child Abuse and neglect. Child sex trafficking and commercial sexual exploitation: health care needs of victims. Pediatrics. 2015;135:566–74.
9. Goldberg AP, Moore JL, Barron CE. Domestic minor sex trafficking: guidance for communicating with patients. Hosp Pediatr. 2019;9:308–10.
10. Smith L, Vardaman SH, Snow M. The national report on domestic minor sex trafficking: America's prostituted children. 2009.
11. Greenbaum VJ. Commercial sexual exploitation and sex trafficking of children in the United States. Curr Probl Pediatr Adolesc Health Care. 2014;44:245–69.
12. Hardy VL, Compton KD, McPhatter VS. Domestic minor sex trafficking. Affilia. 2013;28:8–18.
13. United Nations Office on Drugs and Crime (UNODC). Global Report on Trafficking in Persons. Vienna: United Nations; 2018.
14. Powell CL, Bennouna C. Sex trafficking in the USA. In: Chisolm-Straker M, Stoklosa H, editors. Human trafficking is a public health issue: a paradigm expansion in the United States. Cham: Springer International Publishing; 2017. p. 43–66.
15. Greenbaum J, Kellogg N, Isaac R. The commercial sexual exploitation of children: the medical provider's role in identification, assessment, and treatment: APSAC practice guidelines. 2013.
16. Estes RJ, Weiner NA. The commercial sexual exploitation of children in the US, Canada and Mexico. abolitionistmom.org; 2001.
17. Basson D, Rosenblatt E, Haley H. Research to action: sexually exploited minors (SEM) needs and strengths. WestCoast Children's Clinic: Oakland, CA; 2012.
18. Violence Against Women Reauthorization Act of 2013. Sect. Stat. 54–160, 113–4, 127 2013.
19. Roby JL, Vincent M. Federal and state responses to domestic minor sex trafficking: the evolution of policy. Soc Work. 2017;62:201–10.
20. Justice for Victims of Trafficking Act of 2015 [Internet]. 114–22 2015. Available from: https://www.congress.gov/bill/114th-congress/senate-bill/178.
21. Wayman RA. Safe harbor laws: policy in the best interest of victims of trafficking. ABA Midyear Meeting.
22. Geist D. Finding the Safe Harbor: protection, prosecution, and state strategies to address prostituted minors. Legis & Pol'y Brief. 2011;4.
23. Roby JL, Vincent M. Federal and state responses to domestic minor sex trafficking: the evolution of policy. Soc Work. 2017;62:201–10.
24. Marcus A, Riggs R, Horning A, Rivera S, Curtis R, Thompson E. Is child to adult as victim is to criminal? Sex Res Soc Policy. 2012;9:153–66.
25. Chang KSG, Hayashi AS. The role of community health centers in addressing human trafficking. In: Chisolm-Straker M, Stoklosa H, editors. Human trafficking is a public health issue. Cham: Springer International Publishing; 2017. p. 347–62.
26. Nawyn SJ, Birdal NBK, Glogower N. Estimating the extent of sex trafficking. Int J Sociol. 2013;43:55–71.
27. United States Department of State. Trafficking in Persons Report [Internet]. U.S. Department of State; 2019. Available from: https://www.state.gov/wp-content/uploads/2019/01/282798.pdf.
28. Bigelsen J, Vuotto S. Homelessness, survival sex and human trafficking: as experienced by the youth of covenant house New York. New York: Covenant House; 2013.
29. Reid JA, Baglivio MT, Piquero AR, Greenwald MA, Epps N. Human trafficking of minors and childhood adversity in Florida. Am J Public Health. 2017;107:306–11.

30. Greenbaum VJ, Titchen K, Walker-Descartes I, Feifer A, Rood CJ, Fong H-F. Multi-level prevention of human trafficking: the role of health care professionals. Prev Med. 2018;114:164–7.
31. Jones N, Gamson J, Fisher S, Fucella P, Lee V, Zolala-Tovar V. Experiences of youth in the sex trade in the Bay Area. Center Court Innovat. 2016.
32. Greenbaum J, Bodrick N, Committee on Child Abuse and Neglect, Section on International Child Health. Global human trafficking and child victimization. Pediatrics. 2017:140.
33. Chisolm-Straker M, Stoklosa H, editors. Human trafficking is a public health issue: a paradigm expansion in the United States. Cham: Springer; 2017.
34. Seng MJ. Child sexual Abuse and adolescent prostitution: a comparative analysis. Adolescence. 1989;24:665–75.
35. Stoltz J-AM, Shannon K, Kerr T, Zhang R, Montaner JS, Wood E. Associations between childhood maltreatment and sex work in a cohort of drug-using youth. Soc Sci Med. 2007;65:1214–21.
36. Cochran BN, Stewart AJ, Ginzler JA, Cauce AM. Challenges faced by homeless sexual minorities: comparison of gay, lesbian, bisexual, and transgender homeless adolescents with their heterosexual counterparts. Am J Public Health. 2002;92:773–7.
37. Le PD, Ryan N, Rosenstock Y, Goldmann E. Health issues associated with commercial sexual exploitation and sex Trafficking of children in the United States: a systematic review. Behav Med. 2018;44:219–33.
38. Gerassi LB, Nichols AJ, Cox A, Goldberg KK, Tang C. Examining commonly reported sex trafficking indicators from practitioners' perspectives: findings from a pilot study. J Interpers Violence. 2018;886260518812813.
39. Varma S, Gillespie S, McCracken C, Greenbaum VJ. Characteristics of child commercial sexual exploitation and sex trafficking victims presenting for medical care in the United States. Child Abuse Negl. 2015;44:98–105.
40. Goldberg AP, Moore JL, Houck C, Kaplan DM, Barron CE. Domestic minor sex trafficking patients: a retrospective analysis of medical presentation. J Pediatr Adolesc Gynecol. 2017;30:109–15.
41. Hossain M, Zimmerman C, Abas M, Light M, Watts C. The relationship of trauma to mental disorders among trafficked and sexually exploited girls and women. Am J Public Health. 2010;100:2442–9.
42. Kelly MA, Bath EP, Godoy SM, Abrams LS, Barnert ES. Understanding commercially sexually exploited youths' facilitators and barriers toward contraceptive use: I Didn't really have a choice. J Pediatr Adolesc Gynecol. 2019;32:316–24.
43. Ijadi-Maghsoodi R, Bath E, Cook M, Textor L, Barnert E. Commercially sexually exploited youths' health care experiences, barriers, and recommendations: a qualitative analysis. Child Abuse Negl. 2018;76:334–41.
44. Chung RJ, English A. Commercial sexual exploitation and sex trafficking of adolescents. Curr Opin Pediatr. 2015;27:427–33.
45. Walker K. Ending the commercial sexual exploitation of children: a call for multi-system collaboration in California.
46. Chicago Alliance Against Sexual Exploitation. Know the facts: commercial sexual exploitation of children. 2018 [cited 2019 May 14]. Available from: http://media.virbcdn.com/files/59/FileItem-150155-KtF_CSEC.pdf.
47. Macias-Konstantopoulos W, Ma ZB. Physical health of human trafficking survivors: unmet essentials. In: Chisolm-Straker M, Stoklosa H, editors. Human trafficking is a public health issue: a paradigm expansion in the United States. Cham: Springer; 2017. p. 185–210.
48. Rafferty Y. Child trafficking and commercial sexual exploitation: a review of promising prevention policies and programs. Am J Orthop. 2013;83:559–75.
49. Berckmans I, Velasco ML, Tapia BP, Loots G. A systematic review: a quest for effective interventions for children and adolescents in street situation. Child Youth Serv Rev. 2012;34:1259–72.

50. Gerassi LB, Colegrove A, McPherson DK. Addressing race, racism, and commercial sexual exploitation in practice through an action-based research partnership. Action Res. 2018;17:147675031880754.
51. National Research Council. Confronting commercial sexual exploitation and sex trafficking of minors in the United States. 2013.
52. Spangenberg M. Prostituted youth in New York City: an overview. ECPAT-USA: New York, NY; 2001.
53. Black and Missing Foundation, Inc. Black and Missing in America: a Look at racial disparities in human trafficking cases. 2018 [cited 2019 Jul 1]. Available from: http://www.blackandmissinginc.com/.
54. Banks D, Kyckelhahn T. Characteristics of suspected human trafficking incidents, 2008–2010. US Department of Justice, Office of Justice Programs, Bureau of Justice Statistics: Washington, D.C; 2011.
55. Mitchell KJ, Finkelhor D, Wolak J. Sex Trafficking cases involving minors [internet]. Durham: crimes against children research center, University of New Hampshire; 2013. Available from: http://www.unh.edu/ccrc/pdf/CV313_Final_Sex_Trafficking_Minors_Nov_2013_rev.pdf.
56. Gragg F, Petta I, Bernstein H, Eisen K, Quinn L. New York prevalence study of commercially sexually exploited children. New York State Office of Children and Family Services: Rensselaer, NY; 2007.
57. rights4girls. Domestic Child Sex Trafficking and Black Girls. 2019 [cited 2019 Jul 1]. Available from: http://rights4girls.org/wp-content/uploads/r4g/2019/05/Black-Girls-DCST-May-2019-1.pdf.
58. National Council of Juvenile and Family Court Judges. Reducing Demand for the Commercial Sexual Exploitation of Minors in Your Community [Internet]. 2017 [cited 2019 Oct 3]. Available from: http://www.ncjfcj.org/Reducing-Demand-Webinar.
59. Carey C, Teplitsky L. Commercial sexual exploitation of children (CSEC) in the Portland metro area: Portland State University; 2013.
60. Louisiana Department of Children and Family Services. Human Trafficking, Trafficking of Children for Sexual Purposes, and Commercial Sexual Exploitation. 2018.
61. Curtis R, Terry K, Dank M, Dombrowski K. Commercial sexual exploitation of children in New York City, volume one: the CSEC population in New York City: size, characteristics, and needs [Internet]. The John Jay College of Criminal Justice: New York, NY; 2008. Available from: https://www.ncjrs.gov/pdffiles1/nij/grants/225083.pdf.
62. Zurbriggen EL, Collins RL, Lamb S, Roberts TA, Tolman DL, Ward LM. APA task force on the sexualization of girls. Am Psycholog Ass. 2007.
63. Bryant Y. Relationships between exposure to rap music videos and attitudes toward relationships among African American youth. J Black Psychol. 2008;34:356–80.
64. Ward LM, Hansbrough E, Walker E. Contributions of music video exposure to black adolescents' gender and sexual schemas. J Adolesc Res. 2005;20:143–66.
65. Stephens DP, Few AL. The effects of images of African American women in hip hop on early adolescents' attitudes toward physical attractiveness and interpersonal relationships. Sex Roles. 2007;56:251–64.
66. Stephens DP, Phillips L. Integrating black feminist thought into conceptual frameworks of African American adolescent women's sexual scripting processes. Sexualities Evolution Gender. 2005;7:37–55.
67. Roberts DE. Deviance, resistance, and love. Utah L Rev. 1994;
68. Roberts DE. Prison, foster care, and the systemic punishment of black mothers. UCLA L Rev. 2011;59.
69. Kruger A, Harper E, Harris P, Sanders D, Levin K, Meyers J. Sexualized and dangerous relationships: listening to the voices of low-income African American girls placed at risk for sexual exploitation. West J Emerg Med. 2013;14:370–6.
70. Butler CN. The racial roots of human trafficking. UCLA L Rev. 2015.
71. Kangaspunta K, Sarrica F, Jesrani T, Johansen R. Global report on trafficking in persons.

72. Centers for Disease Control and Prevention. The social-ecological model: a framework for prevention [Internet]. Centers for Disease Control and Prevention. 2015 [cited 2019 Sep 24]. Available from: https://www.cdc.gov/violenceprevention/publichealthissue/social-ecologicalmodel.html.
73. Baldwin SB, Eisenman DP, Sayles JN, Ryan G, Chuang KS. Identification of human trafficking victims in health care settings. Health Hum Rights. 2011;13:E36–49.
74. Macias Konstantopoulos W, Ahn R, Alpert EJ, Cafferty E, McGahan A, Williams TP, et al. An international comparative public health analysis of sex trafficking of women and girls in eight cities: achieving a more effective health sector response. J Urban Health. 2013;90:1194–204.
75. Peters K. The growing business of human trafficking and the power of emergency nurses to stop it. J Emerg Nurs. 2013;39:280–8.
76. Greenbaum VJ. Child sex trafficking in the United States: challenges for the healthcare provider. PLoS Med. 2017;14:e1002439.
77. Dovydaitis T. Human trafficking: the role of the health care provider. J Midwifery Womens Health. 2010;55:462–7.
78. Jülich S. Stockholm syndrome and child sexual abuse. J Child Sex Abus. 2005;14:107–29.
79. Briere JN, Elliott DM. Immediate and long-term impacts of child sexual abuse. Futur Child. 1994;4:54–69.
80. Sanchez RV, Speck PM, Patrician PA. A concept analysis of trauma coercive bonding in the commercial sexual exploitation of children. J Pediatr Nurs. 2019;46:48–54.
81. Reid JA, Jones S. Exploited vulnerability: legal and psychological perspectives on child sex trafficking victims. Vict Offenders. 2011;6:207–31.
82. Anderson PM, Coyle KK, Johnson A, Denner J. An exploratory study of adolescent pimping relationships. J Prim Prev. 2014;35:113–7.
83. Mays AR, Chafee T, Chulani VL. Commercial Sexual Exploitation of Children (CSEC): Addressing the Healthcare Provider's Role in Identifying the Health Needs and Providing Support for Commercially Sexually Exploited Children [Internet]. [cited 2019 May 13]. Available from: https://prh.org/arshep-ppts/#best-practices.
84. Raghavan C. Trauma-coerced bonding and victims of sex Trafficking: where do we go from here? Int J Emerg Ment Health. 2015;17.
85. Sigman G, Silber TJ, English A, Epner JE. Confidential health care for adolescents: position paper of the Society for Adolescent Medicine. J Adolesc Health. 1997;21:408–15.
86. Committee on Adolescence. Achieving quality health services for adolescents. Pediatrics. 2016;138.
87. Sapiro B, Johnson L, Postmus JL, Simmel C. Supporting youth involved in domestic minor sex trafficking: divergent perspectives on youth agency. Child Abuse Negl. 2016;58:99–110.
88. Kalergis KI. A passionate practice. Affilia. 2009;24:315–24.
89. Duncan PM, Garcia AC, Frankowski BL, Carey PA, Kallock EA, Dixon RD, et al. Inspiring healthy adolescent choices: a rationale for and guide to strength promotion in primary care. J Adolesc Health. 2007;41:525–35.
90. Goldenring JM, Rosen DS. Getting into adolescent heads: an essential update. Contemp Pediatr. 2004.
91. Zimmerman C, Watts C, Health OW. WHO ethical and safety recommendations for interviewing trafficked women. 2003.
92. Gerber MR, editor. Trauma-informed healthcare approaches: a guide for primary care. Cham: Springer; 2019.
93. Elliott DE, Bjelajac P, Fallot RD, Markoff LS, Reed BG. Trauma-informed or trauma-denied: principles and implementation of trauma-informed services for women. J Community Psychol. 2005;33:461–77.
94. Ijadi-Maghsoodi R, Cook M, Barnert ES, Gaboian S, Bath E. Understanding and responding to the needs of commercially sexually exploited youth: recommendations for the mental health provider. Child Adolesc Psychiatr Clin N Am. 2016;25:107–22.

95. Substance Abuse and Mental Health Services Administration. Trauma-Informed Approach and Trauma-Specific Interventions [Internet]. Trauma Informed Approach and Trauma Specific Interventions. 2016 [cited 2019 May 14]. Available from: http://www.bharp.org/wp-content/uploads/2016/10/Trauma-Informed-Approach-and-Trauma-Specific-Interventions-_-SAMHSA.pdf.
96. Alpert EJ, Ahn R, Albright E, Purcell G, Burke TF, Macias-Konstantopoulos WL. Guidebook on Identification, Assessment,' ' and Response in the Health Care Setting. Massachusetts General Hospital, Massachusetts Medical Society; 2014.
97. Wilson MR. Medical, legal and social science aspects of child sexual exploitation—a comprehensive review of pornography, prostitution and internet crime edited by Sharon Cooper, Richard Estes, Angelo Giardino, Nancy Kellog and Victor Vieth, GW Medical Publishing Inc, Missouri, 2005. 1200pp. ISBN 1-878060-37-6 (Volume 1 and 2 Casebound), £175.99. Child Abuse Rev. 2007;16:274–6.
98. Ells M. Forming a multidisciplinary team to investigate child abuse. SSRN J. 2000.
99. Workowski KA, Berman SM. Centers for disease control and prevention sexually transmitted disease treatment guidelines. Clin Infect Dis. 2011;53(Suppl 3):S59–63.
100. Reid JA. Exploratory review of route-specific, gendered, and age-graded dynamics of exploitation: applying life course theory to victimization in sex trafficking in North America. Aggress Violent Behav. 2012;17:257–71.
101. Miller E, McCaw B. Intimate partner violence. N Engl J Med. 2019;380:850–7.
102. Greenbaum VJ, Dodd M, McCracken C. A short screening tool to identify victims of child sex trafficking in the health care setting. Pediatr Emerg Care. 2018;34:33–7.
103. McElvaney R, Greene S, Hogan D. To tell or not to tell? factors influencing young people's informal disclosures of child sexual abuse. J Interpers Violence. 2014;29:928–47.
104. Chang KS, Lee K, Park T, Sy E, Quach T. Using a clinic-based screening tool for primary care providers to identify commercially sexually exploited children. J App Res Children: Informing Policy Children Risk. 2015;6.
105. Isaac R, Solak J, Giardino AP. Health care providers' training needs related to human trafficking: maximizing the opportunity to effectively screen and intervene. J App Res Children: Informing Policy Children Risk. 2011;2.
106. Polaris. Referral Directory [Internet]. National human trafficking hotline. [cited 2019 Oct 4]. Available from: https://humantraffickinghotline.org/training-resources/referral-directory.
107. Health, Education, Advocacy, Linkage. HEAL trafficking and hope for justice's protocol toolkit [Internet]. 2019 [cited 2019 Oct 4]. Available from: https://healtrafficking.org/2017/06/new-heal-trafficking-and-hope-for-justices-protocol-toolkit-for-developing-a-response-to-victims-of-human-trafficking-in-health-care-settings/.
108. Andretta JR, Woodland MH, Watkins KM, Barnes ME. Towards the discreet identification of commercial sexual exploitation of children (CSEC) victims and individualized interventions: science to practice. Psychol Public Policy Law. 2016;22:260–70.
109. Greenbaum VJ, Livings MS, Lai BS, Edinburgh L, Baikie P, Grant SR, et al. Evaluation of a tool to identify child sex trafficking victims in multiple healthcare settings. J Adolesc Health. 2018;63:745–52.
110. Enrile A. Ending human trafficking and modern-day slavery: freedom's journey. Thousand Oaks: SAGE Publications, Inc.; 2018.
111. Grace AM, Lippert S, Collins K, Pineda N, Tolani A, Walker R, et al. Educating health care professionals on human trafficking. Pediatr Emerg Care. 2014;30:856–61.
112. Beck ME, Lineer MM, Melzer-Lange M, Simpson P, Nugent M, Rabbitt A. Medical providers' understanding of sex trafficking and their experience with at-risk patients. Pediatrics. 2015;135:e895–902.
113. Moore JL, Baird G, Goldberg AP. Sex trafficking assessment and resources (STAR) for pediatric attendings in Rhode Island. R I Med J (2013). 2016;99:27–30.

114. Titchen KE, Loo D, Berdan E, Rysavy MB, Ng JJ, Sharif I. Domestic sex trafficking of minors: medical student and physician awareness. J Pediatr Adolesc Gynecol. 2017;30:102–8.
115. Stoklosa H, Grace AM, Littenberg N. Medical education on human trafficking. AMA J Ethics. 2015;17:914–21.
116. Stoklosa H, Dawson MB, Williams-Oni F, Rothman EF. A review of U.S. health care institution protocols for the identification and treatment of victims of human trafficking. J Hum Traffick. 2017;3:116–24.
117. Atkinson HG, Curnin KJ, Hanson NC. U.S. state laws addressing human trafficking: education of and mandatory reporting by health care providers and other professionals. J Hum Traffick. 2016;2:111–38.
118. The New York State Senate. Identification and Assessment of Human Trafficking Victims. Article 28. Sect. 2805-Y 2019.
119. Blanco. Texas H.B. No. 2059. May 20, 2019.

Chapter 5
Adolescents and Labor Trafficking

Corey J. Rood, Stephanie Richard, Laura T. Murphy, Julia Einbond, Alison Iannarone, Alessandra Amato, and Hayoung Lee

C. J. Rood (✉)
Department of Pediatrics, University of California Irvine School of Medicine, Orange, CA, USA

S. Richard
Coalition to Abolish Slavery & Trafficking (CAST), Los Angeles, CA, USA

L. T. Murphy (✉)
Helena Kennedy Centre for International Justice, Sheffield Hallam University, Sheffield, UK

J. Einbond (✉) · A. Iannarone
Covenant House New Jersey, Newark, NJ, USA

A. Amato
Trafficking in Persons Program, Refugee & Immigrant Center, Asian Association of Utah, Salt Lake City, UT, USA

H. Lee
Internal Medicine and Pediatrics, Louisiana State University School of Medicine, New Orleans, LA, USA

K. E. Titchen, E. Miller (eds.), *Medical Perspectives on Human Trafficking in Adolescents*, https://doi.org/10.1007/978-3-030-43367-3_5

Labor Trafficking – A Review

Corey J. Rood, Stephanie Richard, and Laura T. Murphy

Introduction

Mary, a young Mexican girl, was forced to peddle tamales on the street and was sexually assaulted in her family's home. While she was peddling on the street, a woman noticed bruises on her body and called the police. Police dropped Mary off at the local homeless shelter where she waited for help for over 2 months before being identified as a child trafficking victim by a staff member.

Jessica was 17 when she was recruited to sell magazines in the southern United States. She was forcibly transported and made to work in various locations in the United States and finally escaped when she was 18. She went to a police department for help. The police department considered her homeless and did not identify this as a labor trafficking case.

Liz and *Marty*, two American youths, were homeless after their families kicked them out of their homes. They answered a website advertisement for au pair services. Once they were flown to the host family's home, they were forced to work every day and sexually assaulted by the father of the household, who used drugs to sedate them.

Marco, 16, was forced to smuggle drugs into the United States. He was violently beaten and forced to watch as a friend was killed in front of him. Marco was arrested for selling drugs and sentenced to time in juvenile hall instead of being identified as a victim of human trafficking.

In Ashland, Ohio, a federal jury convicted three individuals of engaging in a labor trafficking conspiracy after the group held a cognitively disabled woman and her child against their will and forced them to perform manual labor [1]. In addition to beatings and threats with vicious animals, the traffickers also threatened the mother with the possibility that authorities might take her child away [2]. The traffickers forced the mother to hit her child while they recorded video so that they could threaten to show the video to authorities in order to have the child removed.

At its core, the crime of human trafficking is about exploitation for labor or services. The labor or commercial sexual service is the element needed for this crime that distinguishes it from other crimes against children. People often forget that human trafficking of adolescents includes *both* labor and sex trafficking. Medical and mental health professionals must be vigilant in understanding both sides of the commercial exploitation of children so that no vulnerable and exploited child remains unidentified and unassisted.

Adolescent labor trafficking is often less identified and understood today partly because reports and media coverage across the country highlight only child sex trafficking and focus on the link between child sex trafficking and the child welfare system [3]. In comparison to child sex trafficking, the issue of child labor trafficking in the United States is less researched and less frequently highlighted by the media. However, the limited evidence available demonstrates the need for those who work with vulnerable children to pay equal attention to this issue. For example, in Florida 24 US-citizen children were involved in a labor trafficking scheme through which they were forced to sell items door to door until they were identified by an off-duty Florida Department of Child and Families worker [4]. A similar scheme was identified in Colorado, where an anti-trafficking organization helped minors who were trapped in magazine sales crews [5]. Adolescent labor trafficking victims have been identified in a diverse array of industries, including agricultural work, restaurant service, hair braiding, domestic work, forced peddling, and a range of illegal work activities [6]. For example, in California, a newspaper reported the horrific tale of a girl who ran away from foster placement and was then kidnapped, confined in a metal box, sexually assaulted, and only allowed outside to cultivate marijuana for her captors [7]. Adolescent labor trafficking victims are more likely to be identified if protocols and screening are put in place in medical and mental health facilities for both child labor and sex trafficking victims. However, child labor trafficking victims will continue to be exploited and abused if those best positioned to help them continue to ignore this issue, believe this does not occur in the United States, or focus only on identifying sex trafficking.

Who Is a Victim of Adolescent Labor Trafficking?

Commercial sexual exploitation and forced labor are both included in the federal definition of human trafficking. The Trafficking Victims Protection Act (TVPA) of 2000, Section 103(9) defines "severe forms of trafficking in persons" as:

A. Sex trafficking in which a commercial sex act is induced by force, fraud, or coercion, or in which the person induced to perform such act has not attained 18 years of age
B. The recruitment, harboring, transportation, provision, or obtaining of a person for labor or services, through the use of force, fraud, or coercion for the purpose of subjection to involuntary servitude, peonage, debt bondage, or slavery [8]

On the surface, identifying labor trafficking victims appears more complex than identifying sex trafficking victims, because the legal definition does not include all minors engaged in labor. According to US law, an adolescent who is working is not necessarily considered a victim of labor trafficking, as would be the case with any minor involved in the commercial sex trade. However, put most simply, any child providing labor or service through force, fraud, or coercion is a victim of labor trafficking. Therefore, the key information for practitioners to grasp is the legal definitions of *force, fraud, and coercion* [9, 10].

It may be easiest to identify cases of labor and sex trafficking that involve *force*, which can be defined as physical violence or physical restraint. Force is the mechanism of control that people commonly associate with human trafficking – violent beatings, people forcibly restrained when not working. These and other forms of violence are included in the definition of "force."

Other cases involve people who have been lured into work through *fraud*, by which we mean false or misleading contracts, trickery, or false promises. Some adolescent labor trafficking victims are told they will be paid, but then they perform the work without receiving remuneration. For a case of fraud or unpaid wages to be considered trafficking, typically the person has to believe that they cannot walk away from the job. In these cases, fraud may be accompanied by threats or psychological trickery that convinces the worker that they are beholden to remain in the job and will not be allowed to walk away from the job. This usually involves some degree of coercion as well.

Indeed, adolescent labor trafficking victims, like sex trafficking victims, often have cell phones, attend school, work in environments with unlocked doors, or might be left alone for periods of time because the trafficker has instilled a fear in the victim so great that they cannot leave or disobey their trafficker's orders because of the invisible barriers of psychological *coercion*. For this reason, some people describe human trafficking as a "prison without walls."

This type of coercion can start with set rules, veiled threats, monitored phone use, threats about immigration status or calling the police, connections with dangerous individuals, isolation, or threats to family, friends, or others around the victim. The adolescent victim, vulnerable to adult power and influence, subjectively believes that serious harm will occur to them if they do not continue to perform labor or services at the trafficker's request and feels it is impossible to refuse to work or leave the bad work situation.

Although the legal definition of coercion is complex, in practice a simple framework can guide the identification of child labor trafficking cases.

Two important points about coercion, especially in child and youth labor cases, are:

1. The definition of coercion explicitly includes "threats," "abuse of the legal process," or a "scheme or plan" that causes someone to keep working [11]. This definition is broad enough to cover a range of means by which a trafficker will exploit a child's labor or services.
2. The definition of coercion centers around the idea of "serious harm," and this is defined as a broad range of harm that can be nonphysical and includes financial and reputational harm. The legal definition also specifically takes into account the circumstances and background of the victim, so a minor labor trafficking victim will generally not need to demonstrate the same degree of coercion as an adult victim [12].

Non-legal practitioners may find it challenging to distinguish between child labor exploitation and child labor trafficking. Child labor exploitation includes unpaid wages, unsafe working conditions, and specific prohibition on ages and hours when children can work [13]. The key distinction between labor exploitation and labor trafficking is whether the child has decided to work or if a third-party has manipulated the child into believing they must work or else suffer some kind of harm. Medical and mental health practitioners should not worry about trying to distinguish between child labor exploitation and child labor trafficking. The red flags for each are similar, and the same steps should be followed to provide support and protection for the child.

Labor trafficking happens to both foreign nationals and citizens of the United States. In fact, someone may first be smuggled – illegally transported across a border – and may even agree to pay a debt for the smuggling, but the voluntary crossing of a border can become labor trafficking if that child or youth is later made to perform some labor or service under force, fraud, or coercive practices.

Epidemiology

Unfortunately, we do not have a clear portrait of how prevalent child labor trafficking is in the United States. Studies have provided unreliable ranges of numbers of children who are at risk of trafficking, but the truth is that there are no effective surveys that capture this crime and no studies that have successfully quantified the number of victims. Very few adolescent labor trafficking cases have been prosecuted at the federal level to date, and only a few law enforcement agencies have accurately identified the cases that they have encountered.

That said, adolescent labor trafficking is indeed a form of victimization that requires the attention of medical professionals. Because labor trafficking is forced labor, it may occur in any industry. The Polaris Project in 2017 listed 17 different "types" or sites of labor trafficking occurring in the United States alone. Those included sites where adolescents seek their first jobs, including the entertainment industry, landscaping, restaurants and food service, traveling sales crews, carnivals, peddling and begging, domestic work, agriculture, construction, and forestry [14]. In addition, it is not unusual for work in illicit trades, such as the drug trade, stealing, or other gang-related work, to be compelled through force or coercion. Young people are sometimes forced to engage in this illicit work by a family member, neighbor, or friend, who does not allow them to choose the work or to leave it. It is important to understand these often-complex dynamics and check our own personal biases that sometimes lead us to conclude that a juvenile has chosen to engage in criminal activities, when in fact they may be a child labor trafficking victim. In many cases, labor and sex trafficking overlap, particularly in situations in which adolescents who are forced to sell sex are also forced to sell drugs or steal for their traffickers.

No conclusive research has proven that trafficking affects racial/ethnic minority communities (African American, Latin American, or Native American) more than white, as most studies of trafficking are focused on people who are already marginalized in some way and therefore face increased vulnerability to trafficking regardless of race/ethnicity. As poverty and other vulnerabilities fall along the fault lines of communities marginalized on the basis of race/ethnicity in the United States, it is likely that some racial/ethnic minorities are likely to be disproportionately affected by trafficking. [See section "Labor Trafficking – Forced Criminality" for more details regarding labor trafficking of adolescent populations within illicit trades.]

Risk Factors

Children and youth who immigrate to or seek refuge in the United States experience a particularly high vulnerability to labor trafficking for a number of reasons. Whether documented or undocumented, young people traveling across borders often seek work to support themselves and their families. Those whose families arrive on legal temporary H2A and H2B work visas are contractually tied to the employers who sponsor them. Some employers take advantage of fears surrounding immigrant legal status and deportation to force immigrants to work without pay or with limited pay, to convince them that they cannot leave, to force them into illicit work, or to compel their children to work alongside them [15]. Unaccompanied minors crossing the borders are at increased risk of labor trafficking, because they lack a protective support system and are wary of law enforcement and fear deportation [16]. [See section "Labor Trafficking – Vulnerability of Immigrant and Refugee Youth" for more details regarding labor trafficking among the immigrant adolescent population.]

Adolescents who are US citizens also are at risk for labor trafficking, and a number of factors influence this risk. These risk factors are very similar to sex-trafficked youth, as youth do not choose the type of commercial exploitation into which they are recruited. Therefore, young Americans who are economically, socially, or educationally marginalized, as well as those who struggle to find employment because of disability, sexuality, gender identity, addiction, or socioeconomic background are vulnerable to traffickers. Young people who have left school, who have criminal histories, who identify as transgender, or who lack adult guidance may feel they have few formal employment options, leaving them to seek riskier work. A history of extreme poverty, homelessness, or engagement in the foster system can often mean a history of extreme deprivation, and getting basic needs met becomes an everyday challenge that may leave a young person vulnerable to exploitation. Homeless youth in particular are vulnerable to offers of lucrative work that sound "too good to be true." [17] Evidence suggests that lesbian, gay, bisexual, transgender, or questioning (LGBTQ) youth may be up to five times more likely than heterosexual and cisgender youth to be victims of trafficking, due to increased susceptibility that comes with rejection and alienation often experienced by LGBTQ youth [18]. [For more on LGBTQ youth and human trafficking, see Chap. 11.]

Substance use may also leave young people vulnerable, or traffickers may directly develop this addiction in their victims and exploit it for their own benefits. Some adolescents may engage voluntarily in illicit trades to maintain their drug habits; however, their addiction also renders them vulnerable to those who sell/supply drugs and who may force them to commit crimes for their own profit. This vulnerability may be the coercive means a trafficker uses to force youth to engage in the illicit trade themselves, and youth must be carefully screened to recognize third-party exploitation. [See Chap. 13 for more on substance use and human trafficking.]

An individualized education program (IEP) may also be a warning sign of vulnerability to trafficking. Some youth with developmental deficits and low cognition have trouble discerning dangerous situations and may become involved with people who exploit them.

Clinical Presentation

The healthcare setting (including primary care, dental, mental health, and emergency rooms) is a place where patients and clients can present when in need of physical and/or psychological assessment, healing, and access to necessary immediate supportive services to break free of traffickers' control. Human trafficking exacts a significant physical and psychological toll on its victims that all too often brings both labor and sex trafficking victims to the doors of a medical institution. Labor-trafficked persons may present alone or may be accompanied by other victims and/or their traffickers. Healthcare professionals have a unique opportunity to identify all forms of potential commercial exploitation for sex and labor, answer questions about personal health, provide treatment interventions, help navigate resources and referrals, and report to agencies who are better equipped to investigate potential victimization and crimes.

Lederer et al. found in 2014 that of the 107 female sex trafficking survivors they surveyed, ages 14–60 years, nearly 88% made at least one visit to a medical provider during their period of victimization [19]. In 2016, Chisolm-Straker et al. expanded this investigation to include survivors of labor trafficking. Interviews with 173 human trafficking survivors of all ages from the United States showed that 68% of those survivors sought medical attention while being trafficked. The most common location for medical presentation was the emergency department, but other locations ranged from mental health professionals to primary care. In addition, 27% received dental care [20] (See Table 5.1). Chief complaints included physical injury, reproductive health concerns, infections, substance abuse, suicidality, and other mental health concerns.

The most common physical complaints reported by trafficking survivors include neurological complaints such as headaches, migraines, dizziness, neuropathies, and chronic pain. Other common complaints include severe weight loss, malnutrition, loss of appetite, acute and/or chronic physical injury, cardiovascular and pulmonary complaints, gastrointestinal complaints, dental problems including tooth decay and loss, and chronic overuse of joints and back. Many survivors report being victims of physical violence including being hit, kicked, punched, beaten with an object, threatened with a weapon, or strangled [19–26].

The United States Preventive Services Task Force (USPSTF) and other leading medical institutions such as the World Health Organization (WHO) and the

Table 5.1 Medical facilities most often frequented by trafficking victims

Facility location	% Sex trafficking victims presenting to health care (Lederer et al. [19])	% Sex and labor trafficking victims presenting to health care (Chisolm-Straker et al. [20])
Any visit to medical care	87.8	68
Emergency department	63.3	55.6
Planned parenthood	29.6	No data
Primary care provider	22.5	47.8
Urgent care clinic	21.4	No data
OB/GYN	19.4	25.6
Public health clinic	19.4	No data
Dental	No data	26.5
Other	13.3	13.6
Unknown	No data	0.9

American Academy of Pediatrics (AAP) recommend routine assessment and care for immigrant/refugee, homeless, incarcerated, and underserved populations. Such recommendations and best practices can be applied to the medical assessment and management of minor and young adult victims of human trafficking [21, 25–29]. Victims of labor trafficking in particular may suffer from chronic exposure to the elements, industrial exposures to caustic chemicals and poisons, physically exhaustive work conditions, poor living and sleeping accommodations, and malnutrition. General health concerns for these populations should guide health care professionals to evaluate for immunization status, cognitive and/or developmental disabilities, poor oral hygiene, chronic musculoskeletal and neurological complaints or limitations, cardiovascular or respiratory complaints, anemia, vitamin and mineral deficiencies, and exposure to such communicable diseases as tuberculosis [19–26].

Although often subtle, psychological health consequences of the physical and psychological trauma of exploitation are pervasive. The effects of such trauma on the developing adolescent body and mind can be consequential. Most studies looking at the psychological effects of exploitation have surveyed only sex trafficking survivors. Those survivors self-report diagnoses that include post-traumatic stress disorder (PTSD), suicidality, depression, anxiety, eating disorders, shame or guilt, nightmares, and more. Victims who are willing to disclose non-prescription substance use have reported dependence on various substances including tobacco, alcohol, marijuana, cocaine, crack cocaine, methamphetamine, heroin, other opiates, ecstasy, and/or PCP. Highly addictive substances such as cocaine, methamphetamines, heroin, and opiates are often used for two leading reasons: by traffickers to control their victims, and by trafficked persons to cope with their own physical and psychological trauma [19–26]. [See Chap. 9 for more on the intersection of human trafficking and psychological health.]

Although similar data for labor trafficking victim is not available, practitioners who serve labor trafficking victims report similar medical and mental health issues.

Medical Management Approach

Health recommendations for victims and survivors of sex and labor trafficking overlap greatly. Unique medical recommendations for best practices are available for assessing and managing victims of acute sexual assault, more often seen with sex trafficking but not exclusively. Many service providers have observed that sexual assault or rape may be one of the most common means of controlling female labor trafficking victims.

The complex trauma experienced by survivors of trafficking often causes hesitancy, anxiety, and even reluctance to disclose the details of their exploitation and victimization. However, trafficked persons may be willing to disclose current details about their situation if such candor will improve the medical care they will receive. Approaching these patients in a trauma-informed, patient-centered, culturally sensitive manner is crucial [19, 25, 29, 30]. According to the Substance Abuse and Mental Health Services Administration (SAMHSA), an institutional program, organization, or health system that is trauma-informed "realizes the widespread impact of trauma and understands potential paths for recovery; recognizes the signs and symptoms of trauma in clients, families, staff, and others involved with the system; and responds by fully integrating knowledge about trauma into policies, procedures, and practices; and seeks to actively resist re-traumatization." [31] It cannot be emphasized enough that the medical encounter should be structured in such a way that puts the patient or client at the center of the evaluation, uses trauma-informed history taking and exam techniques, and provides an overall environment that is inviting, calm, and safe. Furthermore, the goal of the encounter is not disclosure: it is to provide high-quality health care, rapport building, and trust.

After rapport building and informed consent, victims may still be reluctant to disclose exploitation especially if threats of harm have been made or actual harm has occurred to them or their friends and family. In the medical setting, the primary care professional or therapist should consider further targeted history gathering when contextual information and risk factors suggest trafficking. Particular vulnerabilities that pertain to labor trafficking include homelessness, running away or being kicked out, immigration or refugee status, undocumented and unaccompanied minors, and involvement with any other forms of exploitation. Using open-ended questions that solicit a narrative description from the patient may facilitate greater understanding for the medical team. Even after obtaining a complete, factual history, the lack of a disclosure of victimization does not rule out trafficking. If the medical team continues to be reasonably concerned about exploitation in any form,

Table 5.2 General, non-acute medical management of minor victims of trafficking [28, 32]

Medical approach to minor victims of human trafficking
1. Introduce self and team, build rapport, and discuss limits of confidentiality.
2. Obtain fully informed consent for examination and testing.
3. Complete medical and social history, review of systems, and physical examination.
4. Evaluation of hydration, nutrition, and growth; include head circumference or BMI as indicated.
5. Documentation of old/recent injuries.
6. Anogenital examination, with photo- or video-documentation of injuries/concerning findings if possible.
7. Assessment of development; include screening for motor, cognitive, and speech delays.
8. Assessment of vision and hearing.
9. Assessment of dental hygiene and oral health.
10. Evaluation of immunization records and starting appropriate catch-up immunizations during the same visit.
11. Assessment for anemia, lead, tuberculosis, and other potential exposures (chemical or infectious); consider other testing for vitamin/mineral deficiencies if indicated; consider testing for infectious diseases that are endemic in the patient's home country if indicated.
12. Assessment for mental health concerns.
13. Screen for urine and/or serum alcohol and drugs of abuse, as clinically indicated.
14. Test for pregnancy and sexually transmitted infections as indicated; include gonorrhea (GC), chlamydia (CT), trichomonas (trich), HIV, Hepatitis B & C, and syphilis (exposure history should guide anatomical site testing for GC, CT, and trich).

this concern should be shared with the patient and with the appropriate agencies for further investigation if the patient is a minor. [For more on mandated reporting, see Chap. 18.]

The general, non-acute medical management of victims of trafficking (Table 5.2) is much like other initial medical clinic patient encounters. A thorough and complete medical history is needed, and it is recommended that this occur with the patient alone. While disclosure is not the goal and all patients should receive information about resources available to them, a validated (if available) or thoroughly vetted method to assess for symptoms related to depression, suicidality, and trauma as well as exposures to human trafficking and related situations (e.g., living in a shelter, not being able to leave a job) is highly recommended. Healthcare professionals should not rely solely on responses to screening questions to guide therapeutic interventions and referrals to resources. Of course, with any screening method, there must be a response system in place to provide immediate interventions, referrals, and resources for all positive screens. Following the history, and with the patient's consent, a complete physical examination should be performed, which should include a trauma-informed and trauma-sensitive anogenital examination. [See Chap. 16 for detailed information on conducting a trauma-informed gynecologic exam.] It is highly recommended, especially when working with a potentially exploited patient population, that a chaperone (second licensed medical professional) accompany any provider performing an anogenital or breast exam. This protects both medical professionals and patients alike.

Reasons for Limited Disclosures

Adolescent Hesitance to Disclose

The examples provided in this chapter show the diverse ways that traffickers use force, fraud, and coercion to exploit adolescents and youth. Many individuals who are being trafficked will not self-identify as victims, since they often experience intense shame and distrust of authority figures [6]. Self-identification is also difficult for adolescent labor trafficking victims, similar to child sex trafficking victims, because many victims feel emotionally bonded or physically dependent on their traffickers [33]. Both labor- and sex-trafficked minors are often arrested for the crimes their traffickers force them to commit and get caught up in the juvenile justice system [34].

Trafficked Persons May Not Self-Identify

These factors often contribute to an adolescent's lack of apparent interest or psychological capacity to escape the situation of trafficking. Survivors report that they do not typically self-identify as victims of human trafficking and often state that they do not know what "human trafficking" is. They also may feel complicit in their own enslavement – especially if they believe they have agreed to do the work or to pay off a debt.

Trauma Bonds

Many young people experience what mental health professionals call "trauma bonding," which is to say that they feel connection, loyalty, or even love toward the person who is trafficking them. Trauma bonds can be formed when children seek attachment in the face of extreme danger, or "when there is no access to ordinary sources of comfort, people may turn towards their tormentors." [35] In labor trafficking cases, this commonly occurs when someone is told they are part of the "family" and have to work or commit crimes for the family, or when a young person is caring for small children of a trafficker and forms a connection to this family.

Familial Trafficking

When a trafficker is a family member or close friend, children often find it difficult to resist the wishes of their elders or close relations. They come to believe that they will get in trouble or be considered defiant if they walk away or that they will leave the safety of the persons providing their daily basic necessities – food, shelter, clothing. If they feel they have nowhere else to turn or no other opportunities for work, they may avoid leaving or reporting abusive working conditions unless someone else provides them with outside support and options.

Threats and Fear

Sometimes, if they are involved in illicit work, such as in the drug trade, trafficked persons will fear walking away from their criminal connections because of threats about reporting to the police or other law enforcement. They may owe debts incurred in the course of the work [17]. Furthermore, they may have been explicitly threatened or had the safety of their loved ones threatened, which coerces them into remaining in the trafficking situation. For all of these reasons, children not only do not identify themselves as victims of trafficking but are also fearful of escaping and/or disclosing their abuse.

Screening and Identification

The identification of victims of trafficking, especially labor trafficking, is admittedly quite difficult for medical professionals. Unless risk factors and clinical indicators are identified from the history and physical examination, these patients often go unidentified and return to their exploitative situations. Therefore, awareness and recognition of various clinical indicators of trafficking will speed identification. Such clinical indicators may be the victim's physical presentation, present or past medical or social history, and/or physical examination findings. Additional evidence may be found in laboratory testing for sexually transmitted infections (STIs), drugs or alcohol, immunization status, tuberculosis testing, or radiologic imaging. Table 5.3 provides a list of potential trafficking risk factors or "red flags" that medical professionals should key into as potential signs of trafficking victimization [25]. Medical professionals should use such indicators to help guide their history taking, examination, and laboratory and radiologic screening. Also, in their day-to-day practice, it is a good idea for medical professionals to ask all adolescents if they engage in any kind of work, if it affects their health, and a pointed question about whether any third party receives payment for the adolescent's work.

Assessment Tools

Medical professionals may have a difficult time initiating a conversation around exploitation and exposure to violence. Resource information about healthy relationships that includes human trafficking information can be offered to all youth. Offering such universal education upfront ensures that youth receive information

Table 5.3 Potential "red flag" indicators of human trafficking [25]

Medical presentation	Medical & social history	Physical findings	Other concerns
Accompanied by over-bearing and/or unrelated person ("friend" or "uncle") Companion does not allow the minor or youth to answer medical questions Changing or unknown demographic information Suicidality Acute physical or sexual assault Drug intoxication or sleep deprivation causing disorientation or sedation Preventable work-related injury, injury caused by employer or employer's staff	Past suicidality Runaway, throwaway, or homeless Significant school truancies or absences Child maltreatment including physical or sexual abuse, or neglect Exposure to intimate partner violence as a child, or teen dating violence Involvement with Child Protective Services or the Juvenile Justice System Substance abuse history Self identifies as LGBTQ and any of the above Has a mental health diagnosis and any of the above	Evidence of inflicted trauma Withdrawn, scared, fearful, and/or timid around accompanying person Signs of substance use or withdrawal Stated age is older than appearance and unable to verify with valid I.D.	New to country (immigrant, refugee, or undocumented) Doesn't speak English Concerning work or living conditions Doesn't know city or state of physical location Little or no pay; long hours; not allowed to leave, sleep at work Threatened or physically injured by employer or employer's staff History of drug smuggling or selling/ often called "drug mule"

even though they may not disclose exploitation on a screening form or during a medical history [36].

A standardized tool to assess labor trafficking may help to start the conversation and may also identify risks or exposures that the medical team has previously missed. Such tools are *not* a replacement for trauma-informed care and the building of healthcare provider–patient rapport and trust. While there are no magic-bullet questions, and keeping in mind that the goal of the healthcare professional and patient interaction is *not* disclosure, several key questions about human trafficking may provide important insights. In general, assessment questions should use youth-friendly terminology and should avoid using the term "human trafficking" (an often misunderstood and unclear term) to identify potentially trafficked adolescents.

As of this writing, few studies have assessed the validity of trafficking screening and assessment tools with adolescent and youth populations for both labor and sex trafficking. Some have been validated solely with adult populations but could be applicable to adolescents and youth [8, 37–41]. Finding the right time and the right tool may be important to effective assessment. Medical professionals should make sure any tools they consider adopting can assess both labor and sex trafficking. The following are a few examples of recommended validated tools.

Researchers with John Jay University and the Urban Institute validated the Human Trafficking Screening Tool (HTST), a 6-question short tool as well as a 19-question longer version that screens for both labor and sex trafficking experiences [42]. Though some of the questions are relevant primarily to sex trafficking, they all effectively screen for exploitation at work and can be asked as a screening tool using yes or no answers or as a longer assessment (See Table 5.4).

Covenant House New Jersey in partnership with researchers from Mt. Sinai Hospital tested the validity and sensitivity of a shorter version of the previously validated HTIAM-14. Their Quick Youth Indicators for Trafficking screening tool (or QYIT) had 87% sensitivity and is useful for non-expert intakes as well as more in-depth counselor and social worker assessments. The QYIT questions allow for rapport building that may encourage youth to disclose abuses. These yes/no questions may be used at any stage in working with youth [43] (See Table 5.5).

These, and other screening tools, are useful for assessing for labor trafficking. Regardless of the tool, it is important that questions are asked by the appropriate personnel and in a private setting. The tools suggested here can be utilized on intake

Table 5.4 Human trafficking screening tool [42]

1. Did someone you work for ever refuse to pay what they promised and keep all or most of the money you made?
2. Did you ever trade sexual acts for food, clothing, money, shelter, favors, or other necessities for survival before you reached the age of 18?
3. Were you ever physically beaten, slapped, hit, kicked, punched, burned, or harmed in any way by someone you worked for?
4. Have you ever been unable to leave a place you worked or talk to people you wanted to talk to, even when you weren't working, because the person you worked for threatened or controlled you?
5. Did someone you work for ever ask, pressure, or force you to do something sexually that you did not feel comfortable doing?
6. Were you ever forced to engage in sexual acts with family, friends, clients, or business associates for money or favors by someone you work for?

Table 5.5 Quick Youth Indicators for Trafficking (QYIT) screening tool

1. It is not uncommon for young people to stay in work situations that are risky or even dangerous, simply because they have no other options. Have you ever worked, or done other things, in a place that made you feel scared or unsafe?
2. Sometimes people are prevented from leaving an unfair or unsafe work situation by their employers. Have you ever been afraid to leave or quit a work situation due to fears of violence or threats of harm to yourself or your family?
3. Sometimes young people who are homeless or who have difficulties with their families have very few options to survive or fulfill their basic needs, such as food and shelter. Have you ever received anything in exchange for sex (e.g., a place to stay, gifts, or food)?
4. Sometimes employers don't want people to know about the kind of work they have young employees doing. To protect themselves, they ask their employees to lie about the kind of work they are involved in. Have you ever worked for someone who asked you to lie while speaking to others about the work you do?

by any member of hospital or clinic staff, so long as the questions are only asked in a yes/no/don't know fashion. Staff who are untrained in counseling or social work should not engage youth in prolonged conversations about experiences of exploitation. In a clinical, counseling, or case management setting, the questions can be asked first as yes/no/don't know, and then the youth can be asked to expand on their answers to determine the extent of the exploitation. Regardless of the venue or the interviewer, the conversation about these issues should be non-judgmental. Services should be offered to anyone who is identified as a trafficking victim, regardless of the kind of work they engaged in. Remember too that exploitative labor situations that are not tantamount to trafficking can still be traumatic or can negatively affect youth, so they should be assisted with services and counseling, as well.

A standardized screening instrument for adolescents and youth should be worded as simply and concretely as possible, trying to keep to a fifth-grade reading level. Questions should be prefaced with informed verbal consent and review of the limits of confidentiality. The patient or client should be counseled regarding the nature of the questions, how honesty can help providers make correct medical decisions, and that they will still receive medical care even if they refuse to answer any or all of the questions. It is recommended that the patient answer these questions alone without the influence of a caregiver, accompanying friend or family, caseworker, clergy, law enforcement, or victim advocate.

Patients come from all walks of life, cultures, nationalities, and backgrounds. It is best practice for medical institutions to use professional interpreting and translating services so that patients can communicate their care needs and can best understand the extent of their personal health services and management. Do not use an interpreter from the family, friend, or another individual accompanying the patient to your institution. Keep in mind that an accompanying person could be the trafficker or indirectly involved with the exploitation or violence. In addition, many communities are small and tightly woven, so information about an exposure or perceived "conduct" of an individual may leak to the community and cause serious collateral trauma and stigma.

Conclusions

Despite our ever-evolving knowledge of the victimization and growing criminal enterprise that is labor trafficking, there remains a significant void of evidence-based research to determine best practices for health professionals working with these populations. Medical professionals are uniquely positioned to advocate for patients and clients, many of whom are all too often relying on us to recognize the signs of exploitation and to open the conversation that will recognize, accept, and believe their disclosures. Baldwin et al. (2014) described the effects of psychological coercion in human trafficking and found that all interviewed survivors experienced nonphysical coercive tactics at the hands of their traffickers. Such manipulative tactics were used by traffickers to remove the dignity and autonomy from their victims. All too often these psychological coercive methods were mixed with physical and sexual assault to cause even more damage and produce even more control [44]. Even in the absence of robust evidence to support the application of trauma therapy modalities to youth survivors of labor trafficking, there are a few modalities that mental health providers are initiating. [See Chap. 9 for more information on these modalities.] Working as a multidisciplinary medical and therapy team to assess and address the comprehensive health needs of survivors will be the best approach for survivors to find their path to recovery and enhance their long-term resilience.

Labor Trafficking – Forced Criminality

Julia Einbond, Alison Iannarone, and Corey J. Rood

Introduction

Labor trafficking by forced criminality has recently been recognized as a common form of labor trafficking in the United States, and yet it is under-identified and overlooked in the United States and worldwide [45, 46]. This form of labor trafficking encompasses all labor trafficking whereby the work is conducted in an illicit industry or can otherwise be classified as a crime. Labor trafficking by forced criminality may occur as a single exploitation, for example, forced drug sales or gang activities, or as multiple exploitations, such as forced theft while being trafficked for sex. Traffickers instill in their victims fear of law enforcement and use the threat of arrest to coerce trafficked persons to commit further crimes, thus deepening the labor trafficking victimization or transforming what began as consensual illicit activity into labor trafficking. This type of trafficking is low risk for traffickers, who benefit from convincing victims they are criminals and would be subject to prosecution if they report.

Trafficked persons experiencing such labor trafficking do not typically present with the qualities of an "ideal victim," since having committed a crime is a prerequisite to this type of trafficking [47]. In many instances, because of misidentification, these trafficked persons are not treated from a victim-centered approach. This current reality contravenes human rights principles and clear US federal government guidance that individuals who commit crimes as a direct consequence of victimization should not be held liable [48]. A growing list of states have passed "safe harbor legislation" that provides legal mechanisms to seal, expunge, or vacate prior convictions for crimes related to human trafficking victimization. However, these laws tend to be written with sex trafficking in mind (most do so explicitly), leaving survivors of labor trafficking, who are not properly identified by law enforcement, largely without recourse [49, 50]. For youth, this often means entanglement in the juvenile justice system, with the added traumas of incarceration.

Medical personnel have a unique opportunity to identify victims of this type of trafficking, because they have no mandate to determine or report an individual's culpability for a crime. The proper identification of trafficked persons by medical personnel would increase the number of victims receiving support for their trauma and would assist law enforcement to begin their engagement from a victim services perspective. The increased provision of victim-centered services would lead to more trafficked persons feeling empowered to bring attention to their experiences and therefore allow law enforcement to bring legal action against more labor traffickers.

Definitions

Labor trafficking by forced criminality, also known as labor trafficking in illicit activities, is listed as one of 25 known typologies of human trafficking by the Polaris Project [51]. In guidance from the US State Department, forced criminality is listed as a known characteristic of human trafficking whereby the victims are forced to commit crimes as a part of their victimization. The nature of the crime or crimes committed is irrelevant to the determination of trafficking. The determination rests on the force, fraud, or coercion used as the means to motivate the criminal act. The United States recognizes traffickers' use of victims in illegal industries as a "common pattern" [52]. Outside of the United States, the European Union (EU) has also recognized the prevalence of this crime and broadened its definition of human trafficking. EU Directive (2011) specifically lists exploitation for the purpose of committing criminal activities as an "other" form of human trafficking.

Illicit activities commonly identified in this form of trafficking are drug and arms sales (or other roles in manufacture, transportation, or other drug and arms trafficking), theft (pickpocketing, shoplifting), and gang-related activities. Trafficking by forced criminality may occur as instances of single exploitation (e.g., drug sales) or multiple exploitation (e.g., drug sales during sex trafficking victimization). Multiple exploitation cases are more commonly identified owing to the increased likelihood that persons trafficked for sex will be seen as victims, but the single exploitation cases are no less trafficking crimes and are likely to involve a broader profile of trafficked persons, including more males [53, 54].

U.S. guidance warns that "trafficked individuals who are forced to commit a crime are commonly mistaken for criminals," leading to failure by law enforcement and judicial officers to treat these trafficked individuals as victims and prosecute the traffickers [48]. The EU Directive contains an explicit non-punishment provision: "National authorities are entitled not to prosecute or impose penalties on victims of trafficking in human beings for their involvement in criminal activities… [which are committed as a result of their trafficking]." Yet the EU recognizes that this provision is underused [46]. Non-profit and academic research has begun to show the breadth of this still largely invisible crime, now believed to be the most prevalent form of labor trafficking in the United States.

Vignette Examples

(a) Multiple exploitation sex and labor trafficking: *Latasha and Natalie*

Latasha and Natalie were both in foster care and homeless before they heard about the "rooming house" where they could stay. Once they arrived, they learned the rules of the house. Men would come, and the girls had to perform sex acts on them. They also had to try to sell the men drugs. If the men did not buy drugs, or even if they did, the girls were told to try to steal the men's cash when they were not looking. If the girls tried to leave, the woman who ran the house would get men to beat them up, or she would do it herself.

(b) Forced drug sales: *Brandon*

Brandon was a teenager who stood on the streets with his backpack on his shoulder and a box of candy in his hands offering the candy for sale. He wasn't really trying to sell the candy. Instead, inside the backpack was crack cocaine a drug dealer had given him to "move" (sell). Once, he made a mistake counting the money he owed the dealer, and the punishment landed him in the hospital where he had metal pins placed to repair his jaw. The dealer told Brandon he would make sure he went to jail for life for his drug dealing if he quit selling. He knew that if he quit, he could not get a job anyway, because all he had ever learned to do was sell drugs.

(c) Gang-related criminal enterprises: *Jasmine*

Jasmine reports being "beaten in" to the gang, meaning that her initiation required that she survive a severe beating from several other young initiates. She also says that in order to exit the gang, she would have to be "raped out." This has kept her dealing drugs for them even after it "got hectic" around the time she turned 15. Jasmine does not share many details, but she says selling drugs is nothing compared to the other things the gang has made her do.

(d) Long-term consequences: *Mary*

Mary was adopted at birth. She spent several years as a child in and out of treatment facilities. She left the last treatment facility to live with her biological mother whom she had never met. She quickly found out that her mother was addicted to drugs and that it would not be safe to live with her. Her mother's boyfriend started giving her drugs, and she would take them. The drugs were the only thing that made staying at her mother's house bearable. Soon, her mother's boyfriend threatened her that she would be killed if she did not bring in enough money selling drugs. One night while going to the store, she was picked up by the police and charged with possession of marijuana. The judge told her she would not have a record on the condition that she complete a mandatory drug class, and she was allowed to walk out of court with no jail time. However, presented with an opportunity to leave her mother's house, she did not attend the mandatory class and instead moved to another state with a friend. Years later, she went to find employment, and an open warrant from her former state of residence showed up on her record. It was hard to vacate this charge even with legal support, because she had not completed the mandatory drug class in the state where she was charged.

Impact on Survivors and Solutions

At first glance, none of the examples above may sound like labor trafficking. Frequently when people think about labor trafficking they assume several things: it is a violent crime; only undocumented people get trafficked; it cannot be trafficking if the person consented to be in their initial situation; trafficked persons are physically unable to leave their situations; labor trafficking is only a problem in developing countries; traffickers target victims they do not know [55]. When trafficking is not identified by professionals who encounter these individuals, the victims commonly remain under the control of their traffickers or are prosecuted for the crimes they were forced to commit. In either circumstance, the victims do not access the protections to which they are entitled and instead are re-victimized.

The most immediate and effective way to improve the care of survivors of labor trafficking by forced criminality is to increase the identification of this form of trafficking. Professionals can increase identification by (1) increasing knowledge of this type of labor trafficking, (2) recognizing that victims are not criminals, (3) using scientifically validated assessment tools to identify potential trafficking situations, and (4) creating child- and youth-friendly environments where young people can form trusting relationships with professionals where they might feel more comfortable revealing their victimization(s).

Increasing Knowledge of Labor Trafficking by Forced Criminality

In a qualitative research study to determine the cause for under-identification of labor trafficking by forced criminality, Villacampa and Torres (2017) found that the top reason is lack of awareness of this type of trafficking [47]. Latasha and Natalie are typical sex trafficking victims: a trafficker using threats of violence forced them to perform commercial sex acts. The same force compelled Latasha and Natalie to sell drugs and steal, crimes that were directly related to the sex trafficking. This pattern where sex trafficking and labor trafficking intersect is the example of labor trafficking by forced criminality that law enforcement and judicial actors tend to identify and have the greatest familiarity [47]. The other examples are all single trafficking exploitation cases, and research has shown professionals are less likely to be able to identify these as human trafficking [47]. In these cases, traffickers used force, fraud, or coercion to compel the survivors to commit crimes for the traffickers' gain. In some cases, such as Brandon's, the force was a physical threat, while in others, such as with Mary and Jasmine, coercion was applied through drug dependency and fear.

Recognizing that Victims Are Not Criminals

Without education and training to recognize trafficking via forced criminality, police have a tendency to focus first and foremost on familiar crimes that share some of the same features, such as drug dealing, theft, and gang violence [47]. The risk of focusing first on the underlying crime and not recognizing the exploitation is that victims of labor trafficking by forced criminality are prosecuted for crimes rather than protected as victims. Research shows that law enforcement is commonly unaware of protections available for victims in this context [47]. A trafficked person's best chance for receiving protections is if the law enforcement officer immediately recognizes the victimization and communicates this to their supervisor and even their local prosecutor. Once a conviction or plea deal has been reached, even for low-level crimes not involving prison time, it can limit a victim's future legitimate employment prospects and be very difficult to undo.

Using Scientifically Validated Screening Tools

Validated tools that assess labor trafficking include forced criminality. The use of validated tools are critical to helping identify labor trafficking because they do not require the trafficked person initially to reveal their full story. For a patient who is unaware or confused about their victimization and reasonably wary about confessing to a crime, the option of giving a yes/no answer to a question that does not elicit information about underlying crimes safeguards them from inadvertently making an admission that could be used against them in a future legal case. The Quick Youth Indicators for Trafficking (QYIT) is a four-question screening tool validated for use with the homeless youth population [56]. Since the tool was designed with young survivors in mind, it is written in youth-accessible language and uses desensitizing language to help the youth feel that neither the asking of the questions themselves nor a yes answer to any of them would single them out as bad or unique. As of this writing, the candidate questions for the tool are currently undergoing testing for validation in the hospital emergency room context [57].

Reluctance to Disclose Victimization

Upon scoring positively on a screening tool, or otherwise presenting with "red flags" (e.g., presenting with gang-related tattoos), victims of forced criminality may remain reluctant to disclose their trafficking experience. As with the case of Brandon, a common feature of this type of trafficking is the trafficker's coercion through threats that the victim will be criminally prosecuted for crimes they committed should they report. Even for low-level crimes that do not typically carry prison sentences, arrests may lead to criminal records, costs associated with judicial fines and fees, unintended biases, and reputational damage. The real possibility that victims will be treated as criminals by uninformed law enforcement and judicial actors shifts the balance of risk for reporting from the trafficker to the victim. Added to the coercion is the victim's own limiting mindset that he or she *is* a criminal, not a victim. This mindset is the result of psychological coercion, causing victims to believe they chose to commit crimes and therefore are responsible for the crimes they committed. In fact, research shows that trafficked homeless youth had higher odds, almost six times greater likelihood, of being arrested than homeless youth who were not trafficked [58]. Arrest may have occurred before or after the trafficking began. Sometimes the first crime was compelled by the trafficker, but more often the victim is "groomed" by being enticed to take part in some consensual low-level illicit activity. Forms of coercion and control used by traffickers to groom victims can vary widely as illustrated by the promotion of drug use and dependency employed by Mary's trafficker or the gang activities used by Jasmine's trafficker.

Creating Child- and Youth-Friendly Environments

Professionals who encounter trafficked persons through positive screening tools or other red flags should be particularly sensitive to symptoms of internalized psychological coercion among child and youth survivors. Studies have shown youth survivors of human trafficking often have a history of childhood trauma, such as an emotional, physical, or sexual abuse, witnessing violence in the home, or experiencing family legal problems [56]. In the homeless youth population, additional personal factors have been identified that increase risk for exploitation including having an individualized education program (IEP) or 504 plan, history of arrest, experience in foster care, mental health issue(s), history of suicidality, and/or having a disabling condition [58]. These associated factors support the hypothesis that complex trauma is at the core of the trafficking experience. Complex trauma is defined as exposure to multiple traumatic events, often of an invasive, interpersonal nature. These events are severe and pervasive and usually occur early in life. Early childhood trauma has a measurable effect on a child's brain development and the ability to form secure attachments and coping skills [59].

Individuals with complex trauma may demonstrate nonverbal clues before being able or willing to disclose their experiences, such as nervousness, avoiding eye contact, staring into the distance, sweaty hands, and evasiveness in interviews [47]. For young victims, youth-centered approaches and environments tailored to promote safety and trust are important. In Mary's case, her history of adoption, rejection by her adoptive family, and involvement with the law created a desperate need for physical safety. A safe physical environment can be created by service providers, children's advocacy centers, and other facilities to give some power and control back to the young person as the professional asks difficult questions about their experiences.

A safe emotional environment can be created by taking a trauma-informed approach, which shifts a professional's perspective from "what is wrong with this person?" to "what has happened to this person?" [60] This shift in perspective shows a victim compassion and empathy while allowing them the opportunity to build rapport in a non-judgmental environment. The trauma-informed approach increases their comfort in sharing their experiences with professionals.

Case Presentations

Case 1:

Brandon is a 19-year-old male presenting to a homeless shelter looking for a place to stay. During the intake process, Brandon is screened for prior human trafficking experiences using the Quick Youth Indicators for Trafficking (QYIT) tool (see Table 5.5). You, the licensed clinical social worker, are informed that he scores the highest possible QYIT score, 4 out of 4. This alerts you that he is very likely to be a survivor of human trafficking. You meet with Brandon for a full trafficking assessment.

You use a longer human trafficking protocol created by the VERA Institute and adapted by Covenant House New York to elicit Brandon's story [61, 62]. You know from the QYIT that Brandon has worked in a place that has made him feel scared or unsafe. You ask Brandon, "Did you ever witness another employee being hurt or threatened?" He responds, "Yes," and says, "One time one guy didn't have all of his money right and I was forced to jump him with other guys. I knew this would happen to me if I was in that situation."

After discussing confidentiality and the limits of confidentiality, you review with Brandon the questions he answered affirmatively on the QYIT to learn more of his experience. When you ask him if he was afraid to leave or quit a work situation due to fears of violence or other threats of harm to him or his family, he responds, "I was in the streets. I knew if I left they would think I was snitching and then they would want to kill me because they know I have good information." You then ask what did he think would happen if he tried to leave? He responds, "I thought I would be killed."

You then ask Brandon, "Have you ever worked for someone who asked you to lie while speaking to others about the work you do?" He responds, "Yes, I was told to tell people I was a window washer. I was told to lie so they wouldn't get in trouble for me having drugs."

At this point, you have determined Brandon's experience meets the definition of labor trafficking. You ask Brandon if he feels comfortable sharing his story and he says yes. He shares:

> When I was a teenager, I stood on the streets with my backpack on my shoulder and a box of candy in my hands, offering candy for sale. I wasn't really trying to sell the candy; inside the backpack was crack cocaine a drug dealer had given me to move. Once, I made a mis-

> take counting the money I owed the dealer and my punishment landed me in the hospital where I had metal pins placed to reset my jaw. The dealer told me I would go to jail for life if I quit. I was finally able to leave when my foster care worker moved me to a new foster home hours away from my old neighborhood.

You ask Brandon if he told anyone at the hospital that his jaw was broken because he was being forced to sell drugs. He says, "No." You ask him if anyone at the hospital asked him if he would be safe where he was staying after he left the hospital? He says, "No, no one asked me a lot of questions because my face was all swollen."

At this point in the conversation, you shift to conduct a biopsychosocial assessment to learn more about Brandon, begin to build rapport with him, and figure out how best to support him with services. You allow Brandon a safe space to share his personal history, including his family history and the experiences that led him to Covenant House. You tell Brandon he can share as much information as he feels comfortable sharing so that he retains choice and control over the conversation. While he shares specifics of his childhood, you ask the Adverse Childhood Experience (ACE) questions to explore Brandon's childhood trauma exposure [63]. At the end of the assessment you confirm that he has a score of 7 of 10 on the ACE questionnaire, indicating he has experienced multiple forms of trauma that cumulatively are likely to affect his lifetime health outcomes negatively if left untreated [64]. You further learn that he has experienced 9 of 11 factors associated with human trafficking among homeless youth, including emotional abuse, physical abuse, being arrested, foster care, witnessing violence in the home, mental health issues, history of suicidality, familial legal problems, and having a disabling condition. In telling you about his childhood, Brandon connects his adverse childhood experiences with his entry into the drug industry that ultimately became his prison:

> I was placed in foster care when I was four years old. My mother and siblings had been homeless and sleeping on park benches before I was removed for neglect. In my first placement at a children's shelter, I was emotionally, verbally, and physically abused. I started selling drugs when I was seven. I thought that selling drugs would make me not feel like a victim anymore.

You note that Brandon is at high risk of being trafficked again based on the extent of his previous trauma and his lack of treatment. You learn Brandon is currently experiencing trouble sleeping, nightmares, poor appetite, lethargy, not wanting to be around others, hopelessness, irritability, and passing suicidal thoughts. He is also having headaches from "thinking too much, feeling worried a lot," and having self-reported "panic attacks." He is also smoking marijuana frequently.

You recommend that he meet with you for individual therapy weekly and have an assessment with the psychiatrist. You offer Brandon the opportunity to speak to the staff attorney and talk about pressing charges against his traffickers, but Brandon declines. You assure him that it is up to him and he can always change his mind in the future if he decides he wants legal help.

You meet with Brandon again before his first therapy session, because he comes into your clinic under the influence of drugs. During this conversation, Brandon reveals that he is not only smoking marijuana regularly, but he is also buying benzodiazepines on the street. You discuss with Brandon your concerns about his health and his substance use, and how it will affect his ability to make progress on his housing goal.

Brandon accepts a referral to a substance abuse program to detox from his benzodiazepine addiction and address the underlying reasons for his drug use. You agree to continue weekly therapy sessions.

Over the course of the next year, Brandon cycles in and out of residential treatment for multiple short stays each lasting less than 30 days. He is inconsistent with treatment and unable to address his ongoing substance use. After his last stay, Brandon turns 22 and is no longer eligible for services at the homeless shelter where you work.

One year later, Brandon stops by to say hello. He tells you through his wide grin that he had realized you were right about the illicit substances, and he stopped using them. Since he has been in recovery, he has been able to maintain consistent employment for the first time. He has saved over $4000 and is waiting to rent his first apartment.

Discussion Questions

1. What do you think the reason is that Brandon did not share his substance use with you during your first meeting? Is there something you could have done differently to have helped him feel comfortable enough to have shared during that first visit?

When adolescents first meet healthcare professionals, they are trying to figure out if you are a trustworthy adult. It may have been more difficult for Brandon to build a trusting relationship with you, because he has not had adults in his life who were consistently safe. Dr. Kenneth Ginsburg explains that there are key elements adolescents need to hear to extend their trust to you: what can you do for me, what this visit will be like, why do you need to ask personal questions, honesty, and service with respect and without judgment [60]. In the case of Brandon, these key elements could have been explained to him in a more straightforward manner touching on specifics about common risky behaviors like substance abuse to ensure he knew he was in a safe environment where sharing would not harm him.

2. What referrals for treatment would you make for Brandon at the point he aged out of your facility or clinic?

Due to Brandon's high level of trauma history, as indicated by his score of 7 on the ACE questionnaire, and his addiction, one of the known potential negative long-term health outcomes associated with untreated childhood trauma, you would recommend a referral to a Mental Illness and Chemical Addiction (MICA) program. A program that would address both his mental health and his substance use would give him the opportunity to help prevent or mitigate some of the further long-term consequences of ACEs from occurring [65]. Ideally, this program would also be able to provide trauma-focused treatment.

3. Are there any other medical providers that he needs while in your care?

Brandon needs help in establishing a primary medical provider and dental provider if he does not currently have them. Often, children who age out of the foster system and do not transition smoothly into adult independent living may find themselves disconnected from regular healthcare especially if homeless. Homeless youth frequently lose contact with their medical and dental providers, especially if those providers were associated with the foster system or a prior foster home or shelter. A homeless youth with a history of being trafficked should be reconnected with healthcare, medical and dental, as soon as possible. A family medicine clinic, free or low cost clinic, or public health clinic may be an appropriate option for Brandon. He will require catch-up vaccinations, full screening for infectious disease and environmental exposures, review of his health history and medications, screening for nutritional deficiencies, and assessment of his current vitals and physical exam. He may have some of his own health concerns, and reestablishing care will provide him with the opportunity to have those concerns addressed. Additional guidance can be found in the policy statement (2013) on homeless adolescents from the American Academy of Pediatrics [66].

4. How did a caring relationship with the social worker impact Brandon? How did clearing health obstacles impact Brandon's path to success?

Caring-adult relationships have been identified as the greatest source of resilience in youth [67]. For youth who have experienced severe trauma, caring relationships are especially important as a protective factor against the long-term negative health outcomes associated with trauma [60]. Recent research completed by Covenant House New Jersey has also shown that these same caring relationships serve as a protective factor against human trafficking for youth who have experienced multiple childhood traumas and their outcomes [58]. In Brandon's case, his relationship with the social worker allowed him to have a caring adult in his life to help him begin to overcome obstacles. [For more in-depth perspectives on success and resilience, refer to Chaps. 19 and 21.]

Case 2:

A 16-year-old girl named Jasmine is transported just after midnight to the emergency department at your Level 1 trauma center with a gunshot wound to the eye, significant bleeding, and signs of shock. The trauma team resuscitated her in the operating room with packed red blood cells, intravenous fluid boluses, and vasopressors. While being resuscitated, trauma surgery worked to control her active bleeding by repairing a laceration on her right thigh and scanning her for intracranial and cervical injury. Ophthalmology worked to repair her open globe trauma, resulting in enucleation and subsequent blindness in that eye. After a long recovery in the pediatric intensive care unit, and with no serious intracranial injury, she was eventually moved to the step-down neurotrauma medical unit.

You are the nurse on the floor working the evening shift. Examination of Jasmine's general appearance reveals a patch over her left eye, dressing over the wound on her right thigh, and an old burn scar on her left shoulder. Further examination reveals several scars indicative of healing lacerations on her right thigh and what appears to be a healed abrasion or burn scar on her left shoulder. Blood tests reveal recent marijuana use. Sexually transmitted infection testing for hepatitis B & C, HIV, syphilis, gonorrhea, chlamydia, and trichomonas is positive only for *Trichomonas vaginalis*, and pregnancy test is negative.

After a lengthy hospital stay and some good rapport building, Jasmine discloses to you that she was shot after a male acquaintance made an aggressive sexual advance on her and she resisted. The social worker for the unit is able to complete an assessment, which reveals a history of foster care since childhood after mother's suicide, and gang involvement beginning around 11 years of age when she "escaped" a group home. You visit Jasmine several times over the next two nights while you are monitoring her eye recovery. One of the times you walk into the room, Jasmine is sleeping but yelling "get off me, get off me." It is clear that she is having a nightmare and you gently shake her to wake her up. Jasmine is having a hard time breathing and is sweating. You offer Jasmine a glass of water and the space to talk about what happened. She refuses to talk about it and insists that she is "fine."

The next day, Jasmine seems "off." You ask, "Is everything ok?" She assures you that it is but is visibly shaking as she responds. You sit down in the chair next to her and let her know that you are there if/when she wants to talk, or she can speak to the social worker again if she feels more comfortable. Jasmine turns her head away from you and does not respond. You leave the room. You ask the social worker to check in on her again, but Jasmine will not engage with her either.

Over the next 2 weeks you continue to monitor Jasmine's medical progress, but she has not talked much to you since the night she was having the nightmare. One day, while you are changing Jasmine's bandage, she starts to talk to you. She expresses feeling anxiety about returning to her life. You validate the anxiety she must be feeling as her discharge date from the hospital approaches. She continues to explain that the guy who made the sexual advances toward her is a member of the same gang she is in and was encouraged by other men in the gang to sexually assault her. Her cousin is the "boss," and she has to pay him a portion of everything she makes selling drugs. Jasmine shares that her initiation into the gang required that she survive a severe beating from several other young initiates. She also says that in order to exit the gang, she would have to be raped by gang members. This has kept Jasmine dealing drugs for the gang and prevented her from leaving. Since losing her eye, she has become more reflective about her chances of surviving life with the gang, and she now wants to create an exit strategy. She asks if you can help her do that. You know that it is not your role to create safety plans with patients, but you also know that you do not want this girl to feel abandoned. After telling Jasmine that you would like to get guidance from other experts to be able to help her, you share these new disclosures and concerns with the unit social worker.

Law enforcement officers wait for Jasmine to be released from the hospital, because she returned fire when she was shot. Police have indicated that, upon release, she will be taken directly from the hospital to juvenile detention and potentially charged with attempted murder. You know Jasmine is a victim of trafficking, but you don't know whether to give this information to these officers. Instead, you decide to call Child Protective Services and inform them of the situation, because in your state this falls under a child maltreatment mandate to report. The caseworker makes this high priority and is headed to the hospital to intervene. You also call the National Human Trafficking Hotline and explain the situation. They urge you to tell Jasmine she can talk to a lawyer for free, and they give you phone numbers for the local juvenile defender's office anti-trafficking specialist and a local non-governmental organization that specializes in legal advocacy.

Discussion Questions

1. What type of helping professional is needed most urgently to address Jasmine's physical safety? How does patient confidentiality and HIPAA limit you from connecting Jasmine to available resources?

A trauma-informed hospital system will promote confidentiality about a patient's experiences to the greatest extent possible [68]. A reasonable guarantee of privacy and confidentiality is necessary to encourage trafficked persons to seek treatment, and it is important for survivors to maintain feelings of power and control over their experiences and plans. When there is a need to break confidentiality, the patient should be informed as soon as possible (ideally before any details are disclosed) and allowed to participate in information sharing as much as she or he chooses. Knowing how much information to elicit about trafficking experiences and what to do with that information can be a barrier to providing confidential healthcare [69].

Because Jasmine is under 18, you are required by law as a mandated reporter to report her victimization (or child abuse) to child protective services. If Jasmine were 18 or older, you would not have this obligation and thus would only report Jasmine's victimization with her express consent. A positive practice in trauma-informed hospital systems is to have victim services specialists already identified and available (onsite or in the local community) to counsel trafficking survivors about their options in a safe and confidential setting. If such an advocate is not available, or if Jasmine refuses to speak to this resource, your best option is to do as the nurse did: provide the phone number for the National Human Trafficking Hotline (888-373-7888), a service available 24/7, should Jasmine decide to accept help. [See Chap. 18 for more about mandatory reporting.]

2. Is there any medical follow-up that Jasmine needs?

Upon discharge from the hospital, Jasmine will be provided a list of follow-up appointments and care techniques for her injuries. She should follow those recommendations closely. Much like adolescents and youth who are homeless, those involved in gangs may not have established primary medical and dental providers. Jasmine will need assistance establishing ongoing regular medical and dental care.

This may include a pediatrician, adolescent medicine specialist, family medicine provider, and/or an obstetrics and gynecology provider. If she is arrested and placed in juvenile detention, Jasmine's follow-up appointments and ongoing medical assessment needs should be communicated with any medical professionals at the detention center so that they can help facilitate compliance with recommended care.

3. What mental health plan would you recommend for Jasmine, anticipating that she is likely headed to juvenile detention?

You will want to link Jasmine with a psychiatrist and therapist such that she may be given any prescriptions and plan for mental health care prior to being placed in juvenile detention, since research suggests that the juvenile justice system to date has had difficulty in addressing the numerous mental health needs of youth in detention [70].

Labor Trafficking – Vulnerability of Immigrant and Refugee Youth

Alessandra Amato, Hayoung Lee, Stephanie Richard, and Corey J. Rood

Introduction

The United States Department of Homeland Security (DHS) defines a *migrant* as a person who leaves his or her country of origin to seek residence in another county [71]. Every year, millions of people migrate to the United States. According to the United Nations Department of Economic and Social Affairs, more than 49 million individuals migrated into the United States at mid-year of 2017 [72]. Migration can occur in various forms. Broad categories of migrants include those with authorization of entry, migrants without authorization of entry, asylum seekers, and refugees. Both documented and undocumented migrants have specific vulnerabilities to trafficking.

Research measuring prevalence and incidences of various forms of human trafficking in the United States by industry type and methods of recruitment of victims is limited. Currently, the National Human Trafficking Hotline (NHTH) maintains one of the most extensive data sets on the issue of human trafficking in the United States. According to the 2017 annual report, recent migration/relocation was the number one risk factor for human trafficking, followed by substance use, runaway/homeless youth, mental health concern, and involvement in the child welfare system [74]. Industries involved with labor trafficking include, but are not limited to, agriculture, farms, animal husbandry, domestic work, landscaping service, hospitality, restaurant/food service, construction, education, forestry/reforestation, traveling carnivals, and even health care [78]. The healthcare industry includes nursing homes and home nurse aid agencies. Victims of human trafficking in North America have been found to originate from as many as 96 different countries spanning the continents of Africa, Europe, South Asia, and South America. However, according to the 2017 annual report, the most common nationalities of victims of labor trafficking identified in the United States (listed in descending order) are Mexico, Philippines, Guatemala, India, Jamaica, South Africa, Peru, Nigeria, Brazil, and Columbia [78].

Human Trafficking Versus Human Smuggling

Recognition of the difference between human trafficking and human smuggling is important, but the two crimes intersect. In brief, human trafficking is a crime against a person, whereas human smuggling is a crime against a border. More specifically, *human trafficking* is a crime in which a human being is exploited through force, fraud, or coercion for the purpose of commercial sex acts or a form of labor/servitude [82]. The presence of force, fraud, and coercion are not required elements when an individual induced to engage in commercial sex is under the age of 18 [82]. The confusion regarding the distinction between trafficking and smuggling is caused by the common misunderstanding that trafficking means "movement." Although many victims of trafficking are physically relocated, movement is not a requirement of trafficking [82]. In fact, individuals can be and have been trafficked within their very own homes, towns, and communities.

In contrast, *human smuggling* occurs when a person voluntarily makes an agreement with a smuggler to facilitate their illegal entry into a foreign country [82]. Also referred to as *migrant smuggling*, this crime involves movement and the crossing of international borders. Payments for smuggling can be made to the smuggler in full prior to the movement or in installments with full payment made after the successful crossing of the international border. International data on human smuggling is limited due to a lack of collection and publication of reports on human smuggling trends. Some data based on arrival and apprehension show certain trends of human smuggling. Between 2000 and 2017, humans were smuggled to the United States from China (n = 69,000), Pakistan (n = 24,000), Bangladesh (n = 24,000), India (n = 24,000), Somalia (n = 9200), Brazil (n = 9200), El Salvador (n = 9200), Guatemala (n = 9200), Honduras (n = 9200), Cuba (n = 9200), and Mexico (n = 3200) [83].

Importantly, human smuggling can *lead* to sex or labor trafficking. Consent to being smuggled into the country and agreement to pay the debt for smuggling does not prevent an individual from becoming a victim of human trafficking but rather increases their vulnerabilities for exploitation. Trafficking crimes occur when labor or services, including sex acts, are performed under force, fraud or coercion or in the case of a minor, inducement into commercial sex. Healthcare professionals should understand that smuggling can be a red flag for identifying trafficking and should refer cases for further screening.

Types of Migration

Migrants with Authorization of Entry

Migrants with authorization of entry include immigrants and nonimmigrants. A legal *immigrant* is an *alien,* or an individual who is not a citizen, admitted to the United States as a lawful permanent resident. According to the 2016 Yearbook of Immigration Statistics, the United States admitted more than 1.18 million legal immigrants, of which approximately 22% were under the age of 19 years [73]. *Nonimmigrant migrants* with the authorization of entry are granted temporary residence in the United States. Visas, including H-4 and F-2, are available for children of H-1B and F-1 visa holders, respectively, but do not grant eligibility to work. Approximately 13% of nonimmigrant migrants are 19 years of age or younger. Of note, according to the United Nations Office of Drugs and Crime, 25–40% of migrants without authorization initially enter the country with a visa and overstay [77].

Data from NHTH can offer insight into the demographics and characteristics of victims of labor trafficking. For example, agricultural workers with H-2A visas had the highest rates of report to the NHTH between January 2015 and December 2017 with possible concerns for potential human trafficking [78]. Furthermore, nearly half of the victims of labor trafficking reported to the NHTH from January 2015 to December 2017 were foreign nationals holding legal visas. Although it is challenging to make conclusions based on these data alone because individuals may have a variety of reasons for contacting NHTH, it is important to note that – contrary to common belief – a significant portion of foreign national victims of human trafficking in the United States may be individuals who entered the country *legally* and who were recruited and exploited through legal pathways.

Healthcare professionals in their social history taking should inquire about immigration status in a non-threatening manner while interviewing foreign national patients. Questions such as

- Where are you from?
- What brought you to the United States?
- How long have you been in the United States?
- Where do you work?

may help establish rapport, and responses may disclose red flags for exploitation. However, healthcare professionals should keep in mind that patients may be reluctant to disclose their migrant status due to fear of being reported to law enforcement and deported even when there is no violation of their legal status. Therefore, prefacing this line of questioning with the caveat that the clinician's goal is to provide help and assistance to the patient is key and that the information will be confidential.

Migrants Without Authorization of Entry

Many migrants from countries around the world, including children and young adults, enter the United States without documentation to flee violence and poverty and seek a better life. Under these circumstances, children and young adults are especially vulnerable to becoming victims of trafficking. For example, a migrant heading to the United States from Central or South America would likely cross the Mexican–American border. Before making it to this point, thousands of migrants have suffered assaults, robbery, and abduction by criminal gangs. According to the Mexican National Human Rights Commission, as many as 20,000 migrants are kidnapped every year, and 6 in 10 women and girls are raped during their journey to the United States [76]. Some are killed during this journey, and others report severe mistreatment from immigration officials and police.

Youth and children may or may not be accompanied by a parent from Central and South America while fleeing violence in their home country (See *Case 1: Story of Hector*). These youth (1) could have left their home country because they were fleeing labor or sex trafficking, (2) could have been trafficked en route to the United States for labor or sex, and/or (3) could be trafficked at the US border and forced to engage in drug smuggling or sales (often referred to as *drug mules*). Therefore, when indicated, unaccompanied children and youth should be assessed for their entire experience for trafficking, not just trafficking that may have occurred in the United States.

An added complexity is that these youth are often forced to engage in criminal activity orchestrated by violent gangs, compounding the medical and mental health trauma they experience. Identification becomes even more difficult as these youth feel complicit in their own abuse and in criminal acts. [The dynamics of human labor trafficking and forced criminality are discussed in greater detail in section "Labor Trafficking – Forced Criminality".] This dynamic for immigrant youth in labor trafficking is important to highlight, because they face not only the fear of being undocumented immigrants, but also the fear of being seen as criminals and not youth victims.

Asylum Seekers and Refugees

An *asylum seeker* or *refugee* refers to an immigrant who is found to be unable or unwilling to return to his or her country of origin because of persecution or a well-founded fear of persecution based on race, religion, nationality, membership in a particular social group, or political opinion [71]. Approximately half of the world's refugees are children [85]. Although the terms *asylum seeker* (or *asylee*) and *refugee* are commonly used interchangeably by the general public, there are important legal and procedural differences between the two migrant types. An *asylee* is an individual who meets the international definition of refugee and seeks a request for protection status when they are *already present* in the United States or at a port of entry [71]. In contrast, an individual applies for *refugee* status *while outside* of the United States and enters the Unites States in this status. The limit to the number of individuals obtaining asylum and refugee status and eligibility for adjustment to permanent residence status also differ between the two migrant types. There has been no limit on the number of individuals granted asylum status each year. As such, the United States has been one of the world's largest recipients of new individual asylum applications [80]. In contrast, the President establishes the number of individuals granted refugee status per year based on geographic region [71]. Since 1975, three million refugees from across the world have resettled in the United States [79]. Both refugees and asylum seekers are eligible to transition to lawful permanent resident status after 1 year of continuous presence in the United States [71]. However, a limit of 10,000 asylum seekers are granted permanent resident status per fiscal year [71].

Case Presentations

Case 1: Story of Hector

Hector is a 17-year-old Spanish-speaking boy presenting to your foster care medical clinic for the first time. Prior to seeing Hector, a staff member notifies you that Hector only speaks Spanish, and they have requested a medical Spanish-English interpreter to be present for this visit. With the interpreter you learn the following history.

Hector immigrated without legal documents to the United States from Honduras when he was 15 with his father and older sister for better work opportunity to provide for their family, which includes seven children. The three of them each paid $7000 USD to make the journey into the United States, knowing that another $7000 USD would be owed upon arrival. Hector traveled in a car trunk for days not knowing where he was going. During the journey, his father was caught and deported back to Honduras.

Hector and his sister made it to the United States now unaccompanied and found a "simple place" to live with "simple jobs" to pay rent. After about 6 months, Hector was kicked out of the house. He started living with some friends who worked in roofing and construction. Hector began this work, but he was not receiving the money he was initially promised. He began to receive threats of violence against himself and his family back home, with whom he was rarely allowed to communicate, if he did not continue to work. He worked more than 12 hours a day, 6 days per week.

One day, Hector was driving without a license and was involved in a collision. Although he thought about fleeing the scene because he was undocumented and unlicensed, he stayed at the scene. He was arrested and taken to jail. Hector had a difficult time communicating his story and situation to the officers due to the language barrier. He was placed in juvenile detention before being transferred to the care of child protective services. He is now in an adolescent group home where he is required to have an intake medical examination in the foster clinic where you are the attending provider.

You gather a full medical history from Hector. This is the first time he received medical attention in the United States. Hector lacks medical records and cannot remember if he received any vaccinations as a child. He complains of back pain since he fell off a roof 2 months ago. He also endorses headaches, joint pain, and chronic cough. He does not take medications or have any known medical problems. He endorses using alcohol to manage pain and anxiety but does not drink regularly. He endorses marijuana and occasional cigarette use but denies other illicit drugs. He is sexually active with females and openly stated that he purchased commercial sex work in the recent past, rarely wearing condoms. His medical screening reveals moderate depression and anxiety which he attributes to the lack of contact with his family in Honduras and sister in the United States. He denies suicidality.

Discussion Questions

1. What aspects of human smuggling and human trafficking did Hector experience?
2. How are events Hector experienced contributing to his presenting mental health concerns?
3. What is your differential diagnosis?
4. What vaccines, labs, imaging, and referrals would you order?
5. How does Hector's case reveal problems in using criminal justice language instead of public health language when discussing human trafficking? Can a "victim" of human trafficking also be a perpetrator of human trafficking?
6. What other medical, legal, educational, and social resources should be considered for Hector?

The Resettlement Process

Among migrants entering the United States, refugees go through the most rigorous vetting process. The resettlement process is initiated primarily by the United Nations High Commissioner for Refugees (UNHCR) and consists of 14 steps including several interviews with American officials, vetting and security screening through the FBI, the Department of Homeland Security (DHS), the U.S. Department of Defense (DOD), and medical screenings conducted by the International Organization for Migration (IOM) [81]. Historically, the screening and vetting process has taken on average 2 years, although the applicant's location, local circumstances, and policy changes can create longer waiting periods, sometimes up to a decade. During this time, applicants continue to live in either refugee camps or urban settings in neighboring countries from the one they fled. In the meantime, many are denied access to education, employment, medical care, and other basic human rights. With no legal protection, displaced individuals are ever more susceptible to sex and labor exploitation.

Trauma Associated with Displacement

Regardless of immigration status, migrants face unique challenges that affect their health. The demand for mental health professionals has been increasing to support the needs of migrants as the connection between their unique experiences and mental health is better understood [85]. Therefore, healthcare professionals must be aware of the unique circumstances and experiences of refugee and asylum seekers, especially children and young adults.

While some migrants leave their country of origin voluntarily, displaced migrants such as refugee and asylum seekers leave their country of origin involuntarily. Therefore, most experience traumatic stress due to intense events that threaten or harm their emotional and physical well-being. Such events can include violence, sexual assault, forced labor, and lack of food, water, and shelter in their country of origin and/or during migration.

Refugees' experiences surrounding displacement can be categorized into three phases: preflight, flight, and resettlement [85]. The preflight phase refers to the time prior to departure from the country of origin. A social upheaval and increase in chaos, leading to threats and fear for safety, is the initial experience prior to displacement. During the flight phase, refugees face uncertainties about their future as they are displaced from their home. They are often dependent on external sources to meet basic needs and are vulnerable to smuggling or trafficking. Migrants may experience living in refugee camps, separation from family, loss of community, traveling long distances, inadequate food, and detention confinement. During this phase, refugees can be forced or pressured to engage in commercial sex to meet basic needs [84]. The journey of the migrant is not over upon entering the United States. Once refugees resettle in the new country, they face challenges of adjustment to new cultures, languages, and lifestyles. Social and cultural integration, acculturation, and isolation can increase vulnerability to becoming trafficked [85].

Recruitment and Control

Migrant youths seeking work rely on recruiting agencies to link them with employment in the United States. These agencies, however, may recruit individuals under false promises of work. Once the migrant arrives at the determined destination, they may discover that work expectations and conditions differ from what was agreed upon. Migrant youths also may run out of money during the journey to employment, and many engage in commercial sex in order to survive [75]. Traffickers also use the Internet and social media platforms to recruit for labor trafficking. The Internet is used to promote fake or misleading job advertisements nationally and internationally [75].

Control over victims is a key component of optimizing profit from trafficking. Therefore, traffickers will use various means to maintain control and power over victims. However, specific ways traffickers control foreign nationals is by withholding documents, threatening to report them to law enforcement, promising that they can get the individual a visa or lawful status, and/or deceiving them into believing they must work to pay off an accumulated debt (i.e. debt bondage). Ultimately, the foreign national victim becomes dependent on the trafficker due to the use of strategic physical, financial, and/or emotional force, fraud, and/or coercion [86].

As mentioned, debt bondage is a common method labor traffickers use to control victims. Some migrants arrive in the new country to find that they have accumulated a debt with their smuggler or employer. The debt continues to accrue without signs of liquidation: therefore, its payment in full can be drawn out by the trafficker indefinitely. For example, traffickers tell the migrant that additional payments (often exorbitant) must be made for accommodations, tools, and food, and for interest on the initial transportation debt. This form of debt bondage commonly keeps migrants under the control and servitude of the trafficker for months to years.

Government Support

Foreign, unaccompanied, refugee, minor victims of trafficking can receive comprehensive services they need either through the state's individual child welfare system or through the federal system's Office of Refugee Resettlement (ORR). The ORR has a program designed specifically for refugee children called the Unaccompanied Refugee Minors (URM) program [87]. The services offered to trafficked children through URM are distinct from services offered to unaccompanied immigrant (alien) children (UAC) [88] who, unlike refugee children, frequently lack immigration status.

Additionally, under the Trafficking Victims Protection Act (TVPA) of 2000 [89], both non-US citizen adult and child trafficking victims are eligible for federal benefits to the same extent as refugees [90]. For potential child victims of trafficking, the TVPA requires federal, state, and local officials to notify the Department of Health and Human Services (DHHS) within 24 hours of discovering a foreign national child under the age of 18 who may be a victim of sex or labor trafficking. This is to ensure that the child receives appropriate specialized assistance [91]. More information about this program can be obtained by emailing ChildTrafficking@acf.hhs.gov or calling their information line (1-202-205-4582) [92]. The DHHS also offers monthly webinars for practitioners to learn more about these issues [93].

When developing protocols for referrals and services for foreign national trafficked children, healthcare professionals should be aware of strengths and weaknesses of both the federal and state options available for children in their individual states [94].

Finally, foreign national children of trafficking almost always have specialized immigration service needs. The TVPA established two immigration statuses for victims of trafficking: a temporary legal status called "continued presence" and a nonimmigrant visa under the Immigrant and Nationality Act (INA) called a "T-visa." In general, other forms of relief for trafficking victims, including special immigrant juvenile status (SIJS), asylum, and U-visas for victims of certain crimes are not the preferred form of relief for trafficked children, but these are often utilized because healthcare professionals are less familiar with the specialized relief provided to trafficking victims [95].

Case 2: Story of Carlos

Carlos is a 21-year-old Spanish-speaking young man who presents for an evaluation of a right-foot injury. You are a clinician volunteering at the medical clinic that provides free primary care services to uninsured individuals.

When you enter the patient room with an interpreter, you find Carlos sitting on the chair with sandals on his feet and crutches next to him. Carlos tells you that he hurt his foot while working at the ranch. A metal piece of machinery fell on his right foot a week ago. You ask him, "What led you to come in today, instead of a week ago?" Carlos responds, "My patron didn't want to take me to the hospital when the accident happened. He gave me some cream and bandages for the wound, and medications for pain. But I was in a lot of pain. When I asked for better treatment, my patron became violent and threatened to have me deported."

You quickly evaluate his foot to rule out the need for emergent intervention. There is an area of ecchymosis on the dorsal aspect of his right foot with some healing abrasion, but no open wounds or evidence of necrotic tissue. Cap refill is <2 seconds and sensation is intact. Active and passive range of motion of toes and ankle is limited due to pain. He has point tenderness over the proximal aspect of the third metatarsal around the tarso-metatarsal joint. He denies fever. Given a lower suspicion for vascular compromise, nerve injury, compartment syndrome, osteomyelitis, or the need for immediate surgical referral, you continue to gather additional history. You ask him, "Do you feel safe where you work?"

Carlos responds, "I did not feel safe at the time." Carlos informs you that he left Peru 3 years ago after accepting a job offer on a sheep ranch outside your local town. He was granted a temporary work visa. However, when he arrived at the ranch, Carlos was forced to sleep on the ground with the sheep, did not have access to a toilet or running water, was forced to work long hours without breaks, did not receive any days off, and was being fed "once on a good day." Carlos continues, "When my work visa expired, my patron told me that he would take care of it, but he never agreed to show me any proof that the documents had been renewed. Especially after the accident, I was scared for my life. He wanted to kill me. I would have never survived out there. Therefore, I took the chance and ran away from the ranch with my expired documents. However, I had to leave all my belongings behind. I was never paid." Carlos is now working with an immigration attorney on a T-visa and rents a bedroom from a survivor leader with a local anti-trafficking program. You ask him, "How are you coping with everything you've experienced?" Carlos reports, "I am having trouble sleeping at night, thinking about the abuse and the fear I experienced. I am trying to stay positive. I am very thankful for being connected to many resources."

Concerned about a metatarsal fracture, a possible concurrent injury to the adjacent ligament complex and PTSD, you coordinate with social worker for an x-ray of the patient's foot, an appointment with orthopedics for evaluation, possible physical therapy, and a mental health evaluation.

Discussion questions
1. How did the trafficker try to keep Carlos in "bondage"?
2. What other possible legal outcomes could Carlos have faced prior to meeting the attorney?
3. What experiences qualify Carlos for T-visa?

Continued Presence

Federal law enforcement officials can petition the Department of Homeland Security to grant trafficking victims continued presence in the United States if the victim's presence is necessary for prosecutorial efforts [96]. Continued presence is a temporary form of relief. Persons receiving continued presence may remain only so long as the Attorney General determines that his or her presence within the United States is necessary. This status cannot be adjusted to permanent residency in the United States [97].

T-visa

Alternatively, victims of severe forms of trafficking can self-petition for a T-visa. Persons with T-visas may apply for permanent residency after a period of 3 years or when the criminal case is closed [98]. To be eligible for a T-visa, an adult trafficked person must

- Be a victim of a severe form of trafficking in persons
- Be physically present in the United States or at a port of entry
- Have complied with any reasonable request for assistance in the investigation or prosecution of acts of trafficking
- Suffer extreme hardship involving unusual and severe harm if removed [99]

Victims of trafficking who have not attained 18 years of age are not required to comply with requests for assistance in the investigation or prosecution of acts of trafficking [100].

Reunification of Family Members/Repatriation

Trafficked persons, when applying for a T-visa or after a T-visa has been granted, may file immigration petitions for their immediate families – spouses and children – to join them in the United States. In the case of victims under 21 years of age, the parents of the victim and any unmarried siblings under 18 are also eligible to come to the United States or receive status in the United States if they are already present [101]. The US government funds the IOM to provide specialized services for trafficking victims seeking to reunite with their family members or to return to their home country if they do not want to remain in the United States [102]. Especially important for child victims is that the IOM can offer support for family members in their home country applying for passports and visas necessary to enter the United States. Also, after a visa is granted, the IOM can help with payment for airline tickets and coordinating the sometimes-complex needs of families seeking to reunify. To apply for this support or learn more about these services, contact TIPDC@iom.int. At the time of this writing, federal policies related to refugee status, asylum, T-visas, and related immigration policies are in flux, creating added uncertainty about the resources and supports available to foreign nationals, including those who have been trafficked.

Accessing Medical Care in the United States

Refugees who are resettled to the United States qualify for immediate short-term health insurance called Refugee Medical Assistance (RMA), available for up to 8 months. Some refugees also have access to Medicaid, the Children's Health Insurance Program (CHIP), and the health coverage options available under the Affordable Care Act (ACA). Other groups eligible for the same benefits and services are: (1) asylees, (2) Cuban and Haitian entrants, (3) Amerasians, (4) special immigrant visa holders from Iraq and Afghanistan, (5) Lawful Permanent Residents, and (6) certified victims of human trafficking [103].

Foreign national adult victims of severe human trafficking become certified through the US DHHS once their T-Visa or continued presence status has been approved. Under the TVPA, individuals with a Certification Letter become eligible to apply for the same benefits and services as refugees (e.g., RMA, Medicaid, CHIP, Food Assistance, Refugee Cash Assistance, Match Grant) [104]. Foreign-born minors are eligible for the same benefits and services with few variants. For minor victims, it is not required that they wait for the legal status to be approved to apply for these services. Agencies who assist minor victims may contact the Office on Trafficking In Persons (OTIP) Child Protection Specialist via email at childtrafficking@acf.hhs.gov to discuss a case and be guided on how to submit a Request Assistance for a Foreign Child Victim form (RFA). It is recommended that OTIP be contacted within 24 hours of a child victim identification. OTIP will first issue an Interim Assistance Letter and later an Eligibility Letter (the equivalent of a Certification Letter for adults) [104].

Victims of labor trafficking may experience significant illnesses, work injuries, and physical abuses that require access to health care for diagnosis and treatment. Many may be under-vaccinated, have chronic malnutrition, or be carrying chronic infections or other diseases [105, 106]. Individuals without medical health coverage through DHHS or public health insurance can take quite some time to enroll in health coverage. Therefore, when possible, victims should be referred to free clinics that will treat them while uninsured. Victims also may need to access therapy services in the aftermath of exploitation and trafficking. It is critically important that mental health service professionals be trained and experienced in working with trafficking victims and persons with severe trauma. [See Chap. 9.] They should be culturally sensitive with appropriate access to professional interpretation services. Healthcare professionals should be well aware that health insurance and a lack of local clinicians are two leading barriers to most trafficking survivors receiving the immediate care they need. A more complete description of medical care recommendations can be found in the section above "Labor Trafficking – A Review".

References

Labor Trafficking – A Review

1. Department of Justice U.S. Attorney's Office Northern District of Ohio. Ashland woman sentenced to nearly four years in prison in forced-labor case [Internet]. 2014 [cited 2019 Oct 4]. Available from: https://www.justice.gov/usao-ndoh/pr/ashland-woman-sentenced-nearly-four-years-prison-forced-labor-case.
2. Department of Justice U.S. Attorney's Office Northern District of Ohio. Three Ashland residents arrested for human trafficking [Internet]. 2013 [cited 2019 Oct 4]. Available from: https://www.justice.gov/usao-ndoh/pr/three-ashland-residents-arrested-human-trafficking.
3. Guidance to states and services on addressing human trafficking of children and youth in the United States. Washington, D.C.: U.S. Department of Health and Human Services, Administration for Children, Youth and Families; 2013.
4. Gallop JD. Police say 24 children rescued from human trafficking scheme [Internet]. Florida Today. 2013 [cited 2019 Oct 4]. Available from: https://www.floridatoday.com/story/news/local/2013/10/29/police-say-24-children-rescued-from-human-trafficking-scheme-two/77199404/.
5. Pierce M. Human trafficking may have knocked at your door. [Internet]. The Denver Voice. 2009 [cited 2019 Oct 4]. Available from: https://www.denvervoice.org/archive/2009/11/1/freature-magazine-crew-human-trafficking-may-have-knocked-at.html.
6. Child trafficking for labor in the United States: overview. Freedom Network; 2011.
7. Serna J. L.A. girl kept in metal box on pot farm for sex [Internet]. LA Times. 2013 [cited 2019 Oct 4]. Available from: https://www.latimes.com/local/lanow/la-me-ln-lake-county-pot-farm-arrest-20130726-story.html.
8. Severe forms of trafficking in persons. 22 U.S.C. § 7102(11).
9. Polaris Project. 2013 analysis of state and human trafficking laws.
10. Debt bondage & involuntary servitude. 22 U.S.C. § 7102(7&8).
11. Coercion. 22 U.S.C. § 7102(3).
12. Forced labor. 18 U.S. Code § 1589.
13. U.S. Department of Labor. Youth & labor [Internet]. [cited 2019 Oct 4]. Available from: https://www.dol.gov/general/topic/youthlabor.
14. Polaris Project. The typology of modern slavery [Internet]. 2017 [cited 2019 Oct 3]. Available from: https://polarisproject.org/sites/default/files/Polaris-Typology-of-Modern-Slavery.pdf.

15. Desai N, Tepfer S. Proactive case identification strategies and the challenges of initiating labor trafficking cases. U.S. Attorney's Bill 25. [Internet]. 2013 [cited 2019 Oct 4]. Available from: https://heinonline.org/HOL/Page?handle=hein.journals/usab65&div=77&g_sent=1&casa_token=&collection=journals.
16. Ataiants J, Cohen C, Riley AH, Tellez Lieberman J, Reidy MC, Chilton M. Unaccompanied children at the United States border, a human rights crisis that can be addressed with policy change. J Immigr Minor Health. 2018;20:1000–10.
17. Murphy LT. Labor and sex trafficking among homeless youth: a ten city study. Modern Slavery Research Project: New Orleans, LA; 2017.
18. Yates GL, Mackenzie RG, Pennbridge J, Swofford A. A risk profile comparison of homeless youth involved in prostitution and homeless youth not involved. J Adolesc Health. 1991;12:545–8.
19. Lederer LJ, Wetzel CA. The health consequences of sex trafficking and their implications for identifying victims in healthcare facilities. Ann Health Law. 2014;23
20. Chisolm-Straker M, Baldwin S, Gaïgbé-Togbé B, Ndukwe N, Johnson PN, Richardson LD. Health care and human trafficking: we are seeing the unseen. J Health Care Poor Underserved. 2016;27:1220–33.
21. Ottisova L, Hemmings S, Howard LM, Zimmerman C, Oram S. Prevalence and risk of violence and the mental, physical and sexual health problems associated with human trafficking: an updated systematic review. Epidemiol Psychiatr Sci. 2016;25:317–41.
22. Varma S, Gillespie S, McCracken C, Greenbaum VJ. Characteristics of child commercial sexual exploitation and sex trafficking victims presenting for medical care in the United States. Child Abuse Negl. 2015;44:98–105.
23. Goldberg AP, Moore JL, Houck C, Kaplan DM, Barron CE. Domestic minor sex trafficking patients: a retrospective analysis of medical presentation. J Pediatr Adolesc Gynecol. 2017;30:109–15.
24. Stanley N, Oram S, Jakobowitz S, Westwood J, Borschmann R, Zimmerman C, et al. The health needs and healthcare experiences of young people trafficked into the UK. Child Abuse Negl. 2016;59:100–10.
25. Greenbaum J, Crawford-Jakubiak JE, Committee on Child Abuse and Neglect. Child sex trafficking and commercial sexual exploitation: health care needs of victims. Pediatrics. 2015;135:566–74.
26. Greenbaum J, Bodrick N, Committee on Child Abuse and Neglect, Section on International Child Health. Global human trafficking and child victimization. Pediatrics. 2017;140
27. American Academy of Pediatrics. In: Kimberlin DW, Brady MT, Jackson MA, Long SS, editors. Summaries of infectious diseases, Red book: 2015 report of the committee on infectious diseases. 30th ed. Elk Grove Village, IL; 2015. p. 288–800.
28. US Preventive Services Task Force. Published recommendations [Internet]. 2018 [cited 2019 Oct 4]. Available from: https://www.uspreventiveservicestaskforce.org/BrowseRec/Index/browse-recommendations.
29. World Health Organization. Refugee and migrant health [Internet]. 2019 [cited 2019 Oct 4]. Available from: https://www.who.int/migrants/en/.
30. Greenbaum J. Introduction to human trafficking: who is affected? In: Chisolm-Straker M, Stoklosa H, editors. Human trafficking is a public health issue: a paradigm expansion in the United States. Cham: Springer; 2017. p. 1–14.
31. SAMHSA's concept of trauma and guidance for a trauma-informed approach; 2014.
32. The American Academy of Pediatrics and Bright Futures. 2017 recommendations for preventive pediatric health care. Pediatrics. 2017;139
33. Kitroeff N. Stockholm syndrome in the pimp-victim relationship [Internet]. The New York Times. 2012 [cited 2019 Oct 4]. Available from: https://kristof.blogs.nytimes.com/2012/05/03/stockholm-syndrome-in-the-pimp-victim-relationship/.
34. Saada Saar M. There is no such thing as a child prostitute [Internet]. The Washington Post. 2014 [cited 2019 Oct 4]. Available from: https://www.washingtonpost.com/opinions/there-is-no-such-thing-as-a-child-prostitute/2014/02/14/631ebd26-8ec7-11e3-b227-12a45d109e03_story.html.

35. van der Kolk BA. The compulsion to repeat the trauma. Re-enactment, revictimization, and masochism. Psychiatr Clin North Am. 1989;12:389–411.
36. Futures Without Violence Futures Without Violence. Hanging out or hooking up: teen safety card [Internet]. [cited 2019 Oct 4]. Available from: https://www.futureswithoutviolence.org/hanging-out-or-hooking-up-teen-safety-card/.
37. WestCoast Children's Clinic. You can't stop something you don't see.
38. Leitch L, Snow M. Intervene: practitioner guide and intake tool. Arlington, VA: Shared Hope International; 2013.
39. Chang K. Using a clinic-based screening tool for primary care providers to identify commercially sexually exploited children. J Appl Res Child. 2015;6
40. San Luis Obispo County. San Luis Obispo County CSEC Collaborative Response Team Commercially Sexually Exploited Children (CSEC) Screening Tool [Internet]. [cited 2016 Feb 4]. Available from: http://www.slocounty.ca.gov/Assets/DSS/Flyers/DSS800CSEC.pdf.
41. Mays A, Harvill Z, Mejia J. Sexually exploited children screening protocol: a multidisciplinary model designed for the clinical and school health setting. Oakland, CA: The Native American Health Center; 2013.
42. Dank M. Pretesting a human trafficking screening tool in the child welfare and runaway and homeless youth systems: Urban Institute; 2017.
43. Chisolm-Straker M, Sze J, Einbond J, White J, Stoklosa H. Screening for human trafficking among homeless young adults. Child Youth Serv Rev. 2019;98:72–9.
44. Baldwin SB, Fehrenbacher AE, Eisenman DP. Psychological coercion in human trafficking: an application of biderman's framework. Qual Health Res. 2015;25:1171–81.

Labor Trafficking – Forced Criminality

45. Gibbs DA, Hardison Walters JL, Lutnick A, Miller S, Kluckman M. Services to domestic minor victims of sex trafficking: opportunities for engagement and support. Child Youth Serv Rev. 2015;54:1–7.
46. RACE. Trafficking for forced criminal activities and begging in Europe: exploratorystudy and good practice examples. Report [Internet]. 2014 [cited 2019 Sep 26]; Available from: http://www.antislavery.org/wp-content/uploads/2017/01/trafficking_for_forced_criminal_activities_and_begging_in_europe.pdf.
47. Villacampa C, Torres N. Human trafficking for criminal exploitation: the failure to identify victims. Eur J Crim Pol Res. 2017;23:393–408.
48. The Department of State Office to Monitor and Combat Trafficking in Persons. The use of forced criminality: victims hidden behind the crime. 2016 [cited 2019 Sep 26]; Available from: Available at https://2009-2017.state.gov/documents/organization/233938.pdf.
49. Castillo R. Vacatur laws: decriminalizing sex trafficking survivors. Am Univ J Gend Soc Policy Law [Internet]. 2016 [cited 2019 Sep 26]; Available from: http://www.jgspl.org/vacatur-laws-decriminalizing-sex-trafficking-survivors/.
50. Vacatur & Expungement Database [Internet]. Vacatur & Expungement Database. [cited 2019 Sep 26]. Available from: https://sites.google.com/a/htprobono.org/vsdatabase/
51. TheTypology of Modern Slavery. [Internet]. [cited 2019 Sep 26]. Available from: https://polarisproject.org/typology.
52. Department of Health and Human Services. Labor Trafficking Fact Sheet.
53. Beasley E. Overlooking men and boys in forced criminality at the border: a content analysis of human trafficking training and awareness materials. Master's Theses; 2018, p. 1077.
54. Farrell A, Pfeffer R. Policing human trafficking: cultural blinders and organizational barriers. Ann Am Acad Pol Soc Sci. 2014;653:46–64.
55. Myths & Facts. [Internet]. National human trafficking hotline. [cited 2019 Sep 26]. Available from: https://humantraffickinghotline.org/what-human-trafficking/myths-misconceptions.
56. Chisolm-Straker M, Sze J, Einbond J, White J, Stoklosa H. Screening for human trafficking among homeless young adults. Child Youth Serv Rev. 2019;98:72–9.

57. Chisolm-Straker M, Singer E, Sze J, Rothman E. Universal screening for trafficking in the emergency department: RAFT development and validation. [under review, personal communication].
58. Chisolm-Straker M, Sze J, Einbond J, White J, Stoklosa H. A supportive adult may be the difference in homeless youth not being trafficked. Child Youth Serv Rev. 2018;91:115–20.
59. Complex Trauma [Internet]. [cited 2019 Sep 26]. Available from: https://www.nctsn.org/what-is-child-trauma/trauma-types/complex-trauma
60. Ginsburg Z, Kinsman S. Trauma informed practice: working with youth who have suffered adverse childhood (or adolescent) experiences. Reaching Teens. 2014;22:180.
61. Simich L, Goyen L, Powell A, Mallozzi K. Improving human trafficking victim identification: validation and dissemination of a screening tool: VERA Institute of Justice; 2014.
62. Bigelsen J, Vuotto S, Addison K, Trongone S, Tully K. Homelessness, survival sex, and human trafficking: as experienced by the youth of covenant house New York. Unknown. 2013;
63. Burke Harris N, Renschler T. Center for Youth Wellness ACE-Questionnaire (CYW ACE-Q Child, Teen, Teen SR). San Francisco, CA: Center for Youth Wellness; 2015.
64. Felitti VJ, Anda RF, Nordenberg D, Williamson DF, Spitz AM, Edwards V, et al. Relationship of childhood abuse and household dysfunction to many of the leading causes of death in adults. The Adverse Childhood Experiences (ACE) Study. Am J Prev Med. 1998;14:245–58.
65. Centers for Disease Control and Prevention. Behavioral risk factor surveillance system survey ACE module data, 2010. Centers for Disease Control and Prevention: Atlanta, GA: US Department of Health …, 2015; 2015.
66. Council on Community Pediatrics. Providing care for children and adolescents facing homelessness and housing insecurity. Pediatrics. 2013;131:1206–10.
67. Shonkoff J, Levitt P, Bunge S, Cameron J, Duncan G. Supportive relationships and active skill-building strengthen the foundations of resilience: Working Paper 13. Working Paper No. 13. 2015;
68. Substance Abuse and Mental Health Services Administration. SAMHSA's concept of trauma and guidance for a trauma-informed approach [Internet]. Rockville, MD: Substance Abuse and Mental Health Services Administration; 2014. Report No.: HHS Publication No. (SMA) 14–4884. Available from: https://store.samhsa.gov/system/files/sma14-4884.pdf.
69. Clawson HJ, Dutch N. Addressing the needs of victims of human trafficking: challenges, barriers, and promising practices. humantraffickinghotline.org; 2008.
70. Desai RA, Goulet JL, Robbins J, Chapman JF, Migdole SJ, Hoge MA. Mental health care in juvenile detention facilities: a review. J Am Acad Psychiatry Law. 2006;34:204–14.

Labor Trafficking – Vulnerability of Immigrant and Refugee Youth

71. Definition of Terms. US Department of Homeland Security. 2018 [cited 2019 May 13]. Available from: https://www.dhs.gov/immigration-statistics/data-standards-and-definitions/definition-terms.
72. United Nations, Department of Economic and Social Affairs. Population Division (2017). Trends in international migrant stock: the 2017 revision (United Nations database, POP/DB/MIG/Stock/Rev.2017).
73. United States. Department of Homeland Security. Yearbook of immigration statistics: 2016. U.S. Department of Homeland Security, Office of Immigration Statistics: Washington, D.C; 2017.
74. 2017 Statistics from the National Human Trafficking Hotline and BeFree Textline. Polaris Project. 2017 [cited 2019 May 13]. Available from: http://polarisproject.org/sites/default/files/2017NHTHStats%20%281%29.pdf.
75. UNODC, Global Report on Trafficking in Persons 2018 (United Nations publication, Sales No. E.19.IV.2).

76. Shetty S. Most dangerous journey: what central American migrants face when they try to cross the border. Amnesty International. [cited 2019 May 13]. Available from: https://www.amnestyusa.org/most-dangerous-journey-what-central-american-migrants-face-when-they-try-to-cross-the-border/.
77. Smuggling of Migrants: the Harsh Search for a Better Life. United Nations Office on Drugs and Crime. [cited 2019 May 13]. Available from: https://www.unodc.org/toc/en/crimes/migrant-smuggling.html.
78. Human Trafficking on Temporary Work Visas, A data analysis 2015–2017. Polaris Project. [cited 2019 May 13]. Available from: https://polarisproject.org/sites/default/files/Polaris%20Temporary%20Work%20Visa%20Report.pdf.
79. This Land is Your Land. UNHCR USA. [cited 2019 May 13]. Available from: https://www.unhcr.org/en-us/this-land-is-your-land.html.
80. Global Trends: Forced Displacement in 2017. UNHCR The UN Refugee Agency. 2017 [cited 2019 May 13]. Available from: https://www.unhcr.org/5b27be547.
81. Security Screening of Refugees Admitted to the U.S – US Resettlement Security Screening Process. U.S. Committee for Refugee and Immigrants. [cited 2019 May 13]. Available from: https://refugees.org/explore-the-issues/our-work-with-refugees/security-screening/.
82. Human Trafficking & Migrant Smuggling: Understanding the Difference. Office of monitor and combat trafficking in persons. U.S. Department of State. 2017 [cited 2019 May 13]. Available from: https://www.state.gov/wp-content/uploads/2019/02/272325.pdf.
83. Smuggling of Migrants. Migration data portal: the bigger picture. 2018 [cited 2019 May 13]. Available from: https://migrationdataportal.org/themes/smuggling-migrants.
84. Wilson AP. Trafficking risks for refugees. 2011. Third annual interdisciplinary conference on human trafficking; 2011 [cited 2019 May 13]. Available from: http://digitalcommons.unl.edu/humtraffconf3/4.
85. Lustig SL, Kia-Keating M, Grant-Knight W, Geltman P, Ellis Heidi, Birman D, Kinzie D, Keane T, Saxe GN. Review of child and adolescent refugee mental health. National child traumatic stress network: refugee trauma task force. White Paper Committee. 2003. Boston, MA [cited 2019 May 13]. Available from: https://www.nctsn.org/sites/default/files/resources//review_child_adolescent_refugee_mental_health.pdf.
86. Human Trafficking Power Control Wheel. Polaris Project. 2010 [cited 2019 May 13]. Available from: https://www.acesdv.org/wp-content/uploads/2014/06/Human-Trafficking-PowerControl-Wheel.pdf.
87. About Unaccompanied Refugee Minors. Office of Refugee Resettlement, State Letter #01–13: The Trafficking Victims Protection Act of 2000, 2001 [cited 2019 May 13]. Available from: https://www.acf.hhs.gov/orr/programs/urm/about.
88. Unaccompanied Alien Children. Office of Refugee Resettlement [cited 2019 May 13]. Available from: https://www.acf.hhs.gov/orr/programs/ucs.
89. Victims of Trafficking and Violence Protection Act of 2000, Public Law No. 106–386, §§ 101–11; Trafficking Victims Protection Reauthorization Act of 2003, Public Lazw No. 108–193.
90. Protection and Assistance for Victims of Trafficking 2001 Public Law No. 22 U.S.C. § 7105(b)(1)(A). Available from: http://uscode.house.gov/view.xhtml?req=granuleid:USC-2000-title22-section7105&num=0&edition=2000.
91. Protection and Assistance for Victims of Trafficking 2001 Public Law No. 22 U.S.C. § 7105. Available from: http://uscode.house.gov/view.xhtml?req=granuleid:USC-2000-title22-section7105&num=0&edition=2000.
92. Fact Sheet: Assistance for Child Victims of Human Trafficking. Office of Trafficking in Persons. 2016 [cited 2019 May 13]. Available from: https://www.acf.hhs.gov/otip/resource/eligibilityfs.
93. Monthly Webinars: Responding to Child Victims of Trafficking. Office of Trafficking in Persons. 2018 [cited 2019 May 13]. Available from: https://www.acf.hhs.gov/otip/resource/monthlywebinars.

94. For a review of the services offered to child victims of trafficking in the federal system see: Child Victims of Human Trafficking: Outcomes and Service Adaptation within the U.S. UnaccomApanied Refugee Minor Programs. 2015 [cited 2019 May 13]. Available from: http://www.usccb.org/about/anti-trafficking-program/upload/URM-Child-Trafficking-Study-2015-Final.pdf.
95. Richard, S. Kim CM, Gonzalez E. T-nonimmigrant visas and adjustment of status for victims of human trafficking: a practical guide to the relevant statutory changes and updated regulations. Thomas Reuter Immigration Briefings. 2017 [cited 2019 May 13]. Available from: https://www.castla.org/wp-content/themes/castla/assets/files/reutgers-immigration-stephanie-richardIB-aug2017-08-17-final.pdf.
96. Protection and Assistance for Victims of Trafficking 2001 Public Law No. 22 U.S.C. § 7105(c)(3). [cited 2019 May 13]. Available from: http://uscode.house.gov/view.xhtml?req=granuleid:USC-2000-title22-section7105&num=0&edition=2000.
97. Protection and Assistance for Victims of Trafficking 2001 Public Law No. 22 U.S.C. § 7105(b)(1)(E)(ii). [cited 2019 May 13]. Available from: http://uscode.house.gov/view.xhtml?req=granuleid:USC-2000-title22-section7105&num=0&edition=2000.
98. Adjustment of Status of Nonimmigrant to that of Person Admitted for Permanent Residence 2012 Public Law No 8 U.S.C. § 1255(l). [cited 2019 May 13]. Available from: https://www.govinfo.gov/app/details/USCODE-2011-title8/USCODE-2011-title8-chap12-subchapII-partV-sec1255.
99. Definitions 2015 Public Law No. 8 U.S.C. § 1101(a)(15)(T). [cited 2019 May 13]. Available from: https://www.govinfo.gov/content/pkg/USCODE-2015-title8/html/USCODE-2015-title8-chap12-subchapII-partIX-sec1367.htm.
100. Definitions 2015 Public Law No. 8 U.S.C. § 1101(a)(15)(T)(i)(III). [cited 2019 May 13]. Available from: https://www.govinfo.gov/content/pkg/USCODE-2015-title8/html/USCODE-2015-title8-chap12-subchapII-partIX-sec1367.htm.
101. Definitions 2015 Public Law No. 8 U.S.C. § 1101(a)(15)(T)(ii). [cited 2019 May 13]. Available from: https://www.govinfo.gov/content/pkg/USCODE-2015-title8/html/USCODE-2015-title8-chap12-subchapII-partIX-sec1367.htm.
102. Darlington E. Return, reintegration and family reunification-condensed version. IOM Prezi. 2015 [cited 2019 April]. Available from: https://prezi.com/tnorijio9zwx/return.
103. Health Insurance. Office of refugee resettlement. 2019 [cited 2019 May 13]. Available from: https://www.acf.hhs.gov/orr/health.
104. Eligibility Letters. Office on trafficking in persons. [cited 2019 May 13]. Available from: https://www.acf.hhs.gov/otip/victim-assistance/eligibility-letters.
105. The American Academy of Pediatrics and Bright Futures. Recommendations for preventive pediatric health care. American Academy of Pediatrics; 2017.
106. U.S. Preventive Services Task Force. Published recommendations. USPSTF, Maryland, USA, updated January 2018 [cited 2019 May 13]. Available at https://www.uspreventiveservicestaskforce.org/BrowseRec/Index/browse-recommendations.

Chapter 6
Technology/Sexting/Social Media

Jessica Whitney, Sofya Maslyanskaya, and Marisa Hultgren

Introduction

Human connection… From the day we are born, we possess an innate need for a sense of belonging and love. Human traffickers in their recruitment efforts exploit vulnerabilities that come from feeling a lack of belonging and love, using these vulnerabilities to build trust and loyalty between themselves and their victims. In this new digital age, perpetrators of trafficking have access to information that helps them target individuals who display signs of vulnerability and then foster a relationship with them. This abundance of information has accompanied an exponential growth of technology, particularly among today's youth, and has dramatically changed the way we interact with each other. For many, it has altered the way we express ourselves, communicate, and share our life stories. This in turn has provided traffickers with a plethora of information at their fingertips that can be used to facilitate illicit activities. It is critical to understand the role technology plays in cases of human trafficking. The ability to identify these digital indicators is a critical component in how we can help protect children, adolescents, and young adults from being exploited. The following case study provides an illustration of the connections between technology and the world of sex trafficking specifically. Cues present in this patient's medical and social history as well as in the physical examination demonstrate why the clinician caring for this patient should be concerned that the patient is at high risk for being exploited. This story serves as a starting point to improve recognition of signs of human trafficking among young people seeking care and to aid in counter-trafficking efforts.

J. Whitney (✉) · M. Hultgren
San Diego State University, San Diego, CA, USA

S. Maslyanskaya
Department of Pediatrics, Children's Hospital at Montefiore, Bronx, NY, USA

K. E. Titchen, E. Miller (eds.), *Medical Perspectives on Human Trafficking in Adolescents*, https://doi.org/10.1007/978-3-030-43367-3_6

Case Presentation

Abby is a 15-year-old young girl who comes into your clinic requesting a comprehensive evaluation for sexually transmitted infections (STIs). You are the health care professional seeing Abby for the first time. She is here with a supervisor from the group home where she resides. Abby has been living in the group home for the last year after being removed from her mother's care by child protective services because of neglect by her mother. Her mother is currently living in a substance use residential treatment facility. Abby has recently returned to the group home after running away for 3 days. According to the group home supervisor, Abby runs away weekly and declines to disclose where she stays when she leaves the group home. The supervisor reports that adolescents in the group home tell her that Abby frequently posts angry messages about her mother on Facebook and Instagram and that Abby has a boyfriend.

During time alone in this clinical encounter, Abby declines to explain where she goes when she runs away from the group home, as this is not related to her need for STI testing. She declines to answer how many sexual partners she has had. She reports that she does not have friends and that she met her boyfriend online. She declines disclosing any information about his age but says that he takes good care of her. She reports daily marijuana use and alcohol use when she is with her boyfriend. She does not want to discuss her mood. In her chart, you are able to see that this is her fifth visit in the last 3 months for STI testing, and she has been treated for chlamydia and gonorrhea twice. You also note two emergency department visits for injuries related to fighting and for a suicide attempt.

On physical examination, her vital signs are within normal limits. Abby is sitting in a chair playing on her cell phone and you see another cell phone charging in a socket in the exam room. When asked about the phones, Abby reports that her boyfriend bought her the new model of the cell phone last week and she likes to have both phones with her. Abby is wearing a new pair of popular sneakers. Examinations of the heart, lungs and abdomen are within normal limits. Skin exam is notable for superficial healed linear lacerations on inner distal arms bilaterally. During the review of systems, Abby reports symptoms of intermittent dysuria. You explain to Abby that a comprehensive genitourinary examination is advisable based on this history and would include a speculum and a bimanual examination. Abby agrees to the pelvic examination. Pubic hair is shaved in Tanner stage 5 distribution with no vulvar lesions. On pelvic exam, there is yellow vaginal discharge from the cervical os with no cervical or adnexal tenderness noted. Microscopic exam of her discharge reveals multiple white cells and an elevated pH. Urine hCG (human chorionic gonadotropin) test is negative for pregnancy.

Based on Abby's history and presentation, you consider the possibility of sexual exploitation and offer comprehensive testing for STI, including chlamydia, gonorrhea, trichomoniasis, human immunodeficiency virus (HIV), syphilis, hepatitis B, and hepatitis C. You decide to treat her presumptively for sexually transmitted infections that could cause abnormal vaginal discharge. You order 250 mg of Ceftriaxone as an intramuscular injection and oral administration of 1 gram of azithromycin and 2 grams of metronidazole.

You are concerned about Abby being at high risk for becoming pregnant (she is not using any contraception) and contracting STIs. You review with Abby contraceptive options that you could provide for pregnancy prevention focusing on longer acting reversible contraceptives including intrauterine devices and contraceptive implants. You also review and provide a prescription for emergency contraception and advise Abby that she could use it within 5 days of sexual activity. You also provide Abby with information on HIV pre-exposure prophylaxis (PrEP). HIV PrEP is a medication that needs to be taken daily with initial monthly monitoring of side effects [1]. You explain to Abby that if she is interested in this type of preventive care, you would like to see her come back in 1 week, after her HIV and Hepatitis B test results are back and once you check her kidney function tests. You further advise her that she will need to come back in 1 month and then quarterly to monitor medication use, HIV status, and kidney function.

Discussion and Case Evaluation

When evaluating a patient, it is important to take note of the presence of indicators of human trafficking that involve the use of technology and social media. The more indicators present, the greater the potential that the patient is being trafficked. Abby's case depicts three major indicators:

1. The interview with Abby's group home supervisor suggests that the patient displays vulnerability over social media, specifically the conflict with her mother and perhaps even sharing about her living in a residential facility. This digital footprint potentially provides traffickers with access to information that makes her an appealing potential victim to target.
2. Abby's explanation of how she met her boyfriend and her relationship with him illustrates a popular online recruitment technique used by traffickers, the "Romeo" scenario which will be described below.
3. The fact that the patient has two phones in her possession is concerning since traffickers often gift phones as a way to monitor victims, facilitate buyer solicitation, and avoid detection by law enforcement.

In this chapter, we discuss how to recognize each of these indicators, provide some background on the uses of technology by traffickers, and explain how and why these technologies are being used in relation to human trafficking. As you continue through the chapter, think about the three indicators identified above and how they relate to the discussion that follows.

Social Media Use in Human Trafficking Defined

Historically the concept of social media has been defined as "an environment in which information was passed from one person to another along social connections to create a distributed discussion or community" [2]. Today when most people think of social media, they picture the online social networking platforms and applications society uses to post and share content as well as communicate with each other through instant messaging and other chat features. These social media platforms, such as Facebook, Instagram, YouTube, TikTok, and Snapchat, are causing a huge cultural shift and dramatically changing the way teens and young adults communicate. They provide a plethora of opportunities for today's youth to build connections and share their accomplishments, interests, and so much more.

Despite the many positives of social media communication, it has a dark side. This dark side comes not only from the perspective of facilitating criminal activity, such as traffickers' use of backpage.com and dating "apps" (mobile phone applications) to solicit purchasers of sex, but also from the fact that it provides traffickers with a whole new victim pool. Social media has become an integral part of the way adolescents build social connections and express themselves, and developmentally as youth seek to define their identities, they may share many details about their lives. As they become more and more comfortable with posting about their personal experiences, and especially demonstrate their vulnerability, young people increase the chances of being found by traffickers. This stems from the fact that in many cases social media allows for easy access to this personal information and facilitates traffickers' ability to communicate with and groom their victims. The content posted online allows traffickers to identify vulnerabilities that they can later use to help them build a connection with their victims during the recruitment process [3].

Social Media and Emotional Vulnerability

The relationship between social media and emotional vulnerability brings us to the first major technological indicator of trafficking demonstrated in Abby's case. Her case highlights a potential opportunity where traffickers may use content posted on social media to their advantage. When interviewed, the patient's group home supervisor disclosed that the patient frequently posts angry messages about her mother online. We cannot discern with any level of certainty whether or not the trafficker in this case used the content the patient posted on social media during the recruitment process. However, highlighting the circumstances in this patient's case as they pertain to human trafficking is meant to serve as an example of technology-related indicators to look for when a patient displays symptoms that may be indicative of human trafficking. Patients like Abby who have poor relationships with their families or have been removed from their home by child protective services and placed in a group home are considered high risk for being trafficked. Traffickers look for vulnerable youth who often post on social media about running away from home and anger they feel toward their families. They can use to their advantage the feelings of loneliness and isolation that many adolescents with a difficult home life experience. Patients rarely share with caregivers what they are posting about themselves online; in this case, the group home supervisor shares with the health care professional information about Abby's running away and the emotionally charged social media posts. When cautioning young people about posting online, it may be helpful to note that there are too many people who are searching the Internet to take advantage of young people who are angry or alone. You might ask, "What strategies do you use for yourself or for your friends to keep what you post online private?"

Emotionally vulnerable adolescents with free access to the Internet and no proper guidance or supervision are particularly susceptible to human trafficking. Although victims of trafficking have a variety of things in common, the most pernicious catalyst into a life of human trafficking is emotional vulnerability [4]. Victims of emotional, physical, and/or sexual abuse present the most compelling target for traffickers. The vulnerability of a child who falls under the above parameters is exacerbated by an unrestricted or unmonitored use of social media. Abby's case is the perfect example of an emotionally vulnerable adolescent who has free access to the Internet with little to no guidance on how to participate safely in an online community. As the market for social media increases among adolescents, the problem is worsening. Social media companies have been known to reduce restrictions and safety precautions to retain their younger audience from moving to other online platforms [5]. This, together with the fact that traffickers often pretend to be minors, creates a fertile environment for online trafficking [6]. To detect potential victims, it is vital that healthcare workers are well informed about the connection between emotionally vulnerable youth, unrestricted internet access, and human trafficking.

Social Media and Online Relationships

This discussion on the exploitation of emotional vulnerability by traffickers leads to the second main trafficking indicator present in Abby's case, the "Romeo" scenario. The "Romeo" scenario, as it is often referred to by law enforcement, is one of the most common recruitment approaches and involves traffickers creating the appearance of a romantic relationship so that their victim will develop an emotional attachment to them. In this scenario, traffickers use social media as a tool to build a victim's trust by fostering what starts out as a loving, intimate relationship [7]. With this method of recruitment, also known as the "lover-boy tactic," the trafficker appeals to the victim's desire for affection using the facade of a boyfriend/girlfriend relationship to build trust and later exploit them for sex [8]. Unlike other methods of exploitation online, these traffickers rarely hide their age from the victim [9].

Since this recruitment method is so common, the next step is to ask ourselves how this relates to evaluating a patient's case for potential signs of sexual exploitation and deciding a course of action. While asking questions about partners, take note of patients who decline to answer questions about their partner's age (if asked) or who report being taken care of financially by a partner they met over the Internet. Additional attention should be paid to patients who also frequently come in for pregnancy testing or STI testing to assess their risk for STI acquisition. Another course of action may involve asking questions or reviewing intake questionnaires that can shed light onto whether or not the patient is experiencing any feelings of loss, depression, anger, or lack of affection. If so, is the patient willing to share additional information on how and to whom they have expressed these feelings, and do their answers suggest that they have posted about them online? In these cases, it may be worthwhile to try to ascertain if there is an older "boyfriend" (or intimate partner) who has been there for them and provided emotional support. Even if there is no disclosure, it may be appropriate to consider a referral to behavioral health services if there are any mental health symptoms, including poor sleep or irritability. Providing mental health professionals with the opportunity to introduce patients to the dangers of using the internet and social media as an outlet for their feelings is a major step toward preventing trafficking.

Social Media and Privacy

Knowing that traffickers use social media technologies to their advantage and understanding how digital information is being used to facilitate underage human trafficking is only the beginning. Cybersecurity professionals often refer to the use of information to exploit vulnerabilities as social engineering, "a method of attack involving the exploitation of human weakness, gullibility, and ignorance." [10] This definition is synonymous with the way traffickers take advantage of social media. They use it to identify vulnerable adolescents and then exploit their weaknesses to build connections with them through online communication that draw them into the world of underage human trafficking. From a technological perspective, cybersecurity is all about evaluating the vulnerabilities that cybercriminals target and determining ways to address and protect against them. A similar approach can be taken to combat the use of social media as a facilitator of human trafficking. We have discussed the "vulnerabilities" by examining the connections between social media and Abby's case: but even more important is understanding the concept of privacy in this new digital age and how to protect ourselves online.

Our digital footprint is everywhere, and understanding where all these data come from and how one can protect oneself against those who wish to use these data in harmful, criminal ways is key. Social media is one of the major culprits in cultivating what technology gurus refer to as "big data." At the time of this writing, two of the major social media platforms used by adolescents that are responsible for the collection of big data are Snapchat and Instagram. These social networking apps are primarily designed for sharing photos and videos with friends as well as for individual and group messaging. For many adolescents, social networking applications have become their primary mode of communication with each other. While this can be a good way to build social connections, there are also many concerns involved with the use of social media in this way. During interviews with survivors of human trafficking, researchers identified the significance of peer recruitment in the grooming process. Survivors spoke about how they themselves participated in the recruitment process by befriending other youth and drawing them into trafficking [11]. Due to the way adolescents communicate, it is likely that part of this ruse involves the two peers becoming friends on social media. This is often where the dark side of social media in relation to the recruitment process starts. Many youths have configured their social media privacy settings so that their profile is made visible to people who are classified as "friends of friends." This can provide teens with the opportunity to expand their social network, but it also leaves their information exposed. With this privacy setting configuration, traffickers can access a potential victim's profile as long as they have a social media account that is part of the recruiter's friend group. They can study the available information and use it as a tool to prepare for grooming their new potential victim. They can like her posts, comment and watch her story, and reach out to her by sending her personal messages. Teens who are desperate for attention that they are not getting from their family may latch onto this display of attention as a sign of affection. Traffickers go "fishing" for their next victims over social media and use these widely popular communication platforms to successfully reel them into trafficking.

It is not uncommon for adolescents to share additional information regarding their current location or places they frequent over these types of social media platforms. They may "check in" on Facebook, post to their "story" on Snapchat somewhere fun or exciting they are visiting, or share pictures through Instagram. Photo apps will conveniently organize digital content based on date and location. This is helpful, but it also introduces one of the big dangers involved with sharing content online: geolocation tagging. Frequently, unless steps are taken to turn off certain features for location services, some mobile devices will embed information about when and where a photo or video was taken into the photo itself. It may seem like retrieving this information out of the photos would be difficult, but publicly available web tools make it easy to find and extract this information. One can upload a photo to an open source web app such as Pic2Map or use Google's image search feature to retrieve its best guess on where the image was taken. While this feature may be nice when organizing hundreds of photos, it can also be used for collecting information about where, when, and how adolescents who may be more susceptible to recruitment efforts can be targeted.

This image tagging is only one of many vulnerabilities presented by the use of social media and mobile devices. Other examples include those handy smartphone notifications that communicate the best route and how long it will take to get to work, home, or a favorite morning coffee place based on current traffic conditions or that convenient list of the nearby restaurants that pops up when trying to decide what to get for dinner.

But we have to ask ourselves, what is it that allows us to search for "things near me?" The answer: the same location services feature that tracks the places we frequent to facilitate and create a log of our last location is the very same feature that traffickers can use to monitor their victims' activities. Providing victims with mobile devices they can monitor is particularly attractive to traffickers and can serve as a red flag that a patient is a potential human trafficking victim.

Knowledge about technology's role in human trafficking can be one of the simplest forms of protection against exploitation and highlights why awareness of privacy settings related to social media and digital content is so important. With this knowledge, we can begin to ask some important questions about social media and privacy: How do you define who your "friends" are when it comes to these apps? What information is hidden within this digital content that makes adolescents even more vulnerable to predators? And how can we advise adolescents on how to protect themselves from these digital threats.

Mid-Chapter Activities

Activity 1. How Vulnerable Are You on Social Media?

If you have a Facebook or other social media account, check your security settings. Who can post to your page? Who can see your friends list? Who can see your content? Friends of friends? Keep in mind that pictures are often geotagged and people can easily access the title of your photos by looking at the metadata attached. Even an innocent picture of a child could include the location where the picture was taken and even the child's name (if it was saved to the original file). It is important to regularly review your security settings on any social media platform.

Activity 2. How Vulnerable Are You Online?

There are many ways predators can find information about you online beyond social media. Try searching yourself on the following websites to see what you find. How could this sort of information (such as previous or current addresses, your mother's maiden name, etc.) put you at risk?

- Google
- Peoplefinders.com
- Zabasearch.com
- Ancestry.com
- Myfamily.com
- Melissadata.com
- Brbpub.com
- Thepaperboy.com
- Intelius.com

Mobile Devices and Sexting

Law enforcement uses a variety of technological detection tools to identify potential trafficking cases and track illicit behaviors. Many of these detection tools involve the use of phone numbers to track and identify suspicious activities that may be indicative of human trafficking. This means that, in general, perpetrators of trafficking are careful when it comes to their digital communication footprint. They will often use encoded messages and symbols, such as emojis, in their online and mobile communications. Emojis are small images, symbols, or icons used in digital communication to express ideas, emotions, and attitudes either in support or in lieu of textual content. They can also be used to provide additional context to the underlying meaning or feelings one's message is meant to convey to its readers. One instance in which these encoded messages and symbols are commonly used is in online escort advertisements to avoid detection by law enforcement. Certain emojis, such as the growing heart emoji, are specifically classified as indicators of underage sex trafficking, and multiple emojis indicative of online human trafficking used in combination with each other are a significant red flag [12]. The graphic below is a representation of what one of these ads might look like. The use of the crown emoji and the word "princess" in this particular example are textual/symbolic indicators that the poster, hypothetically in this case, is under the control of a pimp. The use of the rose emoji at the end would be a subtle indicator of price indicating the required exchange of money for her services.

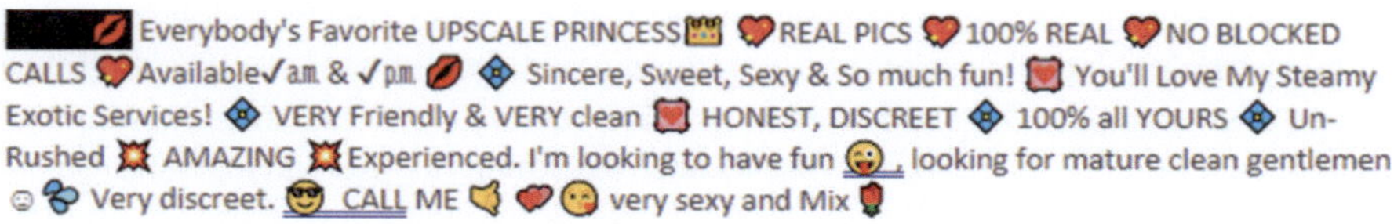
[redacted] Everybody's Favorite UPSCALE PRINCESS REAL PICS 100% REAL NO BLOCKED CALLS Available✓a.m. & ✓p.m. Sincere, Sweet, Sexy & So much fun! You'll Love My Steamy Exotic Services! VERY Friendly & VERY clean HONEST, DISCREET 100% all YOURS Un-Rushed AMAZING Experienced. I'm looking to have fun , looking for mature clean gentlemen Very discreet. CALL ME very sexy and Mix

Traffickers frequently provide their victims with mobile devices to be used for communication between buyers and the advertisement of sexual services using online classifieds, dating apps, and social media as well as to protect their own anonymity [13]. In the case here, Abby had two phones. To the average person, the possession of two mobile phones designated for personal use, especially with adolescents, is in and of itself suspicious behavior. In Abby's case, she specifically disclosed that her second phone was purchased and gifted to her by her older "boyfriend," a red flag when dealing with youth and teens classified as high risk for or showing indicators of being trafficked. Traffickers often bestow gifts upon their victims as part of the lover boy ruse; the underlying reasons for gifting a mobile phone may not be recognized by vulnerable youth. It is likely that Abby truly views the phone as a gift and does not understand the meaning that lies behind accepting it and what its underlying purpose may be. Ironically, many people in this digital age have a dedicated work phone provided by their employer similar to the way in which traffickers provide their victims with phones that are eventually used to communicate with purchasers of sex. While data on the actual profits varies widely, some estimates indicate that sex trafficking brings in $99 billion in revenue for criminal organizations globally each year with an estimated $80,000 profit per victim in developed economies such as the United States [14]. The exact numbers may be unclear, but it is generally accepted that sex trafficking is considered one of the most profitable criminal activities. In summary, mobile devices play a significant role in facilitating these exchanges of sex for money by acting as a marketing tool for traffickers, a monitoring device to control victims, and an access key for buyers seeking an easy way to set a time and place to meet to obtain services.

The use of mobile devices as a facilitator of human trafficking in relation to the exchange of sexual services is not the only concern. Since the advent of the smart phone at the beginning of the twenty-first century, sexting has become a popular activity among smart phone users – so common, in fact, that some contend that sexting may be a normative behavior among young adults and sexually maturing adolescents. Sexting is defined as engaging in the activity of posting, viewing, or sending messages or digital images via mobile devices or the Internet that are either of a sexual nature or have a sexual connotation [15]. One study found that out of 964 teenagers, 27.6% participated in some aspect of creating and sharing this provocative and sexually explicit digital content [16]. Based on numerous studies concluding that about 15% of teens have personally sent a "sext" and the majority of sexting occurs through the act of sending sexually explicit images, [17] the act of sexting is not immediately indicative of an occurrence of sex trafficking. However, one recent study of sexting among more than 500 minor adolescents (<18 years) in a low-income, urban community found that sexting was associated with exploitative and abusive relationships, including sexual abuse and intimate partner violence [18]. Could sexting be an indicator also of human trafficking when it co-occurs with other red flags? For example, a trafficker in one case used sexually explicit, pornographic content a girl had shared during the relationship-building phase of his ruse to later blackmail her into having sexual relations with other men from which he profited [19]. Some states have started to employ legislation to define the differences between minors engaging in sexting and the distribution of child pornography [20], but adolescents still need to be informed about the risks and the potential criminal repercussions. When communicating with patients, it is important to pay attention to whether their behavior or background information suggests that they may have any involvement with sexting. Building their awareness of the possible dangers in engaging in this type of activity is key when trying to lower susceptibility to the trafficker's recruitment efforts in youth already displaying signs of being at high risk for sexual exploitation.

Cryptocurrency, Explained…

What is cryptocurrency? And how does it pertain to human trafficking? The term "cryptocurrency" is a bit misleading since it really does not involve any type of true currency. Instead, cryptocurrency is a process similar to balancing a checkbook or an accounting ledger. Cryptocurrency is a highly sophisticated digital trail of secured transactions that uses virtual keys to validate the transfer of digital assets between two parties. In essence, cryptocurrency allows for all the anonymity of a cash transaction while still taking place exclusively in the cyber sphere. Traffickers use this to securely exchange payment for the transfer of pornographic photos and videos along with live-stream access to sexually explicit activities [21]. Under the Trafficking Victims Protection Act, federal law defines sex trafficking as a commercial sex act, "any sex act on account of which anything of value is given to or received by any person," that has been induced by force, coercion, or involving a minor [22]. It is difficult to define the value of cryptocurrency due to its complexity and the fact that no true exchange of material value occurs.

In January 2019, Congress passed the Fight Illicit Networks and Detect Trafficking Act which requires the United States Government Accountability Office to "carry out a study on how virtual currencies and online marketplaces are used to buy, sell, or facilitate the financing of goods or services associated with sex trafficking or drug trafficking, and for other purposes." [23] While this demonstrates how government entities are beginning to recognize the impact this new digital currency has had on criminal activity, it remains a gray area. Therefore, it is important to be conscious of whether a patient whose condition illustrates they are at high risk for being trafficked mentions their involvement or association with the use of this form of virtual "currency" exchange. These cryptocurrencies can include Bitcoin, Bitcoin cash, Litecoin, Dogecoin, Ethereum, BAT, NEO, and many more. Bitcoin was the first cryptocurrency introduced to market and spiked in value around the end of 2017. There is not really a standard price index for cryptocurrency, but one bitcoin was valued around $17,000 in 2017 and since its peak has ranged in value between $3500 and $9000 [24]. While difficult to address from a legal perspective, it serves as a red flag for prevention efforts when addressing potential cases of sex trafficking.

Conclusion

In recent years, both the recruitment process and exploitation of human trafficking victims have increasingly moved from identifiable physical spaces to the illusive corridors of the Internet. This transition has increased anonymity of both traffickers and purchasers of sex. The medical arena represents a unique space where victims of trafficking come in physical contact with others who can offer help. Therefore, it is vital that healthcare workers increase their fluency in the realm of human trafficking and technology both to identify possible victims and to respond appropriately to red flags.

Discussion Questions

1. How does the use of social media contribute to isolation, loneliness, and self-harm or suicide attempts?
2. What red flags, other than those analyzed in this chapter, were exhibited in Abby's case? And how would you respond to each as an isolated incident?

3. How should you proceed with a patient who exhibits signs of being trafficked? As a mandated reporter, when does it become necessary for you to alert authorities? How should you handle the situation while retaining trust with the patient, protecting their safety, and following proper protocol? [See Chapters 18 and 20 for further information.]
4. What are some dangers in mishandling red flags exhibited by a patient? What risks does it pose to the healthcare provider and the patient if a perpetrator has the ability to record interactions, see emails/messages/texts, and/or control the camera and microphone functions of a victim's phone?
5. What information is hidden within digital content that makes adolescents even more vulnerable to predators? And how can we advise adolescents on how to protect themselves from these digital threats?

Supplemental Materials

1. Geo-location tagging exercise
   (a) https://www.pic2map.com/ [25]
   (b) https://support.google.com/websearch/answer/1325808?co=GENIE.Platform%3DDesktop&hl=en&oco=0 [26]
2. Privacy settings for mobile devices
   (a) https://support.apple.com/en-us/HT207056 [27]
   (b) https://support.google.com/websearch/answer/54068?p=web_app_activity&hl=en&authuser=0&visit_id=636932910356794662-2722802219&rd=1&co=GENIE.Platform%3DAndroid&oco=1 [28]

References

1. Centers for Disease Control and Prevention: US Public Health Service: Preexposure prophylaxis for the prevention of HIV infection in the United States—2017 Update: a clinical practice guideline. https://www.cdc.gov/hiv/pdf/risk/prep/cdc-hiv-prep-guidelines-2017.pdf. Published March 2018.
2. Standage, T. Writing on the Wall: Social Media - the First 2,000 Years. New York, USA; Bloomsbury; 2017.
3. Kunz R, Baughman M, Yarnell R, Williamson C. Social media and sex trafficking process from connection and recruitment, to sales [Internet]. [cited 2019 Sep 24]. Available from: https://f1000.com/work/item/7526106/resources/6900052/pdf.
4. Hultgren MR. "An exploratory study of the indicators of trafficking in online female escort ads." MS [dissertation]. San Diego, CA: San Diego State University; 2015. Available from: https://digitallibrary.sdsu.edu/islandora/object/sdsu%3A1940.
5. Farley M, Franzblau K, Kennedy MA. Online prostitution and trafficking. Albanu Law Rev. 2014;77:1039–67.
6. Yang L. Adolescent sexual behavior in the digital age: considerations for clinicians, legal professionals and educators. J Youth Adolesc. 2015;44:1461–7.

7. Human Trafficking and the Internet∗ (∗and Other Technologies, too) [Internet]. [cited 2019 Sep 25]. Available from: https://www.americanbar.org/groups/judicial/publications/judges_journal/2013/winter/human_trafficking_and_internet_and_other_technologies_too/
8. Smith LA, Vardaman SH, Snow MA. The national report on domestic minor sex trafficking: America's prostituted children. Shared Hope International: Vancouver, WA; 2009.
9. Remington DM. Technology and human trafficking: Utica College; 2016.
10. Smith A, Papadaki M, Furnell SM. Improving awareness of social engineering attacks. In: Dodge RC, Futcher L, editors. Information assurance and security education and training. Berlin, Heidelberg: Springer Berlin Heidelberg; 2013. p. 249–56.
11. Ahn R. The commercial sexual exploitation and sex trafficking of minors in the Boston metropolitan area: experiences and challenges faced by front-line providers and other stakeholders. J Appl Res Child. 2015;6:4.
12. Whitney J, Jennex M, Elkins A, Frost E. Don't want to get caught? don't say it: the use of EMOJIS in online human sex trafficking ads. In: Proceedings of the 51st Hawaii International Conference on System Sciences. Hawaii International Conference on System Sciences; 2018.
13. KM vs Human trafficking: An exploratory study on using emojis for a knowledge driven approach to identifying online human sex trafficking [Internet]. [cited 2019 Sep 25]. Available from: https://digitallibrary.sdsu.edu/islandora/object/sdsu%3A21609
14. International Labour Organization. Profits and Poverty: The Economics of Forced Labour. 2014;
15. Judge AM. Sexting among U.S. adolescents: psychological and legal perspectives. Harv Rev Psychiatry. 2012;20:86–96.
16. Van Ouytsel J, Walrave M, Ponnet K. Adolescent sexting research: the challenges ahead. JAMA Pediatr. 2018;172:405–6.
17. Strasburger VC, Zimmerman H, Temple JR, Madigan S. Teenagers, sexting, and the law. Pediatrics. 2019;143
18. Titchen KE, Maslyanskaya S, Silver EJ, Coupey SM. Sexting and young adolescents: associations with sexual abuse and intimate partner violence. J Pediatr Adolesc Gynecol. 2019;32(5):481–6.
19. Pornography and sexting led to this girl's extortion [Internet]. [cited 2019 Sep 25]. Available from: https://endsexualexploitation.org/articles/pornography-sexting-extortion/.
20. Jerde R. Follow the silk road: how internet affordances influence and transform crime and law enforcement. MA [dissertation]. Monterey (CA): Naval Postgraduate School; 2017. https://apps.dtic.mil/dtic/tr/fulltext/u2/1053310.pdf.
21. Jerde RD. Follow the silk road: how internet affordances influence and transform crime and law enforcement. 2017.
22. Trafficking Victims Protection Act of 2000. 22 U.S. Code §§ 7102(4), (9), and (10). Sect. No. 106–386, 114. Oct 8, 2000.
23. H. Rept. 115-781 – Fight illicit networks and detect trafficking act [Internet]. [cited 2019 Sep 25]. Available from: https://www.congress.gov/congressional-report/115th-congress/house-report/781/1.
24. Global Bitcoin Price Index [Internet]. [cited 2019 Sep 25]. Available from: https://bitcoinaverage.com/en/bitcoin-price/btc-to-usd.
25. Photo Location & Online EXIF Data Viewer – Pic 2 Map [Internet]. [cited 2019 Sep 25]. Available from: https://www.pic2map.com/.
26. Google. Find related images with reverse image search [Internet]. [cited 2019 Sep 25]. Available from: https://support.google.com/websearch/answer/1325808?co=GENIE.Platform%3DDesktop&hl=en&oco=0.
27. Location Services & Privacy – Apple Support [Internet]. [cited 2019 Sep 25]. Available from: https://support.apple.com/en-us/HT207056.
28. Google. See & control your Web & App Activity [Internet]. [cited 2019 Sep 25]. Available from: https://support.google.com/websearch/answer/54068?p=web_app_activity&hl=en&authuser=0&visit_id=636932910356794662-2722802219&rd=1&co=GENIE.Platform%3DAndroid&oco=1.

Chapter 7
Child Abuse

Dana Kaplan, Jordan Greenbaum, and Linda Cahill

Case Presentation

Gabriel is a 7-year-old boy with a mild cognitive deficit, said to be on the autism spectrum. You are his primary care pediatrician. Gabriel presents with a 3-day history of pain on urination. This morning he complained again, and when his mother looked at his penis, she noted some blood-tinged urethral discharge and redness of the foreskin. Exam is notable for painful retraction of the foreskin and purulent, profuse, green penile discharge. No inguinal nodes are palpated. Gabriel tests negative for urinary tract infections with more common organisms but tests positive for gonorrhea of the urethra via urine NAAT; the result is confirmed independently by repeat urine NAAT with an alternate target sequence.

When you ask Gabriel's mother about possible exposure to sexually transmitted infections (STI's), she asserts that to her knowledge, no one in the home has an STI. She herself is tested frequently for STIs, and she reports dating two men, neither of whom has an STI. Gabriel lives with his mother, his 17-year-old sister, Stephanie, and frequently visits his maternal aunt who has seven children. When

D. Kaplan (✉)
Department of Pediatrics, Division of Child Abuse and Neglect, Staten Island University Hospital, Northwell Health, Staten Island, NY, USA

J. Greenbaum
Institute on Healthcare and Human Trafficking at the Stephanie V. Blank Center for Safe and Healthy Children, Children's Healthcare of Atlanta, Atlanta, GA, USA

International Centre for Missing and Exploited Children, Alexandria, VA, USA

L. Cahill
Butler Center for Children and Families, Department of Pediatrics, Children's Hospital at Montefiore Bronx, New York, NY, USA

K. E. Titchen, E. Miller (eds.), *Medical Perspectives on Human Trafficking in Adolescents*, https://doi.org/10.1007/978-3-030-43367-3_7

you ask Gabriel whether anyone has ever touched his "privates" in a way that felt uncomfortable to him, he denies this happening.

When you ask the mother more about his life at home, you discover that Gabriel often sleeps with his 17-year-old sister, Stephanie. The mother does not find this unusual, saying that they have been sleeping together since he was a baby, and they are hard to separate at night.

After discussing Gabriel's case with your clinic social worker, you report the case to the child welfare hotline for suspected sexual abuse given the positive STI testing; law enforcement is notified.[1] In his forensic interview, Gabriel denies that he was ever touched sexually by anyone. His genital exam is normal. The medical team recommends that everyone in all households Gabriel lived in or visited be tested for STIs. Testing takes place over a period of 2 weeks. The only family member who tests positive for gonorrhea is Gabriel's sister Stephanie, who is sexually active.

When questioned by law enforcement as a potential perpetrator of child sexual abuse, Stephanie denies touching Gabriel inappropriately. When asked about the possible source of her gonorrhea infection she discloses having had sex with lots of men at parties. She indicates that her boyfriend pressured her to have sex, telling her he loved her and that he would "do the same thing for her if she asked." She states that she heard he received money and drugs in exchange for her sex acts. She says she did not know the men with whom she had sex and could not identify them. She reports that her boyfriend told her to bring Gabriel to two of the parties when she was babysitting him. When asked if she thought it possible that the child was sexually abused at one or more of the parties, Stephanie states that she does not know because she was not with him at all times while they were there.

Case Resolution

Six months later, while in therapy, Gabriel discloses that a man at one of the parties he attended with his sister "put his thing in my butt" at "a house with deer" and it "hurt." When police investigate, they find mounted stag heads in a bedroom of the house where the parties occurred. Gabriel also discloses that he saw the man give money to his sister's boyfriend before this happened.

[1] In some jurisdictions, notification of law enforcement may happen at the time of the report to the state child abuse reporting hotline. If not, then law enforcement should be notified separately by the medical or other professional (school personnel, mental health counselor or other, for example). A forensic interview and medical evaluation by a child abuse specialist should be scheduled at the local child advocacy center.

Child Sexual Abuse and Commercial Sexual Exploitation/Trafficking

Overlap

Child sexual abuse and commercial sexual exploitation share significant overlap on multiple levels. Both are acts of child abuse. Child sexual abuse occurs when a dependent, developmentally immature minor engages in sexual activities that he/she does not fully comprehend, to which he/she is unable to give informed consent, or that violate the social taboos of family roles [1]. Commercial sexual exploitation of children (CSEC) involves the exchange of a sex act for something of perceived value (e.g., money, shelter, food, luxury items, drugs, or something else), which may go to the child victim or a third party [2]. In some cases of sexual abuse, there are elements of sexual exploitation; for example, the child is given gifts or other items in order to obtain compliance. Research has shown that child sexual abuse earlier in life renders individuals more vulnerable to sexual exploitation later [3–5]. In addition, early sexual abuse of a child is associated with later risk-taking behaviors, such as early age of onset of sexual activity, running away from home, drug use and misuse, and behavioral problems [6, 7]. Many of these factors are also associated with CSEC [8, 9]. Among risk factors for both sexual abuse and CSEC is the presence of cognitive or behavioral disabilities [10]. Thus, Gabriel is at increased risk for sexual victimization.

Interviewing and Information Gathering

Interviewing children for suspected child sexual abuse requires specialized training. The forensic interviewer must be able to assess and accommodate the child's developmental abilities, including language skills, as well as their ability to provide free narrative and capacity to recall contextual details. General healthcare practitioners may lack this specific training but must be aware how to conduct a medical interview of children to get enough information (minimal facts) to make appropriate decisions about reporting to child protective service agencies, referring to counseling facilities, or referring to pediatric clinics specializing in abuse evaluations [11–13]. It is important not to embark on a formal forensic interview without appropriate training as this could lead to poorly phrased questions that suggest an answer or otherwise increase the risk of misinformation. It may also cause unnecessary discomfort to the child if a trauma-informed approach is not used and trust is lacking. Formal protocols for forensic interviewing are available [11–13].

When gathering basic information to determine if a report to authorities is needed, it is important for the clinician to begin with open-ended, general, non-threatening questions to build rapport. Talking about the child's family or what he likes to do allows the interviewer to build trust and assess verbal and developmental skills. Open-ended questions are preferable when asking about abuse experiences as well. In this case, the physician asked the patient if anyone had ever touched him in a way that made him "uncomfortable." The patient is a 7-year-old cognitively limited male who may not know what the word "uncomfortable" means. Furthermore, with grooming in child sexual abuse, the physical contact may not be "uncomfortable" and may feel good. It is important also to consider that in the case of grooming, a child may not identify what happened to him/her as "sexual abuse" or in this case "trafficking."

When questioning young children in a primary care setting to collect information on the possibility of sexual abuse, it may be more appropriate to ask the child who is close to him/her and what those around the child do to show their love for him/her. In the case presented in this chapter, it may be helpful to ask the patient if there is anything he is worried about or if something happened that he does not understand [11–13].

Issues with Disclosure

More than half of sexually abused children do not disclose their abuse until they are adults [14]. Disclosure of child sexual abuse is a process, not an event [15]. In many instances, the process of disclosure includes denial, tentative disclosure, and active disclosure, followed by recantation and reaffirmation [15]. An awareness of the dynamics of this process is important so that the child's statements are not dismissed as unreliable or inconsistent when further details emerge, when there is a denial followed by disclosure, or when a disclosure is followed by recantation [15]. In this case, the patient disclosed penile-anal penetration after an initial denial phase, the details of which were corroborated based on law enforcement investigation. However, the patient tested positive for gonococcal urethritis and this was confirmed on urine NAAT, which would not be consistent with receptive penile-anal penetration and would be more consistent with additional sexual contact. The patient may therefore be in the tentative phase of his disclosure, and with time further details may emerge. Given this information, the patient should be actively engaged in psychological counseling where further details may emerge in the context of an ongoing, therapeutic trusted relationship. It may also be appropriate to have a second forensic interview at a later time. Depending on the disclosure and information regarding the timing of last sexual contact, it may also be appropriate to consider forensic evidence collection if the last sexual contact was within 72–96 hours of presentation to medical care. It is important that the exact timing of forensic kit collection is based on recommendations in the jurisdiction of the evaluation.

Sexually Transmitted Infections

The identification of certain sexually transmitted infections in children beyond the neonatal period strongly suggests sexual abuse. Postnatally acquired gonorrhea, syphilis, chlamydia, and *T. vaginalis* infection, as well as nontransfusion, nonperinatally acquired HIV, are all indicative of sexual contact [16].

Culture of potentially infected sites has traditionally been the diagnostic gold standard for cases of possible sexual abuse/assault and would be indicated in the case of Gabriel's penile discharge [17]. Nucleic acid amplification testing (NAAT) has been in use for years in the sexually active adolescent and adult populations due to its higher sensitivity (100% by transcription mediated amplification, TMA), ability to collect a sample noninvasively, ability to test for both *Neisseria gonorrhea* and *Chlamydia trachomatis* with one sample, and its lower cost compared with culture [17]. The US Food and Drug Administration has not approved the commercially available NAATs for use in prepubertal children because of the low prevalence of STIs in this population (5%). Per the Centers for Disease Control and Prevention (CDC), NAATs can be used as an alternative to culture with vaginal specimens or urine from girls, whereas culture remains the preferred method for urethral specimens or urine from boys and for extra-genital specimens for all children [16]. However, although the CDC still recommends culture for nongenital sites, many clinicians find it difficult to access cultures, as many laboratories have discontinued these tests [17]. NAATs have been evaluated in adult studies for pharyngeal and anorectal infections and have been found to have superior sensitivity for detecting infection at these sites compared with culture, and specificity rates are well within the range of acceptable for clinical practice [17].

When NAATs are used to diagnose infection in prepubertal children or older children and the result could have significance in legal proceedings, confirmatory testing should be performed to exclude a possible false-positive result. This can be accomplished with certain NAAT testing which uses a second, alternate target sequence on the same specimen [17]. Given the forensic value of these tests in asymptomatic prepubertal children, prophylaxis at the time of initial testing, and treatment of an asymptomatic child with an initial positive NAAT should be withheld until a positive test is confirmed with additional testing. In the present case, however, Gabriel is symptomatic and should be treated.

The Physical Exam

It is important to remember that a normal anogenital exam after the disclosure of sexual abuse neither confirms nor excludes a history of sexual abuse or previous penetration, as the absence of anogenital findings after sexual abuse is common

[18, 19]. There are a variety of reasons for the lack of diagnostic findings. Depending on the type of sexual contact, there may be no visualized tissue trauma (e.g., fondling with a hand). In addition, anogenital injuries that do occur tend to be superficial (contusions, abrasions, small lacerations), and these heal relatively quickly. Such injuries may heal completely and without scarring within 72 hours to 2 weeks [20]. With regard to anal penetration, there may be no injury, or there may be nonspecific fissures, which can be seen with expected trauma to the area (e.g., stooling) and can heal within a few days. Therefore, Gabriel's normal anogenital exam, occurring as it did after a delayed disclosure of penile-anal penetration, is not inconsistent with the history.

Safe Discharge Plans

It is important to note that children are more likely to be sexually abused by someone they know rather than by a stranger [21]. Therefore, when an evaluation is occurring in a medical setting, a decision needs to be made about a safe discharge plan, as the perpetrator may reside with the patient or have access to the patient. This decision-making process is often multidisciplinary when cases are reported for investigation. Please refer to Chap. 18 for further discussion on mandated reporting.

Similar to child sexual abuse, in cases of CSEC the child often is recruited by someone they know (e.g., intimate partner, family member, or other relative, peer); however, the child may then be exploited by multiple strangers who purchase the sex acts [3]. In the context of this case, it is also important to consider descriptions in the literature of two categories of adults who sexually abuse/exploit children: "situational" vs. "preferential" child molesters [22]. Situational molesters victimize children sexually, but only under certain circumstances, such as opportunity and lack of a current adult partner. Preferential molesters prefer children as their primary source of sexual gratification [22]. Therefore, a situational molester could have sexual contact with a woman, for instance Stephanie, and then also perpetrate sexual abuse with a young boy, in this case, Gabriel. This could explain why both the patient and his sister tested positive for gonorrhea given that they had sexual contact with the same man at the party.

Neglect

This case also highlights the spectrum of neglect that may be encountered in high-risk scenarios. First, the patient had symptoms of pain on urination for three days prior to his mother bringing him to medical attention, which is concerning for medical neglect. Medical neglect includes failure to act when there are obvious signs of serious illness or failure to follow a physician's instructions once medical advice has been sought [23]. Another form of neglect – supervisional neglect – is the failure to provide age-appropriate supervision by a parent or caregiver [24]. It is not unreasonable to expect a developmentally appropriate 17-year-old to safely watch her 7-year-old sibling, and therefore this in and of itself does not constitute supervisional neglect by the mother. However, this case scenario raises questions about the mother's understanding of the 17-year-old's activities outside the home and calls into question the mother's awareness of the older sister's decision to bring Gabriel to the parties.

Patients May Not Identify as Victims

It is important also to recognize that the 17-year-old sister is herself a victim, though she may not yet conceptualize herself in this way. Common recruitment techniques used with CSE victims involve various forms of psychological manipulation, often within a romantic relationship. Adolescents may feel that they are doing a "favor" or demonstrating their devotion to their partner by agreeing to perform sexual acts with others [25]. They may feel obligated to agree to sex acts since the person asking has "been good" to them [26]. They may or may not be aware of the commercial aspect of the activities and have no perception of exploitation [5]. This holds true for the teenage sister's perception of her sexual encounters. This lack of awareness of their exploitative situation makes recognition of CSEC and effective intervention difficult for health professionals since the trafficked person may deny victimization and refuse any services.

Nonetheless, it is important to offer medical services regardless of a person's readiness to disclose or their insight into their involvement in trafficking. Consideration of the person's STI status and need for pregnancy prevention given high-risk behaviors make it crucial for adolescents to seek the expertise of a specialist who can guide the medical care of at-risk youth. It is also important to recognize the role of mandatory reporting for medical professionals when child abuse and CSEC are suspected. Please refer to Chap. 18 for information about intersections with mandatory reporting.

Questions for Further Exploration/Discussion

1. Do you think there is there a lower age limit on human trafficking? How could infants and toddlers become victims of human trafficking?
2. Would the patient still be a victim herself if she were 19-years-old at the time this occurred? How do we define victims?
3. What are the effects of trauma on neurologic and psychologic development? How might such exposure to trauma contribute to intergenerational trauma?

4. Are all parents of minor victims who become involved in sex trafficking neglectful by default? Are there circumstances where parents may not be considered neglectful?

Resources

https://www.helfersociety.org/
https://www.healtrafficking.org
https://www.apsac.org/
https://www.nationalcac.org/
https://www.nationalchildrensalliance.org/
www.AAP.org

References

1. Jenny C, Crawford-Jakubiak JE. Committee on child abuse and neglect, American Academy of Pediatrics. The evaluation of children in the primary care setting when sexual abuse is suspected. Pediatrics. 2013;132:e558–67.
2. Institute of Medicine (U.S.) Committee on the Commercial Sexual Exploitation and Sex Trafficking of Minors in the United States., Clayton EW, Krugman RD, Simon P, Institute of Medicine (U.S.), National Research Council (U.S.). Confronting commercial sexual exploitation and sex trafficking of minors in the United States. Washington, D.C.: National Academies Press; 2013.
3. Reid JA, Baglivio MT, Piquero AR, Greenwald MA, Epps N. Human trafficking of minors and childhood adversity in Florida. Am J Public Health. 2017;107:306–11.
4. Goldberg AP, Moore JL, Houck C, Kaplan DM, Barron CE. Domestic minor sex trafficking patients: a retrospective analysis of medical presentation. J Pediatr Adolesc Gynecol. 2017;30:109–15.
5. Landers M, McGrath K, Johnson MH, Armstrong MI, Dollard N. Baseline characteristics of dependent youth who have been commercially sexually exploited: findings from a specialized treatment program. J Child Sex Abus. 2017;26:692–709.
6. Lalor K, McElvaney R. Child sexual abuse, links to later sexual exploitation/high-risk sexual behavior, and prevention/treatment programs. Trauma Violence Abuse. 2010;11:159–77.
7. Maniglio R. The impact of child sexual abuse on health: a systematic review of reviews. Clin Psychol Rev. 2009;29:647–57.
8. Greenbaum VJ, Dodd M, McCracken C. A short screening tool to identify victims of child sex trafficking in the health care setting. Pediatr Emerg Care. 2018;34:33–7.
9. Moore JL, Houck C, Hirway P, Barron CE, Goldberg AP. Trafficking experiences and psychosocial features of domestic minor sex trafficking victims. J Interpers Violence. 2017:886260517703373.
10. Reid JA. Sex trafficking of girls with intellectual disabilities: an exploratory mixed methods study. Sex Abus. 2016;30:107–31.
11. Listenbee RL. Child forensic interviewing: best practices. 2015.
12. La Rooy D, Brubacher SP, Aromäki-Stratos A, Cyr M, Hershkowitz I, Korkman J, et al. The NICHD protocol: a review of an internationally-used evidence-based tool for training child forensic interviewers. J Criminolog Res Policy Pract. 2015;1:76–89.

13. Anderson J, Ellefson J, Lashley J, Miller AL, Olinger S, Russell A, et al. the cornerhouse forensic interview protocol: RATAC. 2010 [cited 2019 Apr 29]. Available from: https://www.cornerhousemn.org/images/CornerHouse_RATAC_Protocol.pdf.
14. Smith DW, Letourneau EJ, Saunders BE, Kilpatrick DG, Resnick HS, Best CL. Delay in disclosure of childhood rape: results from a national survey. Child Abuse Negl. 2000;24:273–87.
15. Sorensen T, Snow B. How children tell: the process of disclosure in child sexual abuse. Child Welfare. 1991;70:3–15.
16. Centers for Disease Control and Prevention. Sexual Assault and Abuse and STDs - 2015 STD Treatment Guidelines [Internet]. 2015 [cited 2019 Sep 25]. Available from: https://www.cdc.gov/std/tg2015/sexual-assault.htm.
17. Adams JA, Kellogg ND, Farst KJ, Harper NS, Palusci VJ, Frasier LD, et al. Updated guidelines for the medical assessment and care of children who may have been sexually abused. J Pediatr Adolesc Gynecol. 2016;29:81–7.
18. Adams JA, Harper K, Knudson S, Revilla J. Examination findings in legally confirmed child sexual abuse: it's normal to be normal. Pediatrics. 1994;94:310–7.
19. Adams JA, Farst KJ, Kellogg ND. Interpretation of medical findings in suspected child sexual abuse: an update for 2018. J Pediatr Adolesc Gynecol. 2018;31:225–31.
20. McCann J, Voris J. Perianal injuries resulting from sexual abuse: a longitudinal study. Pediatrics. 1993;91:390–7.
21. U.S. Department of Health & Human Services, Administration for Children and Families, Administration on Children, Youth and Families, Children's Bureau. Child Maltreatment 2017 [Internet]. 2019. Available from: https://www.acf.hhs.gov/cb/research-data-technology/statistics-research/child-maltreatment.
22. Lanyon RI. Theory and treatment in child molestation. J Consult Clin Psychol. 1986;54:176–82.
23. Jenny C. Committee on child abuse and neglect, American Academy of Pediatrics. Recognizing and responding to medical neglect. Pediatrics. 2007;120:1385–9.
24. Hymel KP. Committee on child abuse and neglect. When is lack of supervision neglect? Pediatrics. 2006;118:1296–8.
25. Anderson PM, Coyle KK, Johnson A, Denner J. An exploratory study of adolescent pimping relationships. J Prim Prev. 2014;35:113–7.
26. Edinburgh L, Pape-Blabolil J, Harpin SB, Saewyc E. Assessing exploitation experiences of girls and boys seen at a child advocacy center. Child Abuse Negl. 2015;46:47–59.

Chapter 8
Human Trafficking in the Foster Care System

Catherine G. Coughlin, Robyn R. Miller, Selina Higgins, Kidian Martinez, Christine Dipaolo, and Jordan Greenbaum

Case Presentation

Maya is a sexually active 16-year-old female who self-presents to the adolescent medicine clinic for sexually transmitted infections (STIs) testing. You are the clinician who has been providing care to her for the past six months. At her initial visit, you placed an intrauterine device (IUD) for contraception at Maya's request. After an initial adjustment period with some spotting and lower pelvic pain, she became amenorrheic and was pleased with this method of contraception. At this visit, Maya informs you that she has been experiencing lower pelvic pain and worries that her IUD may be misplaced. Her last sexual partner did not like the fact that she had the IUD and on several occasions attempted to remove it himself. When asked why he did not like the IUD, Maya informs you that she is not sure why. It never really made sense to her since this last sexual partner was exploiting her. She was very

C. G. Coughlin (✉)
Boston Combined Residency Program, Boston Children's Hospital/Boston Medical Center, Boston, MA, USA

R. R. Miller · K. Martinez · C. Dipaolo
Department of Pediatrics, Division of Adolescent Medicine Nemours/A.I. duPont Hospital for Children, Sidney Kimmel Medical College at Thomas Jefferson University, Wilmington, DE, USA

S. Higgins
Office of Child Trafficking Prevention and Policy, NYC Administration for Children's Services, New York, NY, USA

J. Greenbaum
Institute on Healthcare and Human Trafficking at the Stephanie V. Blank Center for Safe and Healthy Children, Children's Healthcare of Atlanta, Atlanta, GA, USA

International Centre for Missing and Exploited Children, Alexandria, VA, USA

K. E. Titchen, E. Miller (eds.), *Medical Perspectives on Human Trafficking in Adolescents*, https://doi.org/10.1007/978-3-030-43367-3_8

matter-of-fact about her reply, as her trafficking status had already been identified by authorities.

Reproductive Coercion

Maya's story illustrates a common presentation of reproductive coercion, as her trafficker tries to interfere in her autonomous reproductive health decision-making. Reproductive coercion can take many forms – interfering with birth control (disposing pills, removing IUDs), manipulating or tampering with condoms, pressuring girls and women to become and remain pregnant, and controlling the outcome of pregnancy – with increased risk for unwanted pregnancies and sexually transmitted infections [1–3]. The goals of coercion are diverse, but qualitative studies reveal that pregnancy may be a way to maintain social and economic security for the abuser, particularly if the abuser anticipates he may become incarcerated soon [4]. When these abusers and traffickers go to jail, the mothers of their children are seen as guaranteed support systems for them while incarcerated and once released. Given the disproportionate incarceration of African American men compared to white men, this may help to explain the higher risk of reproductive coercion for African American women [4, 5]. Additionally, reproductive coercion disproportionately affects women experiencing concurrent intimate partner violence, single women, women of low educational and socioeconomic status, and non-Caucasian women [1, 3, 4]. Reproductive coercion can also serve to increase trauma bonding between victim and manipulator, as the child embodies a concrete representation of the power and control tactics used to control circumstances. Moreover, a child born due to reproductive coercion can become an object of relational conflict for the mother, who may emotionally reject the child. Patterns of emotional rejection result in the development of insecure attachment types that affect social-emotional development and may perpetuate child abuse and/or maltreatment [6, 7].

You are concerned that, despite her previously negative STI screens, Maya currently has an STI that has progressed to pelvic inflammatory disease and Fitz-Hugh-Curtis syndrome. Your differential diagnosis also includes a partially expelled or malpositioned IUD, uterine perforation given the persistent manipulation of the IUD by her trafficker, urinary tract infection, and constipation. Much lower on the differential but more concerning is an ectopic pregnancy secondary to a partially expelled IUD. On exam, you visualize her IUD strings exiting a pink, nonfriable external cervical os. There is no cervical or adnexal tenderness and no pus appreciated exiting the os. There is no vaginal discharge or odor, and her vaginal mucosa is pink without lesions. Her abdomen is soft with mild tenderness in the right lower quadrant but without guarding or rebound. The rest of your exam is benign. Maya presented with her usual somewhat flat affect, but she communicated openly with good eye contact and occasional smiles. Since most STIs are asymptomatic and she is very high risk, you send testing for gonorrhea, chlamydia, trichomoniasis, syphilis, HIV, and hepatitis C. You are reassured by your physical exam that her IUD is in good position but order a pelvic ultrasound that does in fact show a good central uterine position of the IUD and no pregnancy. You hold empiric treatment, since she is now in a therapeutic residential facility with good follow-up. All testing results are negative.

When Maya initially presented to your clinic, she had been living in a foster home where she was not mistreated, yet she was not happy. This foster home represented Maya's seventh placement since entering the system at age six. Maya's story is sadly representative of many youth who have experienced foster care due to caregiver abuse and maltreatment. Born to a 15-year-old mother who continually ran away from home, Maya spent her early years in her alcoholic maternal grandmother's overcrowded household. Maya remained socially isolated within the family until kindergarten, at which time her teacher noted extreme shyness alternating with angry outbursts. Maya's behavior escalated from verbal outbursts to physical manifestations, including walking on classroom desks during the school day. The desk elevation permitted the teacher to view dirt- and blood-encrusted underclothes, which provided a reasonable suspicion of abuse/maltreatment, resulting in a call to the state's child abuse hotline [8].

Investigation uncovered sexual abuse of Maya by the grandmother's partner resulting in protective removal to foster care when the grandmother refused to believe the investigation results and would not take steps to remove the perpetrator from the household. Initially placed in a kinship setting with a relative, the court ordered Maya re-placed after access to Maya by the grandmother's boyfriend occurred at a family event. She attended weekly play therapy sessions but refused to participate after an unforeseen change in therapists occurred. Maya exhibited age-inappropriate hypersexual behavior, extreme temper tantrums, bedwetting, and physical aggression toward the other children in the household. Due to safety concerns for the other children, Maya was re-placed alone in a therapeutic foster home with a highly comprehensive service plan. However, the intense history of insecure attachment, parental abandonment, sexual abuse, emotional neglect, betrayal of trust by her grandmother, and familial and environmental losses resulted in a brief psychotic break resulting in psychiatric hospitalization followed by placement in a residential setting.

After 18 months in residential placement, Maya overtly appeared to have benefited from the therapeutic milieu and stepped down to a less restrictive level of care within the home of a veteran foster parent with an excellent reputation for helping severely traumatized youth. Three other youth resided in the home and Maya quickly attached herself to them, thinking of them as family. Seeking belonging and acceptance, Maya became overly susceptible to the pressure to assimilate with her foster siblings and therefore matched her behaviors and choices to theirs, including running away with them for periods of time.

One night, Maya and one of the other girls in her foster home again decided to run away. The foster sister had a friend she was planning on meeting that night who offered to let her stay with him for a while. She said Maya was welcome to stay with them too, if she wanted. They had fun the first night, "hanging out," drinking, and talking, with the male friend flirting with Maya, telling her how beautiful she was and how he wished they could always be together. When Maya awoke the next morning, her foster sister was gone and the male friend explained that if she wanted to stay with him she was going to have to help him out by earning money for them to live by having sex with other men. Maya felt highly conflicted, as the thought of sleeping with men triggered memories of the sexual abuse, yet he was so sweet and considerate and spoke of their future together. Maya felt she had finally found someone who loved her and would not reject her as long as she complied. Only after being sold to multiple clients did she realize she really did not have a choice about staying with him, as he had begun to exhibit aggression alternating with affection in no predictable pattern. The manipulation of emotions through intermittent punishment and positive reinforcement resulted in the development of a traumatic bond further escalated by fear that he would come after her if she left. Maya referred to this man – her trafficker – as her "pimp" in a very matter-of-fact and emotionless manner. Underlying her flat affect, Maya continually suppressed myriad conflicting thoughts and emotions: love, fear, doubt, guilt, self-blame, and lack of self-esteem. Maya used alcohol, marijuana, and ecstasy daily to escape the reality of her physical and emotional pain. On the days she did not want to use, her trafficker forced her to use, as it made it easier for him to have unprotected sex with her, and to force her to forgo condom use with customers, who paid extra money for this privilege.

Control Tactics

Control tactics used by traffickers vary and may include some combination of psychological manipulation, false romance, isolation, drugs/alcohol, violence, obligation (financial or otherwise), and threats and intimidation, including blackmail, misinformation, and making a child complicit in a crime [9–11]. Many exploited youth become trauma bonded (a concept recently reframed as "trauma-coerced bonded") to their traffickers, through the intermittent use of positive reinforcement and punishment in no discernable pattern [12]. The alternating of compliments and affection with insults and cruelty serves to condition a response focused upon maintaining the feeling of love and belonging at any cost. Psychological manipulation may involve instilling in the child a sense of guilt, shame, stigma, hopelessness, and dependency. It may entail systematic belittlement, criticism and humiliation, paired with episodic praise and gift-giving. Pregnancy may also be used by a trafficker to maintain control over a trafficked female, who is more likely to comply with the trafficker's wishes while pregnant, perhaps fearing a beating and subsequent loss of the fetus. After birth, the trafficker may use the baby as leverage, telling the mother she may only see her baby if she earns her quota, threatening to put the baby up for adoption, or threatening to keep the baby if she tries to leave. Isolation may be physical, involving locked doors, alarms, or video surveillance; or psychological, such as forbidding contact with family and peers, misinforming a child that friends and family no longer want to see her/him, manipulating social media access, or making the child use a different name.

While taking the medical history, Maya revealed that while she was being trafficked, her exploiter "hospital shopped," taking her to different emergency departments for medical attention. She never disclosed to hospital staff that she was being trafficked because of fear of violence by her trafficker. She received STI screening several times; she believes all testing was negative. When asked how she returned to foster care, Maya indicated that to escape her trafficker, she blatantly shoplifted so she would be arrested and placed back into the foster care system. Due to the arrest, Maya was placed in a group home with weekly mental health therapy.

Risk Factors

Foster care is a documented risk factor for trafficking [13, 14]. Children in protective custody may run away from their placement and become involved in commercial sexual exploitation (CSE) out of a need for money, shelter, or drugs while living on the streets, or they may become involved with a trafficker who uses force, deception, or coercion to sexually exploit them. Many sex-trafficked youth are also labor trafficked, as they strive to fulfill their quota in any way possible to avoid the wrath of their trafficker. Labor trafficking amongst exploited youth can take many forms, from being forced to sell drugs to shoplifting items for re-sale [15]. Conversely, some labor trafficking victims are forced into sex work to repay debts owed to the trafficker [16] (see Chap. 5 for more information on labor trafficking and forced criminality).

Many risk factors for CSE overlap with risk factors for foster care placement, including low socioeconomic status, a history of sexual or emotional abuse, a history of running away, and exposure to domestic violence [13, 14, 17]. In fact, youth who have experienced sexual exploitation have been found to have higher rates of adverse childhood experiences (ACEs), and a higher number of ACEs, particularly for sexual abuse and physical neglect [18]. Between 50%–80% of child sex trafficking survivors report a history with the child welfare system [13, 14]. In one study, 59% of trafficking victims had experienced sexual or physical violence prior to being trafficked, and 12% had experienced sexual coercion under the age of 15 [19]. Trafficking is also associated with youth who run away from foster care [20] (see Chap. 12 for more information on homelessness and human trafficking). It is likely that these risk factors work synergistically with a history of child sexual abuse to increase vulnerability to trafficking [14, 21]. Furthermore, traffickers may *target* children in the foster care system, as these children often have a history of trauma, lack family support, and lack adequate parental supervision [14]. However, the exact incidence of foster children involved in CSE or other forms of exploitation is challenging to obtain, due to the subversive and secretive nature of trafficking [22, 23].

Many trafficked persons do not spontaneously disclose their exploitative situation to healthcare professionals. Reluctance to disclose may be related to fear (of retribution from the trafficker, of deportation or arrest, of judgment by providers), shame, feelings of guilt, hopelessness, the presence of the trafficker at the visit, or other factors [24–26]. In one study of trafficked youth, the majority (68%) exhibited features of "Stockholm syndrome," believing that to some degree the exploiter was acting in their best interest and defending the actions of the perpetrator.[1] [13] Many youth do not understand the concept of trafficking, may not view themselves as victims, and may not understand that they are being manipulated or coerced [13, 27].

Clinical complaints themselves may not suggest sex trafficking, although a presentation for a suicide attempt, behavioral issues including signs/symptoms of post-traumatic stress disorder, recurrent STI, acute sexual or physical assault, or issues related to substance misuse may prompt further questioning to assess risk of trafficking [28–30] (see Chap. 9 for more information about psychiatric illness and human trafficking). Similar to our patient in this case, somatic, non-specific symptoms at presentation, including headache, tiredness, dizziness, back pain, abdominal pain, or pelvic pain, are common in trafficking victims [21, 31]. Other "red flags" in the history or presentation may raise a suspicion of human trafficking, such as the presence of high-risk behaviors or other concerning issues identified in the social history [23, 27].

[1] The Diagnostic and Statistical Manual of Mental Disorders (DSM 5) (2013) does not recognize Stockholm Syndrome. The term has been in general usage since inception through a bank robbery in Stockholm in 1973. Prior to DSM 5, it was under consideration to be included under Disorders of Extreme Stress, Not Otherwise Specified. American Psychiatric Association: Diagnostic and statistical manual of mental disorders, Fifth Edition. Arlington, VA, American Psychiatric Association, 2013.

Almost a year later, you are consulted by your hospital's emergency department (ED) to see a 17-year-old girl presenting with abdominal pain, who is said to be known to your service. When you search for the patient in the electronic medical record, you find that the patient is Maya, who had been lost to follow-up. You see that Maya was evaluated in the ED for abdominal pain, vomiting, and diarrhea with a likely diagnosis of viral gastroenteritis. As part of her ED evaluation, a pelvic ultrasound was obtained and revealed that her intrauterine device (IUD) was displaced in the lower cervix. You see that Maya refused a pelvic exam, and you head to the ED to meet her. When you arrive at the ED, you discover that Maya refused to wait for the adolescent medicine consult and was discharged home with her foster mother and instructions to follow up in adolescent medicine clinic.

After several days and three telephone calls, you finally succeed in scheduling an appointment for Maya. On the day of the appointment, Maya does not come to clinic. Your attempt to reach her by phone is unsuccessful.

Building Trust

Engaging with traumatized youth can be challenging, as their capacity for trust has continually degenerated with every negative experience. It is unrealistic to expect that youth will promptly disclose traumatic experiences to a professional with whom they have not developed personal rapport. The need and desire for health care may be overshadowed by a young person's fear, embarrassment, shame, or guilt, as well as mistrust of health professionals.

Several options are available to reach Maya in a way that she may be more likely to perceive as safe. You might contact the Social Work Department to find out if Maya has interacted with a hospital social worker. Some hospitals also have a child abuse liaison, often within the Social Work or Patient Advocate Department. The Liaison has an ongoing working relationship with the child welfare agency and can help to identify staff known to Maya who can assist with outreach. Outreach to the foster care worker with whom Maya has a relationship could serve to encourage Maya to attend appointments and develop trust in her clinician. The child welfare agency can also contact Maya's legal advocate, as, depending on the State's model, children in foster care should have a court-assigned law guardian or a guardian ad litem (GAL) or a court appointed special advocate (CASA), who will work with Maya toward identifying her best interests. (See "Getting Help" below for more on GAL and CASA volunteers). No matter the situation, remain nonjudgmental, and continually maintain recognition of the extensive and sequential trauma Maya has experienced, and continues to experience, while in the psychological captivity of the trafficker.

Identification

Some CSE youth may be overlooked as victims, as they do not fit the stereotype of trafficked persons as foreign-born, female, pre-adolescent/adolescent, and without prior interaction with the criminal justice system [13, 22, 32]. While several studies suggest that most *identified* sex trafficking victims are domestic-born and while females predominate, it is likely that male and transgender victims are overlooked and underrecognized [14, 19, 31]. LGBTQ youth in foster care have an amplified vulnerability to sex trafficking, as they meet the criteria for two of the recognized vulnerable populations. One study reported that some LGBTQ youth experienced violence at the hands of staff and clients at social service organizations and other locations that are intended to be safe [33]. If youth involved with social services do not feel safe, the risk of homelessness and, thereby, survival sex can also escalate [34] (see Chap. 11 for more information about LGBTQ youth and human trafficking).

Given that children in foster care interact with many professionals and agencies, it is vitally important to train first responders, including healthcare professionals, mental health professionals, law enforcement, and child protective service staff, to be able to identify and offer assistance to victims of commercial sexual exploitation [27, 32]. Many first responders are not knowledgeable about the nuances of trafficking, including possible indicators of exploitation.

A lack of first responder knowledge and skills regarding trauma-informed, culturally sensitive, victim-centered care may cause trafficked children to experience distrust, shame, stigma, and embarrassment, further exacerbating their complex trauma [19, 26, 35]. Therefore, it is critical for first responders to receive education and training regarding human trafficking and trauma-informed care so that trafficked children and those at risk may be identified and offered appropriate services [36, 37] (see Chap. 20 for more information about human trafficking education).

Getting Help

First responders also need to know how and where to report juvenile trafficking. Should a provider suspect that a child in foster care has been trafficked, it is vital to make the child's case worker aware of the concern for trafficking. Foster care regulations vary from state to state, so it is imperative that the provider understand the mechanisms for response within their state's child welfare system [8]. Additionally, as mandated reporters, first responders are required to file a new report with the state or county's child abuse hotline with any recently learned information to ensure the trafficking allegations are thoroughly investigated [8]. In many states, child protective investigations pertain solely to parents or other persons legally responsible for the child. However, even if a parent is not the trafficker per se, they may be perpetuating the trafficking through neglect, which is reportable. If a parent is not providing adequately for the child, or if the parent is not either supervising the child or making diligent efforts to protect the child, those are reportable situations. If the parent leaves the child with someone who is trafficking the child, then the question is whether the parent knew or should have known (see Chap. 18 for medicolegal aspects of human trafficking and mandatory reporting).

Multidisciplinary collaboration is essential and is not limited to interaction with the protective investigation team that forms as a result of reporting. In some states, legal counsel is appointed to a child when entering foster care. In New York State, the Family Court appoints an attorney as "law guardian" to serve as the child's legal advocate. The law guardian represents the child's best interest and is counsel independent from that of the parent and of the child welfare agency [38]. In some states, foster children with particularly complex cases may benefit from a guardian ad litem (GAL) or a court-appointed special advocate (CASA); these highly trained volunteers help a foster child when the child's desires are not aligned with the child's best interests. A GAL or CASA volunteer is a unique resource for foster children that may serve as a positive adult role model. A case worker should be able to obtain a GAL or CASA for a patient in foster care. Medical professionals should also refer this child and/or the case worker to a local anti-trafficking organization and notify the National Human Trafficking Hotline (888–3737-888).

Common Denominators

It should be noted that placement in foster care itself should not be considered a per se risk factor for trafficking. The real risk factor in reference to foster care is the actual *reason for being in care*. Children are removed from the custody of their parents due to abusive or neglectful situations which negatively impact their physical and emotional safety. Vulnerability to trafficking stems from those traumatic experiences that resulted in the removal and placement into care (e.g., development of an insecure attachment due to inappropriate caretaker responses which can result in a desire for acceptance and belonging and mistakenly appears fulfilled through the seemingly attractiveness of the exploitive relationship). Susceptibility to trafficking can be exacerbated by factors *relating* to placement, which may serve to intensify feelings of rejection that originated in the home. Foster care, even at its best and most caring, can still be traumatic when a kinship situation is not available and the youth is placed in an unfamiliar environment with strangers. Furthermore, a foster care placement may or may not be sufficiently engaging to meet the particular emotional needs of a child, as it sometimes takes more time for a full assessment of strengths and needs than is available during emergency safety situations. Trafficked children are looking for love and acceptance, and sometimes foster care can sufficiently fulfill the attachment needs for love and belonging, but occasionally it does not. This can sometimes occur with highly traumatized, special need children and more often with older youth who have experienced repeated trauma and rejection and are apt candidates for exploiter deception.

Case Continued

The following day, an inpatient psychiatric facility nurse contacts the office. You soon learn that Maya was admitted to this psychiatric facility after being sexually assaulted vaginally and anally. Maya was initially evaluated in an ED where mental health screening determined that she was suicidal; she was transferred to the inpatient psychiatric facility. Because of concern that Maya's IUD had been expelled, you see her that same day in your adolescent medicine clinic. You discern that the IUD is in a good position based on visualization of IUD strings exiting from external cervical os, but secondary to Maya's complaints of excessive vaginal bleeding, you remove the IUD at her request, insert a hormonal contraceptive implant, and schedule a follow-up appointment in two weeks given the complex social situation and ongoing mental health concerns.

Maya misses the two-week follow-up, and after several attempts to reschedule, she finally returns six weeks later for follow-up and tells you that she has been placed in yet another foster home and has been seen in another ED due to tenderness at the implant insertion site. In the ED, the implant was visualized on x-ray and showed no signs concerning for infection. She returned to her foster home only to run away again. This time, Maya met a man in a city four hours away from her home. They engaged in consensual sex for several days, but this eventually progressed to nonconsensual sex. Once she was able to remove herself from this situation, she again presented to another emergency department and was evaluated and released to the state's foster care system. A human trafficking detective was involved after her last assault and found no evidence of trafficking in his investigation, based upon Maya's denial.

Collaborative and Coordinated Care

Many victims will deny trafficking involvement for a variety of reasons. Although Maya is aware of her situation and identifies her abuser to you as her "pimp" or trafficker, she may be afraid of repercussions from the trafficker, embarrassed or ashamed of the abuse endured, and/or a victim of trauma bonding. First responders should recognize that even though Maya would not disclose her abusive situation to the detective at this time, the empathy and engagement provided during interactions can serve to plant seeds toward a time when she is more comfortable and capable of disclosing (see Chap. 19 for survivor insights about human trafficking).

To best help trafficked youth in foster care, first responders should maintain an awareness of services available, as many states have specialized services that require specific documentation for consideration, e.g., psychiatric evaluation, psychological evaluation (with projective, objective and intelligence tests). and psychosocial assessment which a medical professional can facilitate.

Services can vary from jurisdiction to jurisdiction based upon the resources available, so it is important for all medical professionals to have awareness of what their state/city/county has to offer. For example, in Delaware, the Department of Services for Children, Youth and their Families provides independent living services for youth aged 14 and older who are in foster care. The child will age out at 18 years unless they have Another Plan Living Arrangement (APLA) or they have a board extension. The youth is assigned an independent living worker who will work along with the case worker assigned to the child. The Independent Living Program is geared toward advocating self-sufficiency and responsible living for young adults [39]. These youth receive training in life skills and personal development, mentoring, tuition assistance, and support with transitional living. They may also qualify for rent assistance and other living expenses.

Clinicians who care for victims of trafficking should collaborate with their state child protective service (CPS) agencies. This partnership within their communities can ensure children and adolescents in foster care are receiving adequate comprehensive medical and mental health screenings. It is a federal recommendation that states develop systems of care for children in foster care, and this process can be collaborative between clinicians and CPS. The health care children in foster care receive can sometimes be compromised by lack of health information, consent and confidentiality barriers, time constraints, and challenges to care coordination and communication. The American Academy of Pediatrics recommends the medical home care model for children and adolescents in foster care as it provides high-quality, comprehensive, coordinated health care that is continuous over time, as well as compassionate, culturally sensitive, trauma-informed, family-centered, and child-focused care [40]. In partnership with CPS, the medical professional within the medical home should establish an appropriate timeframe for the appointments to ensure each child's unique needs are met. Through appropriate health care, screening, referral, support, education, and a focus on the child's innate strengths and resilience, clinicians can ensure children and adolescents in foster care receive optimal and developmentally appropriate health care and can further promote healing [41]. If service agencies do not have access to pediatric medical homes, it is recommended that children and adolescents receive care through foster care clinics in the state. Foster care clinics are run by pediatric health care organizations in partnership with CPS, and their overall goal is to provide comprehensive physical and mental health care, as well as specialty care, dedicated to promoting the health and well-being of children and adolescents in foster care. The foster care clinic model is distinguishable from medical and mental health clinics maintained by foster care agencies. Models vary from state to state, so the medical professional should proactively become familiar with the resources available in their jurisdiction.

Across the United States, there have been significant efforts to focus upon a victim-centered approach to better identify, provide for, and protect trafficking survivors. The model focuses upon strengthening legal codes and law enforcement, while improving service provision for survivors [42]. The State Department's 2018 Trafficking in Persons Report encouraged a "more consistent application of victim-centered and trauma-informed approaches in all phases of victim identification, assistance, recovery, and participation in the criminal justice process."[43].

In reference to youth in foster care, 2014 federal legislation, The Preventing Sex Trafficking and Strengthening Families Act, mandated the identification and protection of children and youth at risk for sex trafficking by requiring all states to develop policies and procedures to screen, document, and determine appropriate services for all youth over whom the state has child welfare responsibility [44]. Of note, no such mandate yet exists for youth who are victims solely of labor trafficking, although sex and labor trafficking frequently overlap.

One example of a state response to the federal mandate is the New York's Safe Harbour Program's development of a two-tier screening system and law enforcement referral form [45]. Trafficking identification and service provision are especially crucial in New York State, as it ranked as the fifth highest state in calls to the National Human Trafficking Hotline in 2018 [46]. In 2015, New York City's child welfare agency, the Administration for Children's Services (ACS), became the first public agency to dedicate resources toward identifying and ensuring service provision to youth identified as trafficked or at-risk for trafficking through inauguration of its Office of Child Trafficking Prevention and Policy (OCTPP). ACS offers a comprehensive continuum of services to youth within its foster care system, as well as specialized preventive services for trafficked youth in care, or at home with their families [39, 47]. OCTPP also liaises with a wide variety of community-based providers specializing in services to trafficked and at-risk youth.

Although extricating oneself from a life of human trafficking can be especially difficult in the face of societal poverty, racism, misogyny, and discrimination, our hope is that one day, Maya will be sufficiently empowered to leave her trafficker and move on to a more positively focused life. To do so, she will require affirmation, support, resources, and therapeutic interventions from a multi-system trauma-informed team. As first responders, we have the opportunity to participate in helping youth like Maya learn to mitigate their traumatic experiences through our recognition, collaboration, support, and empathy as well as advocacy for a more equitable future for our youth.

References

1. Hill AL, Jones KA, McCauley HL, Tancredi DJ, Silverman JG, Miller E. Reproductive coercion and relationship abuse among adolescents and young women seeking care at school health centers. Obstet Gynecol. 2019;134(2):351–9.
2. Miller E, Silverman JG. Reproductive coercion and partner violence: implications for clinical assessment of unintended pregnancy. Expert Rev Obstet Gynecol. 2010;5(5):511–5.
3. Grace KT, Anderson JC. Reproductive coercion: a systematic review. Trauma Violence Abuse. 2018;19(4):371–90.
4. Nikolajski C, Miller E, McCauley HL, Akers A, Schwarz EB, Freedman L, et al. Race and reproductive coercion: a qualitative assessment. Womens Health Issues. 2015;25(3):216–23.
5. Miller E, Decker MR, Reed E, Raj A, Hathaway JE, Silverman JG. Male partner pregnancy-promoting behaviors and adolescent partner violence: findings from a qualitative study with adolescent females. Ambul Pediatr. 2007;7(5):360–6.
6. Greenberg MT, Cicchetti D, Cummings EM, editors. Attachment in the Preschool Years: Theory, Research, and Intervention. illustrated, reprint. University of Chicago Press; 1993.
7. Ainsworth MD, Blehar MC, Waters E, Wall SN. Patterns of attachment: a psychological study of the strange situation: Psychology Press; 2015.
8. U.S. Department of Health & Human Services CsB, Child Welfare Information Gateway. Mandatory reporters of child abuse and neglect. [cited 2019 October 4] 2016. Available from: https://www.childwelfare.gov/pubPDFs/services.pdf.
9. Anderson PM, Coyle KK, Johnson A, Denner J. An exploratory study of adolescent pimping relationships. J Prim Prev. 2014;35(2):113–7.

10. Reid JA. Entrapment and enmeshment schemes used by sex traffickers. Sex Abus. 2016;28(6):491–511.
11. Roe-Sepowitz D. A six-year analysis of sex traffickers of minors: exploring characteristics and sex trafficking patterns. J Hum Behav Soc Environ. 2019;29(5):608–29.
12. Raghavan C, Doychak K. Trauma-coerced bonding and victims of sex trafficking: where do we go from here? Inter J Emerg Ment Health Hum Resilience. 2015;17(2):583–7.
13. Shaw JA, Lewis JE, Chitiva HA, Pangilinan AR. Adolescent victims of commercial sexual exploitation versus sexually abused adolescents. J Am Acad Psychiatry Law. 2017;45(3):325–31.
14. Landers M, McGrath K, Johnson MH, Armstrong MI, Dollard N. Baseline characteristics of dependent youth who have been commercially sexually exploited: findings from a specialized treatment program. J Child Sex Abus. 2017;26(6):692–709.
15. Bigelsen J, Vuotto S, Addison K, Trongone S, Tully K. Homelessness, survival sex and human trafficking: as experienced by the youth of covenant house New York. 2013.
16. Camacho H. labor trafficking persists amid outrage over sex trade [Internet]. CityLimits.org. 2014 [cited 2019 Sep 25]. Available from: https://citylimits.org/2014/09/11/labor-trafficking-persists-amid-outrage-over-sex-trade/.
17. McKinney M. Hospitals train staff to spot victims of human trafficking. Mod Healthc. 2015;
18. Naramore R, Bright MA, Epps N, Hardt NS. Youth arrested for trading sex have the highest rates of childhood adversity: a statewide study of juvenile offenders. Sex Abus. 2017;29(4):396–410.
19. Zimmerman C, Hossain M, Yun K, Gajdadziev V, Guzun N, Tchomarova M, et al. The health of trafficked women: a survey of women entering posttrafficking services in Europe. Am J Public Health. 2008;98(1):55–9.
20. Latzman NE, Gibbs DA, Feinberg R, Kluckman MN, Aboul-Hosn S. Human trafficking victimization among youth who run away from foster care. Child Youth Serv Rev. 2019;98:113–24.
21. Seng MJ. Child sexual abuse and adolescent prostitution: a comparative analysis. Adolescence. 1989;24(95):665–75.
22. Chisolm-Straker M, Baldwin S, Gaïgbé-Togbé B, Ndukwe N, Johnson PN, Richardson LD. Health care and human trafficking: we are seeing the unseen. J Health Care Poor Underserved. 2016;27(3):1220–33.
23. Barnert E, Iqbal Z, Bruce J, Anoshiravani A, Kolhatkar G, Greenbaum J. Commercial sexual exploitation and sex trafficking of children and adolescents: a narrative review. Acad Pediatr. 2017;17(8):825–9.
24. Baldwin SB, Eisenman DP, Sayles JN, Ryan G, Chuang KS. Identification of human trafficking victims in health care settings. Health Hum Rights. 2011;13(1):36–49.
25. Ijadi-Maghsoodi R, Bath E, Cook M, Textor L, Barnert E. Commercially sexually exploited youths' health care experiences, barriers, and recommendations: a qualitative analysis. Child Abuse Negl. 2018;76:334–41.
26. Rajaram SS, Tidball S. Survivors' voices-complex needs of sex Trafficking survivors in the Midwest. Behav Med. 2018;44(3):189–98.
27. Cole MA, Daniel M, Chisolm-Straker M, Macias-Konstantopoulos W, Alter H, Stoklosa H. A Theory-based didactic offering physicians a method for learning and teaching others about human trafficking. AEM Educ Train. 2018;2(Suppl 1):S25–30.
28. Edinburgh L, Pape-Blabolil J, Harpin SB, Saewyc E. Assessing exploitation experiences of girls and boys seen at a child advocacy center. Child Abuse Negl. 2015;46:47–59.
29. Greenbaum VJ, Dodd M, McCracken C. A short screening tool to identify victims of child sex trafficking in the health care setting. Pediatr Emerg Care. 2018;34(1):33–7.
30. Hornor G, Sherfield J. Commercial sexual exploitation of children: health care use and case characteristics. J Pediatr Health Care. 2018;32(3):250–62.
31. Greenbaum VJ. Child sex trafficking in the United States: challenges for the healthcare provider. PLoS Med. 2017;14(11):e1002439.
32. Reid JA, Baglivio MT, Piquero AR, Greenwald MA, Epps N. No youth left behind to human trafficking: exploring profiles of risk. Am J Orthopsychiatry. 2018.

33. PolarisProject. Unique obstacles put transgender people at risk of trafficking | polaris [Internet]. Polaris. 2017 [cited 2019 Sep 27]. Available from: https://polarisproject.org/blog/2017/03/10/unique-obstacles-put-transgender-people-risk-trafficking.
34. Dank M, Yahner J, Madden K, Banuelos I, Yu L, Ritchie A, et al. Surviving the streets of New York: experiences of LGBTQ youth, YMSM, and YWSW engaged in survival sex. Urban Institute. 2015.
35. Lederer LJ, Wetzel CA. The health consequences of sex trafficking and their implications for identifying victims in healthcare facilities. Ann Health Law. 2014;23(61).
36. Greenbaum J, Crawford-Jakubiak JE. Committee on child Abuse and neglect. Child sex trafficking and commercial sexual exploitation: health care needs of victims. Pediatrics. 2015;135(3):566–74.
37. Substance Abuse and Mental Health Services Administration. SAMHSA's Concept of Trauma and Guidance for a Trauma-Informed Approach [Internet]. Rockville, MD: Substance Abuse and Mental Health Services Administration; 2014 [cited 2019 Sep 25]. Report No.: HHS Publication No. (SMA) 14–4884. Available from: https://store.samhsa.gov/system/files/sma14-4884.pdf.
38. Somberg D. Defining the Role of Law Guardian in New York State by Statute, Standards and Case Law. Touro Law Rev. 2015;19(2).
39. Congressional Research Service. Youth transitioning from foster care: background and federal programs [Internet]. Congressional Research Service; 2019 May [cited 2019 Oct 4]. Available from: https://fas.org/sgp/crs/misc/RL34499.pdf.
40. American Academy of Pediatrics. Task force on health care for children in foster care. fostering health: health care for children and adolescents in foster care. Am Academy Pediatrics. 2005.
41. Szilagyi MA, Rosen DS, Rubin D, Zlotnik S. Council on Foster Care, adoption and kinship care, committee on Adolescense et al. health care issues for children and adolescents in Foster Care and kinship care. Pediatrics. 2015;136(4):e1142–66.
42. Picarelli JT, Jonsson A. Fostering imagination in fighting Trafficking: comparing strategies and policies to fight sex Trafficking in the U. S. Sweden: DIANE Publishing; 2010.
43. United States Department of State. Trafficking in persons report [Internet]. 2018 [cited 2019 Sep 27]. Available from: https://www.state.gov/reports/2018-trafficking-in-persons-report/.
44. Trafficking PS, Act SF. Public Law 113–183. InUnited States 113th Congress 2014.
45. NYS Office of Children and Family Services. 5-OCFS-ADM-16: requirements to identify, document, report, and provide services to child sex trafficking victims. New York State; 2015.
46. PolarisProject. Hotline statistics | national human trafficking hotline [Internet]. Polaris. 2018 [cited 2019 Sep 30]. Available from: https://humantraffickinghotline.org/states.
47. Casey Family Programs. Addressing child sex trafficking from a child welfare perspective [Internet]. Casey Family Programs; 2015 [cited 2019 Sep 27]. Available from: https://casey-familypro-wpengine.netdna-ssl.com/media/child-sex-trafficking.pdf.

Chapter 9
The Psychiatric Patient

Mary C. Reissinger, Amanda C. Castro, Rachel A. Robitz, and Mollie R. Gordon

Case Presentation

Ella is a 17-year-old transgender female who was admitted to the inpatient psychiatric unit with suicidal ideation. Prior to starting her intake, you review the note from the emergency medicine physician:

> *17-year-old transgender female sex worker presents with black eye and multiple abrasions after being beaten by pimp. She reports suicidal ideation and is exhibiting paranoia. Patient has been evaluated for multiple physical injuries and is now medically clear. Will consult psychiatry for a safety assessment.*

When you begin your assessment of Ella, she initially is hesitant to speak with you. She will only speak with you in the presence of one of the nurses with whom she bonded last night when she was admitted. Throughout the course of the interview, she becomes increasingly relaxed with you and willing to disclose personal information. The patient reports that her suicidal thoughts have worsened over the past two weeks and she now feels "totally hopeless." The patient tells you she does not feel capable of leaving her current situation and describes a recent incident where she attempted to leave her trafficker, but one week later was found by him while waiting at a bus stop. She adds that upon finding her, "he beat [her] up, bad."

M. C. Reissinger (✉) · M. R. Gordon
Menninger Department of Psychiatry and Behavioral Sciences Baylor College of Medicine, Houston, TX, USA

A. C. Castro
Department of Behavioral Health Nemours/A.I. Dupont Hospital for Children, Sidney Kimmel Medical College, Wilmington, DE, USA

R. A. Robitz
Department of Psychiatry and Behavioral Sciences University of California, Davis, Sacramento, CA, USA

K. E. Titchen, E. Miller (eds.), *Medical Perspectives on Human Trafficking in Adolescents*, https://doi.org/10.1007/978-3-030-43367-3_9

The patient states her belief that he is secretly tracking her movement through her cellphone and she does not feel that she can ever escape him. It is important to note that adolescents represent a particularly vulnerable subpopulation of victims of human trafficking. Providing for their basic needs by exchanging sex acts (i.e., survival sex) and bartering are common tactics employed by the perpetrators of trafficking. Food, shelter, drugs, and material items, in addition to attention/affection, help maintain the "trauma bond" utilized by traffickers to continuously exploit their victims.

When queried, the patient informs you that her "mood swings" are currently her most troubling mental health symptom. She explains how she quickly goes from feeling "very hyper [to] angry [to] suicidal." The patient goes on to explain her irritability and how she is easily "set off" by even minor annoyances. She provides one example where she was arrested for punching a hole in the wall of a coffee shop as a reaction to perceiving she was being treated unfairly by the barista. She reports additional clinical symptoms such as difficulty sleeping "through the night [due to violent] nightmares" and excessive anxiety and worry. When you cue her to explain her cognitive symptoms, the patient specifies that when she feels "really, really upset…" she does not feel in control of her thoughts or emotions declaring, "…my mind races. I think of every bad thing and I just lose it." Regarding the frequency of her mood symptoms (e.g., "hyper, can't sleep, angry at everyone, [and] explode at people"), the patient maintains she is "like that most of the time." Further, the patient reports she "sometimes" experiences a "crashing feeling" of low energy followed by increased feelings of guilt (e.g., about mainly her sexual behavior) and low self-worth and generally thinks of herself as "a failure [and] a burden." Throughout the encounter, intrusive and persistent thoughts of suicide are reported as Ella maintains she "can't see any other way out" of her current situation. She denies any access to weapons or guns, and when asked directly, she adamantly denies any thoughts of harm toward others.

Ella's past medical history is notable for chronic headaches treated with ibuprofen and acetaminophen and for which she has never sought specialty consultation. She reports treatment for chlamydia at age 16. The patient denies hormone treatment but expressed some interest; specifically, she plans to speak with a physician about gender-affirming surgery once she reaches the age of 18.

The patient first identified as female as a young child but did not tell her family until she was 15. They were reportedly unsupportive and dismissive and kicked her out of the house. She lived transiently for a couple of months until meeting her would-be trafficker and moving in with him. Ella reports a recent expulsion from school six months ago for "defending [herself]." Ella endorses being a victim of bullying since early childhood.

You review the routine lab work for victims of sexual assault. Laboratory studies for sexually transmitted infections including syphilis, human immunodeficiency virus (HIV), hepatitis serology, urine gonorrhea, and chlamydia are all negative.

Complete blood cell count shows mild anemia, and the complete metabolic panel is within normal limits. Urine drug screen is positive for methamphetamine and cannabis, while blood alcohol is undetectable.

During the mental status exam (MSE), you note that Ella has poor grooming and hygiene. You observe she wears her hair long, and it appears unwashed and generally unkempt. Multiple horizontal scars are visible on the inside of her left wrist. She appears adequately nourished. Upon initiation of the MSE, Ella is markedly guarded, refusing to speak, appearing angry, and not making direct eye contact. However, over time, Ella becomes increasingly cooperative and engaged. She typically speaks in a lowered volume with decreased cadence and limited words. Thought processes, although linear, logical, and goal-directed, are assessed as overtly concrete, negativistic, absolutist, and childlike. Behaviorally, she appears distracted and nervous; while you are speaking, she repeatedly peers out of the office window as if constantly surveilling her surroundings. Further, Ella appears to have limited coping/problem-solving ability and limited capacity for self-soothing.

Ella is admitted to the psychiatric inpatient unit with diagnoses of unspecified depressive disorder and unspecified trauma-related disorder. Considerations for differential diagnosis are as follows: bipolar II disorder, posttraumatic stress disorder (PTSD), acute stress disorder, oppositional defiant disorder, unspecified gender dysphoria, other substance-induced disorder, and borderline personality disorder. Ella agrees to initiate a course of treatment including fluoxetine 10 mg daily for the treatment of her affective symptoms.

The following morning in the nursing report you learn that although Ella initially stayed to herself, by dinner her relatedness to peers on the unit became increasingly familiar and friendly. However, an incident was documented where a nurse approached the patient while she was sitting at a table in the day room, startling her, and apparently Ella's reaction was to raise her voice, yell profanities, and threaten the nurse. Subsequently, nursing staff prepared emergency intramuscular medication for agitation not responding to verbal redirection. As staff approached Ella, she ran into her room, climbed on to the bed, and pulled the covers over her. At that time, the decision was made that since the patient was able to demonstrate the ability to keep herself and others safe, emergency intramuscular medications were no longer medically necessary.

The next morning, Ella appears embarrassed although outwardly she ardently yells, "You best not sneak up on me again!" Later, during daily unit rounds, she denies symptomatic improvement but implores you to discharge her immediately. The patient demands that "it's Saturday" and mentions her belief that the inpatient unit is "making [her] worse [and she will] only feel better if [she] can some fresh air and enjoy the weekend!" After this statement, the patient abruptly terminates the conversation by standing up and demanding to call a friend to "come and get [her] right now."

Improving Communication Strategies with Psychiatric Patients Who Have a Recent or Remote History of Human Trafficking Victimization

A systematic review of the current literature on trauma-informed mental health services compels advocates and clinicians alike to select interventions, conceptualize cases, and formulate treatment plans based upon the guidelines from the National Center for Trauma-Informed Care (NCTIC) [1]. A trauma-informed approach is both intuitive and distinctively practical when caring for patients with a history of human trafficking victimization. Due to the prevalence of trauma-related mental health symptomology amongst survivors of trafficking, it becomes imperative to respond to trauma patients in a manner that denotes flexibility and consistency but is also evidence-based or evidence-informed [2]. Hopper and Gonzalez (2017) found that trafficking survivors like Ella who identify as transgender endorsed more PTSD mental health symptoms than their cis-gendered counterparts, further supporting the need for trauma-informed strategies especially when caring for transgendered survivors and victims of human trafficking. Equally important is the quality of the work environment for the treating multidisciplinary team.

The psychiatric patient's feelings toward people from their past, quite often their abusers, will commonly be misdirected toward treatment team members; consequently, treatment staff tend to respond with feelings and behaviors informed by their own perceptions which are shaped by their past experiences (i.e., transference and countertransference). Such occurrences have the potential to directly impact the quality and effectiveness of the applied treatment [3]. Drawing from the professional experiences of providers who routinely care for survivors of trafficking and the limited research addressing communication and rapport-building strategies with this population, utilizing Rogerian (i.e., person-centered) psychotherapeutic techniques along with the NCTIC guidelines appears to be a pragmatic, relevant, and operative clinical response [4]. When applying person-centered therapeutic techniques, the overarching goals are to convey genuine and accurate empathy through verbal and non-verbal communication and to provide an environment free of judgment or condescension. An example would be a non-directive and thoughtful open-ended question such as, "What do you need to feel better?" or "Please let me know if at any point you are uncomfortable or need a break." This therapeutic orientation assumes a fundamental impetus for personal growth is achieved through a healthy relationship with another person who can demonstrate active listening and accurate identification of your mental and emotional status.

For patients with a history of repeated traumatization, particularly those who have suffered recurrent sexual violence or exorbitant and malicious neglect, the initial encounter represents a singular opportunity for healthcare professionals to be seen as potential allies. In the case example of Ella, the opening progress note which documents the emergency medicine attending physician's findings and referral, appears to indicate significant negative countertransference and the distinct absence of a trauma-informed approach: the minor victim is mislabeled as a "sex worker," and the slang definition "pimp" is used to refer to her trafficker or exploiter. The label "sex worker" implies a volitional component which undermines the criminality and victimization inherent in the situation. "Sex worker" is not only an inaccurate label in this situation but may also serve to stigmatize and interfere with the quality of the patient's medical care. One could reasonably assume that the physician's countertransference is due at least in part to an antiquated and stereotyped generalization about the character qualities of people who engage in the solicitation of sexually based services. Moreover, there exists an even greater risk for being trafficked given the youth's transgender identity which may have been experienced as stigmatizing and socially isolative [3]. In summary, the provider is advised to exercise caution and discretion when choosing trafficking-related terminology as it may affect the professional judgment and objectivity of their colleagues and, as a result, the quality of care for the patient.

Approaches for Assessment and Psychiatric Care

Commercially sexually exploited (CSE) youth most commonly present to healthcare settings directly following an assault or disruption of the relationship with a trafficker, or due to an acute medical symptom [5, 6]. The most common medical presentations include sexually transmitted infections, pregnancy, pelvic inflammatory disease, complications from abortions, and bodily injuries [7]. Psychiatrists may become involved when consulted by other medical disciplines either when acute mental health symptoms become overtly concerning or when the patient is brought in by child welfare workers for symptoms related to trauma, substance abuse/intoxication, anxiety, depression, and PTSD [7]. If electing to be proactive, psychiatrists or other mental health professionals may choose to integrate a human trafficking assessment into their intake or other evaluative process.

Many CSE youth fear asking for or accepting help and are altogether wary of trusting authority (i.e., healthcare systems and professionals): consequently, they often appear reluctant or even ashamed when prompted to discuss personal, often painful, past experiences [8]. In addition, former negative experiences with mental health professionals [9], cultural mistrust of healthcare professionals, and/or fear of law enforcement/immigration officials may be transferred onto members of the treatment team, further inhibiting the potential for an outcry (i.e., disclosure of trafficking victimization) [10]. Other factors making self-disclosure infrequent are fear of retaliation from the trafficker, personal feelings of embarrassment and/or hopelessness, and the trauma bonds formed from an allegiance to the trafficker [10]. Such factors, along with the trafficker's use of coercive psychological techniques to control victims, may create major barriers to connecting these patients with available resources.

Psychological Coercive Techniques

Nonphysical psychological tactics such as deception, intimidation, fear, shame, humiliation, and manipulation are employed by the trafficker in order to control and dominate their victims. The eight methods of psychological coercion identified through research to enforce compliance of trafficking victims include isolation, monopolization of perception, induced debility or exhaustion, threats, occasional indulgences, demonstration of omnipotence, degradation, and enforcing trivial demands [9]. (See Chap. 8 for more on technology as a mechanism for control in human trafficking). Medical professionals must consider a history of such dynamics between their patient and their patient's trafficker during each clinical encounter. For instance, the aforementioned coercive techniques may have exhausted Ella's ability to cope with her environmental demands which ultimately led to a state of exhaustion and exacerbation of mental health symptoms. Both physical and sexual abuse coupled with psychological control tactics may be expected to result in psychiatric sequelae frequently seen in survivors of trafficking such as generalized depression and anxiety, trauma- and other stress-related symptoms, and substance use disorders [11]. If identified and psychiatrically treated, alternative coping strategies and healthier replacement behaviors can be taught to such patients to reduce their risk of further exploitation.

Screening and Assessment

The first step in human trafficking identification is to interview the CSE youth alone and to work on establishing trust and developing an alliance. CSE youth often do not recognize their situations as exploitative. They may feel responsible for their victimization, identify with their trafficker, or possess a limited ability to tell their story [12]. According to Chisolm-Straker et al. (2019), utilizing evidence-based screening tools such as the Quick Youth Indicators for Trafficking (QYIT) and then administering them in a confidential and secure environment – all while using a clinical approach that aims to minimize stress and limit the elicitation of explicit details of traumatic memories – may provide trafficked youth a better chance of being identified [13].

In 2018, Greenbaum et al. developed and validated a screening tool specifically designed for youth in an ED setting that is both short and data-driven. This study found that at least two positive answers in a six-item questionnaire could identify CSE youth with a sensitivity of 92%, a specificity of 73%, a positive predictive value of 51%, and a negative predictive value of 97% [14].

The Role of Psychiatry and Psychiatric Treatment Settings

Gordon and Salami (2018) recommended that providers of psychiatric care utilize an integrated, multi-disciplinary treatment team approach to providing comprehensive care for victims of human trafficking, which encompasses CSE youth. They also emphasized psychiatry's involvement in all levels of care and points of assisting trafficking victims; these include assessing for human trafficking victimization, mental health treatment and medication management, safe reintegration back into the community, and the provision of ongoing care [15]. Further, the authors suggest mental health professionals consider the value of liaising with various systems of care, help connect patients with needed medical and social work services, then act as facilitators to move patients through different services to increase their access to and use of needed resources.

Relative to generalists in psychiatry, child and adolescent psychiatrists are uniquely positioned to screen and identify CSE youth and should be involved with multiple aspects of their treatment whenever possible [7]. Psychiatric inpatient units and community outpatient clinics can provide the therapeutic environment that fosters development of the kind of therapeutic rapport necessary to generate trust and a working alliance between survivors and their healthcare team. In addition, such treatment settings can function as sites for assessment and identification and as a platform for applicable community-based anti-trafficking agency referrals. It is particularly important for patients with a history of trafficking to feel safe and welcomed within a psychiatric setting, as feelings of security may increase the likelihood of a patient's outcry and/or acceptance of help. Psychiatrists who gain patient trust, who acknowledge the potential impact of trauma, and who strive to construct treatment plans that prioritize the autonomy and wishes of the survivor are much more likely to form lasting therapeutic alliances with this distinctive patient population [7, 8].

In certain clinical situations such as acute psychiatric decompensation and imminent threats of harm to self or others, an elevated level of care – such as an inpatient psychiatric unit – may become necessary to ensure patient and/or public safety. The primary focus of treatment in such a highly structured setting is acute stabilization of psychiatric symptoms. In a 2017 paper [8], psychiatric inpatient units, specifically, were discussed as a treatment milieu providing a potential advantage for trafficking victims when compared with other levels of psychiatric or medical care. Inpatient psychiatric units may serve as a crucial location for identification, initiation of biopsychosocial treatment, as well as learning a person's trafficking history in an environment conducive to confidentiality, safety, and patient-centered care [8, 15].

Within an inpatient setting, psychiatrists may better help patients interrupt their cycle of trafficking and prevent re-victimization [15, 16]. One proposed reason for this is the increased amount of time available to initiate the kinds of biopsychosocial interventions which may lead to decreased vulnerability to future exploitation. In addition, psychiatric inpatient settings allow for victims' and survivors' complete separation from the trafficker by maintaining an access-restricted environment. Typically, psychiatric inpatient units provide a good patient-to-provider ratio and make available an integrated, multidisciplinary team of medical and social work staff who can collaboratively support traumatized patients using multiple models of care [8]. There are often a range of treatment providers at different levels with whom the patient may share information pertaining to a potential history of trafficking victimization. This can provide more opportunities for identification, alliance building, and improving patients' trust across healthcare professions, which in turn could lead to increased willingness to engage supportive services offered by the healthcare system.

When applicable, acute inpatient psychiatric settings make accessible medical care across specialties through a consultation model. Because patients with a history of being trafficked may present with complex medical problems and historically have had limited access to quality medical care, all serious and relevant aspects of their healthcare should be assessed and addressed (dental, respiratory, cardiovascular, neurological, gynecological, substance use disorder diagnoses, surgical, etc.). Medical interventions may be easier in a setting where a victim/survivor is separated from the trafficker (who may have previously blocked or restricted the victim's access to care) [8].

Trafficked youth commonly experience psychiatric symptoms as a result of depression, anxiety, substance use, and/or trauma [2, 3, 5]. Often, they are vulnerable to experiencing exacerbations of their mental health symptoms due to repeated exposure to environmental stressors such as violence, terrorization, isolation, and the general lack of autonomy (i.e., servitude) characteristic of trafficking situations. Additionally, complex childhood trauma is believed to predispose individuals to the development of mental health disorders and other vulnerabilities associated with an increased likelihood for future victimization [2, 3, 5]. A recent study of CSE youth found significantly elevated rates of depression, with more than half of the respondents also exhibiting problems with anger, anxiety, and attachment [7]. CSE youth understandably also have an increased tendency to exhibit maladaptive coping skills, including non-suicidal self-injury (NSSI) behaviors, and may present to medical settings for suicidal ideation, plan, or attempt [5, 6, 9]. In the case of Ella, she presented with symptoms of suicidal ideation, self-harm, depression, anxiety, and chronic and/or acute trauma. Consequently, after being treated in the emergency department and medically cleared, an inpatient psychiatric admission was initiated for the purpose of stabilization, safety evaluation, and the initiation of mental health treatment.

A Trauma-Informed Approach

To date, there are no standardized treatment guidelines in psychiatry tailored for CSE youth regarding how best to deliver therapeutic treatment services [17]. In general, it has been recommended by researchers and advocacy groups alike to treat victims of trafficking with a trauma-informed approach. Such an approach has been empirically validated with other marginalized groups who have suffered repeated and prolonged exposure to traumatic events including war, torture, domestic violence, and sexual abuse [6]. To meet clinical criteria for DSM-IV diagnosis, PTSD present as four clusters of symptoms: re-experiencing symptoms, avoidance symptoms, negative changes in mood and brain function, and hyperarousal symptoms. Rafferty (2018) recently outlined a trauma-informed approach to patient care, which emphasizes avoiding re-traumatization of victims by triggering feelings and states of emotional arousal similar to those that were elicited during their trafficking victimization. The author suggests all healthcare professionals be trained in trauma-informed approaches, especially any staff who facilitates the delivery of mental health services [18].

Training mental health staff in the provision of a trauma-informed approach involves teaching dialectic clinical techniques which simultaneously demonstrate to the patient both support and empowerment [13]. Correspondingly, the treatment team should routinely convey overt sensitivity through warm and clear communication that accurately tracks a patient's emotional state. To deliver clinical services in a trauma-informed and trauma-sensitive manner, the trained clinician's feelings and behaviors would include empathic reactions to even difficult patient behaviors such as hostility, hypervigilance/suspicion, self-harm gestures, and acting-out [19]. In summary, a trauma-informed treatment approach would apply to all points of service with an overarching goal of providing necessary medical and psychiatric treatment while mostly avoiding the use of interventions likely to trigger trauma-related symptoms in the patient [13]. If a CSE youth patient is treated in a setting where psychiatric and/or environmental safety emergencies might occur due to the behavior of other patients (e.g., agitation/aggression, mania, psychosis, or other acute mental health symptoms of dysregulation or decompensation), staff must work collaboratively to minimize the youths' exposure to these events in order to reduce the potential for re-traumatization. Victims of violence (e.g., human trafficking victims and CSE youth) can be expected to benefit from a predictable and safe environment [2, 8, 20].

Patient autonomy must be emphasized in the decision-making process related to use of psychiatric medications. Ella's case illustrates that emergency medications may need to be considered when managing an emerging safety risk. The use of emergency psychiatric medication should be carefully considered in any treatment setting but may prove explicitly problematic for the patient–provider alliance when working with CSE youth who show symptoms of severe trauma. Because acute and posttraumatic symptoms can be both psychological and physical in nature, patients who experience severe trauma-related symptoms may enter into a state of acute mental distress with negatively skewed thinking and impaired judgment, impulse-control, and self-awareness [21, 22]. Furthermore, the stimuli which trigger severe PTSD symptoms may in some cases result in full or partial dissociation, hyperarousal, motor agitation/retardation, difficulty with communication, or weakening of reality-testing ability. When acutely triggered, a patient is typically flooded with vivid and painful memories of the trauma which consequently destabilizes their psychological condition. Patients whose trauma-related symptoms coalesce to form marked expression of their trauma may become outwardly expressive (e.g., hypervigilance) or retreat inward (e.g., depression). Assessing a patient while they are experiencing such dysregulated states is difficult and potentially unsafe. Verbal de-escalation should always be attempted first, with oral medications offered only after this approach fails. If psychiatric medications for acute agitation or psychosis must be given by intramuscular route, this should occur with as much autonomy afforded to the patient as possible and based on best ethical clinical practice. Forming trust while using tactics of coercion and ultimatums in this already vulnerable population may prove exceedingly challenging, and treatment should strive to be patient-centered and trauma-informed, although not at the expense of safety for the staff or the patient.

Psychological Treatments

Psychological treatments that are evidence based and well established with traumatized youth include multisystemic therapy for child abuse and neglect (MST-CAN), dialectical behavior therapy (DBT) for teenagers and young adults, and trauma-focused cognitive behavioral therapy (TF-CBT). MST-CAN is an intensive approach for system-involved youth and requires the participation of multiple therapists, a psychiatrist, and a caseworker. Services are delivered in a suitable location, are multimodal in nature, and provide skill building and support opportunities for both the caregivers and the youth. In a 2010 study, MST-CAN was found to be significantly more effective in reducing mental health symptoms, parental distress and the behaviors associated with maltreatment, out-of-home placements, and incidents of re-abuse [23]. The adaptation of DBT for youth is similar in structure and practice to its adult-normed counterpart apart from the caregivers' involvement in treatment. DBT teaches mindfulness, interpersonal skills, emotion regulation, and distress tolerance; the adapted version adds a domain termed "walking the middle path," which acknowledges the worldview differences of parents and children [24]. As a treatment modality, TF-CBT has proven efficacious with survivors of child sexual abuse and may represent a promising potential treatment option for CSE youth [25]. TF-CBT is typically initiated in an outpatient mental health setting, but some inpatient psychiatric centers may offer augmented psychological treatment approaches, initiate psychoeducation related to trauma, and provide coping skills and brief therapeutic support without causing de-stabilization of symptoms [8].

Nguyen et al. discussed the importance of knowing and understanding patients' trafficking histories to inform the treatment plan and associated interventions, and to break the cycle of re-victimization. Clinicians must understand the multiple biopsychosocial factors that influence medical illnesses and psychiatric conditions and must seek to resolve exacerbating environmental stressors. Accessing all available psychological, medical, and social service resources may lead to more long-term solutions and may decrease susceptibility to trafficking victimization in the future

[8, 26]. Too often CSE youth are dismissed as simply troubled, delinquent, and/or mentally-ill in a manner not accurate or representative of the complex trauma and its associated symptoms [27].

Case Resolution

Ella initially struggled to build trust with her providers and exhibited moderate paranoia and hypervigilance, but ultimately, she was able to build a working alliance with a staff nurse and her treating psychiatrist. By disclosing aspects of her trauma history, Ella may have gained access to specialized anti–human trafficking services. Although she nearly required emergent medication via intramuscular route, staff on the unit utilized a trauma-informed approach and were able to verbally de-escalate the situation and minimize the use of unnecessary medication. This de-escalation protected the patient–provider therapeutic relationship, built on trust. Precisely because it is very difficult to examine, interview, or treat an agitated patient, healthcare staff must be trained to use trauma-informed techniques at each level of service. Ella's mental health symptoms were likely exacerbated by or the direct result of her trafficking experience, but similar reactions occur in patients with a history of sexual abuse, rape, torture, and psychosis. Therefore, psychiatric treatment recommendations for CSE youth may be applicable to other clinical situations as well.

Conclusions and Directions toward Future Care Models: Psychiatric Providers Utilizing an Integrated, Multi-disciplinary Treatment Approach

Psychiatrists and mental health treatment settings can serve as important agents of trust building and alliance formation with CSE youth through the provision of therapeutic support, empathic validation, and maintenance of safety as these youth undergo treatment. Interdisciplinary healthcare teams such as medicine, nursing, social work, case management, psychology, and chaplaincy services should consult and work in tandem with psychiatry depending on the individual needs of the patient [8, 9, 14, 21]. Potential resources for patients beyond medical care should include short- and long-term housing, vocational rehabilitation agencies, transportation services, food banks, access to clothing and hygiene products, child protective services, and others [8, 24]. Additionally, treatment team members should align with local immigration and legal aid organizations to advocate for patients who are undocumented or have legal concerns related to their trafficking history [8].

Future areas to be explored in human trafficking-related psychiatric research include [8, 9, 15]:

- Comparing best treatment modalities for patients with psychiatric comorbidities
- Examining how psychiatric illnesses or childhood trauma can exacerbate and perpetuate the risk of becoming a victim of trafficking
- Exploring how psychiatric conditions can complicate the identification of victims and hinder self-disclosure from patients
- Describing how to approach screening services with markedly decompensated psychiatric patients

Psychiatry as a profession can bring awareness to the critical public health issue of human trafficking by (1) promoting education of this topic in residency and fellowship training programs and (2) publishing and sharing research/work with this patient population [15].

References

1. Blanch A. SAMHSA's national center for trauma-informed care changing communities, changing lives [Internet]. National Center for Trauma Informed Care; 2012 [cited 2019 Oct 1]. Available from: https://nasmhpd.org/sites/default/files/NCTIC_Marketing_Brochure_FINAL(2).pdf.
2. Hopper EK, Gonzalez LD. A comparison of psychological symptoms in survivors of sex and labor trafficking. Behav Med. 2018;44(3):177–88.
3. Kiss L, Yun K, Pocock N, Zimmerman C. Exploitation, violence, and suicide risk among child and adolescent survivors of human trafficking in the greater mekong subregion. JAMA Pediatr. 2015;169(9):e152278.
4. Joseph S. Client-centred therapy, post-traumatic stress disorder and post-traumatic growth: theoretical perspectives and practical implications. Psychol Psychother. 2004;77(Pt 1):101–19.
5. Zimmerman C, Hossain M, Yun K, Roche B, Morison L, Watts C. Stolen smiles: a summary report on the physical and psychological health consequences of women and adolescents trafficked in Europe. Lond Sch Hyg Trop Med [Internet]. 2006 [cited 2019 Oct 1]. Available from: https://doi.org/www.lshtm.ac.uk/php/ghd/docs/stolensmiles.pdf.
6. Chisolm-Straker M, Baldwin S, Gaïgbé-Togbé B, Ndukwe N, Johnson PN, Richardson LD. Health care and human trafficking: we are seeing the unseen. J Health Care Poor Underserved. 2016;27(3):1220–33.
7. Ijadi-Maghsoodi R, Todd EJ, Bath EPJ. Commercial sexual exploitation of children and the role of the child psychiatrist. J Am Acad Child Adolesc Psychiatry. 2014;53(8):825–9.
8. Nguyen PT, Coverdale JH, Gordon MR. Identifying, treating, and advocating for human trafficking victims: a key role for psychiatric inpatient units. Gen Hosp Psychiatry. 2017;46:41–3.
9. Baldwin SB, Eisenman DP, Sayles JN, Ryan G, Chuang KS. Identification of human trafficking victims in health care settings. Health Hum Rights. 2011;13(1):E36–49.
10. Rhodes SD, Mann L, Simán FM, Song E, Alonzo J, Downs M, et al. The impact of local immigration enforcement policies on the health of immigrant hispanics/latinos in the United States. Am J Public Health. 2015;105(2):329–37.
11. Najavits LM, Weiss RD, Shaw SR. The link between substance abuse and posttraumatic stress disorder in women. Am J Addict. 2010;6(4):273–83.
12. Fund FV. Turning pain into power: trafficking survivors' perspectives on early intervention strategies. In: Turning pain into power: Trafficking survivors' perspectives on early intervention strategies; 2005.

13. Chisolm-Straker M, Miller CL, Duke G, Stoklosa H. A framework for the development of healthcare provider education programs on human trafficking part two: survivors. J HumTraffick. 2019;17:1–15.
14. Greenbaum VJ, Dodd M, McCracken C. A short screening tool to identify victims of child sex trafficking in the health care setting. Pediatr Emerg Care. 2018;34(1):33–7.
15. Gordon M, Salami T, Coverdale J, Nguyen PT. Psychiatry's role in the management of human trafficking victims: an integrated care approach. J Psychiatr Pract. 2018;24(2):79–86.
16. Macias-Konstantopoulos W. Human trafficking: the role of medicine in interrupting the cycle of abuse and violence. Ann Intern Med. 2016;165(8):582–8.
17. Coverdale J, Beresin EV, Louie AK, Balon R, Roberts LW. Human trafficking and psychiatric education: a call to action. Acad Psychiatry. 2016;40(1):119–23.
18. Rafferty Y. Mental health services as a vital component of psychosocial recovery for victims of child trafficking for commercial sexual exploitation. Am J Orthopsychiatry. 2018;88(3):249–60.
19. Hossain M, Zimmerman C, Abas M, Light M, Watts C. The relationship of trauma to mental disorders among trafficked and sexually exploited girls and women. Am J Public Health. 2010;100(12):2442–9.
20. Ottisova L, Hemmings S, Howard LM, Zimmerman C, Oram S. Prevalence and risk of violence and the mental, physical and sexual health problems associated with human trafficking: an updated systematic review. Epidemiol Psychiatr Sci. 2016;25(4):317–41.
21. Tsutsumi A, Izutsu T, Poudyal AK, Kato S, Marui E. Mental health of female survivors of human trafficking in Nepal. Soc Sci Med. 2008;66(8):1841–7.
22. WestCoast Children's Clinic. Research to action: Sexually Exploited Minors (SEM) needs and strengths [Internet]. WestCoast Children's Clinic. 2012 [cited 2019 Oct 2]. Available from: https://www.westcoastcc.org/wp-content/uploads/2012/05/WCC_SEM_Needs-and-Strengths_FINAL.pdf.
23. Swenson CC, Schaeffer CM, Henggeler SW, Faldowski R, Mayhew AM. Multisystemic therapy for child abuse and neglect: a randomized effectiveness trial. J Family Psycholog [Internet]. 2010;24(4):497–507. https://doi.org/10.1037/a0020324.
24. Freeman KR, James S, Klein KP, Mayo D, Montgomery S. Outpatient dialectical behavior therapy for adolescents engaged in deliberate self-harm: conceptual and methodological considerations. Child Adolesc Social Work J. 2016;33(2):123–35. https://doi.org/10.1007/s10560-015-0412-6.
25. Ramirez de Arellano MA, Lyman DR, Jobe-Shields L, George P, Dougherty RH, Daniels AS, et al. Trauma-focused cognitive-behavioral therapy for children and adolescents: assessing the evidence. Psychiatr Serv. 2014;65(5):591–602.
26. Harris M, Fallot RD. Envisioning a trauma-informed service system: a vital paradigm shift. New Dir Ment Health Serv. 2001;89:3–22.
27. Kerig PK, Ward RM, Vanderzee KL, Moeddel MA. Posttraumatic stress as a mediator of the relationship between trauma and mental health problems among juvenile delinquents. J Youth Adolesc. 2009;38(9):1214–25.

Chapter 10
Human Trafficking in Adolescents and Young Adults with Co-existing Disordered Eating Behaviors

Tonya Chaffee, Kristina L. Borham, Nadia E. Saldanha, Amy Gajaria, and Heidi Strickler

Case Presentation

Case 1: Ana Ana, an 18-year-old young woman, was referred to the adolescent clinic after hospitalization for clinically significant hypophosphatemia, hypokalemia, and prolonged QT. She initially presented to an emergency department (ED) for a pre-syncopal episode after feeling shortness of breath, hand cramping, weakness, and dizziness. Her height was 5′ 3.8″ and her weight on admission was 43.6 kg but her previous maximum weight was noted to be around 50 kg. Upon initial ED evaluation, she was noted to have potassium 2.4 and phosphorous 2 and an abnormal electrocardiogram. Given her presentation, and because of her need for extended electrolyte stabilization including potassium supplementation to correct her

T. Chaffee (✉)
Department of Pediatrics, University of California, San Francisco, Teen and Young Adult Health Center, Zuckerberg San Francisco General Hospital, San Francisco, CA, USA

K. L. Borham
Department of Obstetrics and Gynecology, Walter Reed National Military Medical Center, Bethesda, MD, USA

N. E. Saldanha
Department of Pediatrics, Division of Adolescent Medicine Hofstra Northwell School of Medicine, Cohen Children's Medical Center Queens, New Hyde Park, NY, USA

A. Gajaria
Department of Psychiatry, University of Toronto, Toronto, ON, Canada

H. Strickler
United Healthcare Community & State, Maryland Heights, MO, USA

K. E. Titchen, E. Miller (eds.), *Medical Perspectives on Human Trafficking in Adolescents*, https://doi.org/10.1007/978-3-030-43367-3_10

prolonged QT, there was concern the patient may have an eating disorder. Further lab work-up during her hospitalization was negative for other etiologies of her electrolyte abnormalities. Ana had denied any binging or purging behavior, and reported being happy with her weight, denied knowledge of any weight loss, and was not trying to lose weight.

Further social history obtained included that Ana had immigrated to the United States 2 years before this encounter and that she had reported "lot of responsibilities at home" as well as work on her graduate educational diploma (GED) to get into nursing school. She reported feeling anxious and tired, had trouble sleeping, and felt some social isolation since immigrating. She missed her home country but reported being happy to be in the United States.

Upon discharge from the hospital, her plan was for daily nutritional shakes and a multivitamin to maximize her weight and nutritional status, and after consultation with the adolescent medicine service regarding the concerns of disordered eating, she was to have close follow-up to monitor her weight and a mental health referral to assess for an eating disorder.

Ana missed several scheduled and rescheduled follow-up appointments after her hospitalization and was not reevaluated until 3 months after discharge from the hospital. Of note, Ana was not a native English speaker, and this proved a barrier to her follow-up care and post–hospital treatment plan. At her first follow-up visit to the adolescent clinic, she reported feeling "tired and weak." She denied any sick contacts, shortness of breath, lightheadedness, palpitations, or chest pain. She admitted to not eating regular meals since her hospitalization, and she stopped taking her multivitamin and nutritional shake because she did not like the taste and did not understand the need for them. She did report having regular menses. She never had been sexually active, and she denied drug or alcohol use. At this visit she reported living with her father and three teenage brothers.

On exam Ana was noted to be afebrile, normotensive, and mildly tachycardic and with no orthostatic changes. Her weight had decreased 1 kg since her hospitalization. She showed no stigmata for purging, including normal dentition, no callouses on her fingers, and no parotid enlargement. Labs were obtained to assess her current nutritional status. Given her report of inadequate nutritional intake, and her noted weight loss, Ana was counseled via a medical interpreter about the importance of increasing her caloric intake including three regular meals with two nutritional shakes daily until her next follow-up. A social work consultation was also placed to facilitate a mental health referral.

At her subsequent two-week follow-up visit, all labs were noted to be within normal limits, except for a mild normocytic anemia due to a mild iron deficiency. In the interim, Ana was assessed by the clinic's social worker, who noted that the patient reported history of physical and sexual abuse from a family member in her home country. As a result, she had a history of multiple different living arrangements prior to immigrating to the United States. Ana also reported that she had many responsibilities at home that included cooking, cleaning, and other household tasks. She reported having a difficult time balancing these tasks with her GED studies. She told the social worker that she was living with her stepmother, and not her father and brothers as she had previously reported.

Given her current living situation, and history of sexual and physical abuse, it was determined that her social stressors may have been contributing to her mental and physical health and subsequent challenges in getting enough caloric intake to gain weight. Ana agreed to follow-up and was referred to see a mental health therapist.

At the follow-up visit, Ana reported she had not seen the therapist yet, and her weight was noted to have dropped again. She reported continued regular menses, and she was trying to incorporate more snacks since she had run out of nutritional shakes. Upon further inquiry into her living situation and based on inconsistencies from previous visits, Ana reported that she was not actually living with her stepmother, but a friend of her father's. She subsequently disclosed that she was forced to care for this woman's children all day as well as required to cook and perform many other household chores for her brother and father and was threatened with deportation if she did not comply. She was again referred for a mental health evaluation as well as to a local agency working with human trafficking survivors, but the patient was subsequently lost to follow-up

Clinical Questions to Consider

1. *What are some of the red flags or other indicators that this young woman may be a victim of human trafficking?*
2. *What are some indicators that she does or does not have an eating disorder?*
3. *How can clinicians better identify those who may be trafficked for labor or sex and who may be suffering from disordered eating behaviors due to their trafficking situation?*

Red Flags for Human Trafficking

To date there is very little in the literature to suggest that disordered eating is a specific indicator of human trafficking; however, this chapter highlights two cases – one from the perspective of how human trafficking can present with a disordered eating diagnosis, and a second case that underscores the complexities in treatment and long-term management of a human trafficking survivor with an eating disorder.

As noted in this first case, even before there is any disclosure of trafficking, there are important indicators based on her past medical history and other historical factors that would raise suspicion for possible risks for exploitation in this young woman. Some of these indicators are for both labor and sex trafficking, and others are more specific to labor trafficking. Particular details contained within her social history, e.g., history of sexual and physical abuse, indicate a higher risk for susceptibility to human trafficking [1]. Her unknown immigration status is another such indicator [1]. When caring for patients suspected for trafficking with unknown legal status, it is important to differentiate trafficking from smuggling. Smuggling is defined as "the importation of people into the United States involving deliberate evasion of immigration laws" and is transportation based [2]. Smuggling is usually a consensual agreement to illegally enter a foreign country and is provided as a service to the immigrant [2]. It is important to note that what may begin as smuggling can evolve into trafficking [1] (See Chaps. 3 and 5 for further detail). New immigrants may rely on traffickers to provide basic needs such as food and shelter, as well financial support during their transition period. Traffickers may withhold official identification and travel documentation, and victims may fear accessing care for risk of deportation [1]. In Ana's case, we learn she was not in the legal guardianship of her family and was therefore at risk for being trafficked when she immigrated to the United States. In addition, because she immigrated to the United States as a minor, this put her at even higher risk of being trafficked [3]. Ana was not a native English speaker, and language barriers can limit victims' ability to disclose their situation to a healthcare provider, especially when accompanied by a native English-speaking trafficker [1]. Similarly, Ana's description of her living situation constantly changed, throwing into question the stability of her housing, and this is also considered a red flag for trafficking [4]. Inconsistent histories such as this should be considered a red flag for possibility of being trafficked, as the patient may be trying to avoid, or be fearful of disclosing their trafficking situation [1]. Clinicians should offer information and support regardless of disclosure, and an inquiry about being trafficked should be asked only while the patient is alone with a healthcare provider and using a professional, medically trained translator if the patient is not a native English speaker.

Of additional significance is Ana's history of sexual abuse by her family member. History of sexual abuse is a well-known significant risk factor for human trafficking, particularly child sexual abuse [5]. It has been estimated that 70–90% of commercially sexually exploited youth have a history of sexual abuse and are 28 times more likely to be arrested for prostitution at a later point in life [6].

Although Ana describes undertaking studies to obtain a GED in hopes of starting nursing school, many victims of human trafficking may be given false promises of education and employment when immigrating to the United States. Traffickers subsequently may force their victims to work under inhumane conditions with the expectation of long hours, often unpaid [1]. Victims may be threatened with deportation if they leave or disclose their trafficking situation, or they may be coerced through debt bonds or threats to their family members in their home countries [1, 3]. Ana's disclosure of her desire to pursue education (while a key strength) also demonstrates one of the root causes for vulnerability to exploitation for immigrants, particularly those who come from countries with limited educational achievement and economic opportunities in their home countries [3, 7]. (See Chap. 5 for further information.)

Physical Exam Findings

Known physical exam findings for both sex and labor trafficking include dehydration, electrolyte abnormalities, low BMI, loss of appetite, tooth pain, weight loss, fatigue, and exhaustion [8, 9]. These may result from poor access to healthcare and

Table 10.1 Potential Indicators on Physical Exam of Human Trafficking (From *Adolescent Gynecology Clinical Casebook*)

Health Sequelae of Human Sex Trafficking
Bums, branding, tattoos, and other purposeful and permanent stigmata of "ownership"
Trauma by blunt force, gun, knife, or strangulation
Fractures, dental and oral cavity injuries, and traumatic brain injury inconsistent with the history
Neuropathies and other effects of torture
Scarring, especially from unattended prior injuries
Genital trauma
Repeated unwanted pregnancy and/or forced abortion
Sexually transmitted infections (e.g., chlamydia, gonorrhea, human papilloma virus, hepatitis B and C, and HIV)
Infertility, chronic pelvic pain, cervical cancer, liver failure, HIV-AIDS, and chronic disease states resulting from untreated sexually transmitted infections
Impaired social skills
Long-term effects of inadequate treatment of common childhood diseases
Headaches, chronic pain syndromes, and abdominal complaints
Fatigue
Substance abuse
Infectious diseases usually prevented through routine immunization
Psychological sequelae: feelings of intense stigma, shame, anxiety, and hopelessness, pathologic fear, panic attacks, sleep disturbances, dissociative disorders, depression, post-traumatic stress disorder, and suicidal ideation and/or attempt

Adapted from http://www.massmed.org/Patient-Care/Health-Topics/Violence-Prevention-and-Intervention-Human-Trafficking-(pdf)/

food, irregular eating schedules, and traffickers' use of food as a means of control. Trafficking-related medical conditions such as anemia, communicable diseases, addiction, malnutrition, sleep cycle disorders, and environmental exposures may also lead to the aforementioned physical exam findings [8, 9] (see Table 10.1).

Disordered Eating Behaviors

Weight loss is a common presenting symptom of many organic etiologies including malignancies, malabsorption-related illnesses, and endocrine disorders, among others [10] (see Table 10.2). Once an evaluation has been completed to rule out these causes, as occurred during the inpatient course for this patient, an eating disorder becomes a diagnosis of exclusion for the weight loss. Eating disorders that feature weight loss as defined by the DSM-5 can include anorexia nervosa where there is a clear desire to lose weight and caloric restriction is intentional; atypical anorexia nervosa in which the amount of weight loss and medical complications are similar to anorexia nervosa but in patients with an average or above-average body mass index (BMI) or avoidant restrictive food intake disorder (ARFID) in which the weight loss may be unintentional and undesired but there is a fear of eating due to general anxiety or a specific phobia of choking or allergic reaction or other

Table 10.2 Possible Findings on Physical Examination in Children and Adolescents with Eating Disorders

Anorexia Nervosa	Bulimia Nervosa
Bradycardia	Sinus bradycardia
Orthostatic by pulse or blood pressure	Orthostatic by pulse or blood pressure
Hypothermia	Hypothermia
Cardiac murmur (one third with mitral valve prolapse)	Cardiac murmur (mitral valve prolapse)
Dull, thinning scalp hair	Hair without shine
Sunken cheeks, sallow skin	Dry skin
Lanugo	Parotitis
Atrophic breasts (postpubertal)	Russell's sign (callous on knuckles from self-induced emesis)
Atrophic vaginitis (postpubertal)	Mouth sores
Pitting edema of extremities	Palatal scratches
Emaciated, may wear oversized clothes	Dental enamel erosions
Flat affect	May look entirely normal
Cold extremities, acrocyanosis	Other cardiac arrhythmias

Identifying and Treating Eating Disorder, American Academy of Pediatrics, Policy Statement, Committee on Adolescents. Pediatrics. 2003:111;204. https://doi.org/10.1542/peds.111.1.204

sensory-based avoidance [11]. Ana's first presentation to the emergency room showed findings that are generally present in more severe cases of malnutrition. Whereas many patients with eating disorders will have normal electrolytes and a normal electrocardiogram (EKG), Ana's hypokalemia was significant and is more typically seen in patients with purging but also can be seen in cases of malnutrition. Many eating disorder patients exhibit bradycardia, but prolonged QT is a rarer EKG finding and, in Ana's case, likely due to a profound hypokalemia. Hypophosphatemia may be due to malnutrition but is more common and more worrisome during the refeeding process when the increased nutritional load causes an intracellular shift of ions such as phosphorus due to an increase in insulin. Hypophosphatemia can cause seizures, delirium, coma, and even death [12].

While it was certainly appropriate to consider an eating disorder as the primary etiology of Ana's clinical picture, the severity of her presentation coupled with her lack of a desire to lose weight should have prompted clinicians to investigate what else may have been contributing to her state of severe malnutrition. There can be a fair amount of secrecy due to guilt and shame for many patients with eating disorders, so an initial statement that there is no desire to lose weight may not always be accurate. This patient was willing to make additions to her diet and drink nutritional supplements when available. This supports the probability that her weight loss was unintentional and due to food insecurity related to her trafficking situation. When patients appear motivated to gain weight and are willing to make changes to their diet yet continue to lose weight, clinicians should investigate further and assess for food insecurity. To meet a DSM-5 diagnosis of an eating disorder, inadequate access to nutrition cannot be the primary cause [13]. For this patient, anxiety and stress related to her possible trafficking situation may also have contributed to weight loss, suppressing her appetite. Data is limited with regard to the physical toll of trafficking, but Oram et al. did find that a high percentage of women who were trafficked reported weight loss, loss of appetite, and stomach pain, highlighting the overlap in presentation and the need to look for other red flags to avoid missing a victim of human trafficking [8].

Treatment Plan, Follow-Up

Ana's case presents some of the common difficulties in caring for trafficking survivors: a lack of return to care and adherence to treatment plans, and a lack of trust in the healthcare system that may be exacerbated by language and other communication barriers. While these may be indicators of other psychosocial problems (transportation barriers, personal beliefs about healthcare, working hour conflict, etc.), these are also important risk factors for human trafficking [5, 6]. Clinicians should consider asking about trafficking early in the initial evaluation, as well as providing information regardless of any disclosure (including hotline numbers and available services) [5].

Maintaining an index of suspicion in certain clinical presentations will enhance the clinician's ability to recognize and aid trafficking survivors. A skilled clinician should follow up on abnormal lab values, and any concerning activities and behaviors, and should utilize non-relative medically trained interpreters in obtaining medical and social history and to assess inconsistencies in the medical history. Ongoing informed assessment will help identify concurrent and separate issues from human trafficking. Various assessment tools are available to identify trafficking (see Chap. 3, Table 3.3 and section "Assessment Tools" in chapter 4 for further details).

It is also important to understand that patients may not identify and/or disclose trafficking status even when asked [1, 5]. Many patients do not recognize their situation as a victim of human trafficking, particularly in individuals who have been exploited for long periods of time where the abuse is normalized [1, 5]. Self-identification and disclosure can also be hindered by fear, shame, language barriers, and poor follow-up as reported by survivors [1]. Disclosure can be facilitated by building a long-term, trusting, and non-judgmental relationship with the patient to help provide safety and referral for support [1]. And it is important to remember that disclosure is not the goal, and survivors who do disclose report negative experiences of being dismissed, judged, shamed, not listened to, and denied resources [14]. Instead, a strong clinician–patient relationship will provide a safe space for survivors to receive appropriate trauma-sensitive care. If a disclosure is obtained, varying state laws mandate reporting [15]. Mandated reporting may be required in cases of minor exploitation. Like cases of intimate partner violence and sexual assault, the patient should be allowed to decide the next course of action including for law enforcement involvement as safety of the patient and team is paramount. See Chap. 18 for more about mandatory reporting and medicolegal aspects of human trafficking. See sections "Health Care Settings and Trafficking" in chapter 3 and "Trauma Informed Care" in chapter 4 and "Trauma Informed Care" in chapter 20 and Chap. 21, Figure 21.1 for more about trauma-informed and trauma-sensitive care.

Because human trafficking itself is not a primary diagnosis, it is essential to recognize the signs and address medical conditions that are concurrent with trafficking and consider this in the differential diagnosis. It is also essential to know that the goal of treatment is not to rescue survivors, but to help with safety planning and to provide access to resources. These include, but are not limited to, social work or case management, drug and alcohol rehabilitation, mental health services, housing opportunities, employment and financial assistance, primary care services, immigration and citizenship offices, and legal services. All care should be conducted in a trauma-informed manner and ideally in a multidisciplinary setting as this has been shown to be effective [5, 16]. It is imperative to ensure follow-up care which can be facilitated by case management to ensure medical follow-up including weight checks, reviewing imaging or laboratory studies, and routine care and to facilitate referrals for the often complex psychosocial challenges human trafficking survivors confront.

Case 2: Michael Michael is a 17-year-old African American gay identified male, who presented for psychotherapy due to a recent hospitalization for a suicide attempt by overdose. He had a known history of sex trafficking from age 13–15. He described failing most of his classes in school and then dropping out after ninth grade. He reported multiple male sex buyers many of whom were significantly older than him. He denied ever having a long-term or stable romantic relationship. He had a history of impulsive behavior and was previously diagnosed with post-traumatic stress disorder and severe major depressive disorder. In addition to these diagnoses, he presented with significant disordered eating behavior, including body dysmorphia, binge eating, and excessive exercise. The patient reported seeing himself as overweight and related a need to stay "fit," although his BMI was significantly below normal at 17. Michael also expressed a need to punish himself by not eating or not eating certain foods or excessively exercising. He was also noted to have been diagnosed with multiple sexually transmitted infections (STIs) while being trafficked and subsequently was diagnosed with human immunodeficiency virus (HIV).

Although this young man presented with restrictive disordered eating behavior in the setting of his co-occurring HIV and depression diagnoses, this was not initially considered a separate eating disorder. Michael's eating behaviors had previously been assumed to be "normal" for a teenage boy when the patient was binge-eating or were attributed to depression when the patient was restricting. No clinician considered the presence of a separate eating disorder nor considered that the patient's excessive exercise represented compensatory exercise as part of an eating disorder. In addition, the link between this disordered eating and the patient's trauma and trafficking history had not been explored.

Michael had a history of difficulty in engaging with medical and mental health services. Multiple attempts at outpatient mental health treatment including counseling had been unsuccessful, and he had a history of residential treatment for mental health and behavioral challenges. During his most recent hospitalization, he declined having medical exams and would often exhibit destructive behaviors such as detaching the leads from the monitors, becoming belligerent with hospital staff, and threatening staff. These resulted in another psychiatric admission, which was followed by outpatient therapy.

During therapy, Michael described how he would engage in relationships with abusive partners, often leaving safe situations and then finding himself unable to leave his new abusive situations. He reported being physically and sexually abused by those who were exploiting him in the sex trade as well as suffering abuse from other sexual partners. Michael did seek help out of his trafficking situation, but often the adults around him would not believe him or would blame him for his circumstances.

Questions to Consider

1. *What are some of the long-term mental and physical health consequences of being trafficked that should be considered in individuals who also have eating disorders?*
2. *How can healthcare professionals best care for survivors of trafficking who may have co-existing eating disorders, particularly to try to prevent these long-term health consequences?*

Long-Term Health and Mental Health Consequences to Consider

Care of patients who have been trafficked is challenging, as patients may present with multiple mental health and physical health needs, resulting from extended (sometimes lifelong) exposure to trauma. These needs often become chronic in nature and difficult to address in short-term or acute-care settings. Trauma symptoms are often exacerbated by repeated hospital admissions for crisis because of the lack of control experienced during these admissions. Such crisis admissions can consequently be experienced as re-enacting and revictimizing to the survivors. As a result, youth may begin to internalize a sense that their problems are far too complex to ever be addressed, leading to an increased sense of powerlessness and hopelessness about being able to act on their own behalf and engage in help-seeking or recovery-focused activities.

Michael's case demonstrates several components of complex trauma, which interferes with child and adolescent development and leads to dysfunction in multiple domains [17]. The domains include attachment, biology or physical health, affect regulation, dissociation, behavioral control/emotional regulation, cognition, and self-concept [17]. In terms of Michael's physical or biologic domain, he suffers significant medical infections as a result of being trafficked, including HIV, and he develops an eating disorder leading to malnutrition. Michael in Case 2, unlike Ana in Case 1, demonstrates more classic features of an eating disorder by using restrictive eating and excessive exercise to control his weight with an intentional focus on his body image. Eating disorders have a lifetime prevalence of 0.5–2%. The majority of those affected tend to be female, but more recent data suggest that 10–25% of these patients are male [18]. Because the focus on appearance and a desire to be thin are often associated with being female, many male eating disorder patients may present for care further into their illness when symptoms and signs are more severe [18]. This may mean that young men need more intensive treatment sooner. In addition, data suggest that LGBTQ adolescents have higher rates of body dissatisfaction than their heterosexual peers and are at greater risk for eating disorders [19]. Such may be the case for this patient. Treatment programs may also have a predominantly female population which can also make some male patients uninterested in being involved. Treatment remains the same for both males and females, with the goal of weight restoration and an absence of disordered eating [18]. Treatment occurs for most patients in an outpatient setting, but those with medical instability (severe bradycardia, hypothermia, hypotension, electrolyte abnormalities, EKG changes, among others) will require medical hospitalization for stabilization during the refeeding process [20]. Because eating disorders and other medical conditions resulting from being trafficked, such as HIV, are chronic in nature, they will require longitudinal follow-up in the context of a trusting patient–clinician relationship and with the coordination of medical, nutritional, and psychological care [17, 21].

Michael also demonstrates dysfunction in the domain of cognitive function due to inconsistent attendance in a formal academic environment, resulting in school failure. His school failure may be due to problems relating to authority figures such as teachers and other staff, or because of malnutrition and hunger resulting in poor concentration and poor academic performance. Individuals with active eating disorders who have severe malnutrition and early recovery may demonstrate significant impairment in executive function, as well as polarized thinking [22]. Addressing cognitive concerns, such as school and work performance, requires a collaboration among health, mental health, and education sectors to effectively engage youth. Psychoeducational testing can be key in determining a young person's current academic profile and creating an individualized education plan [17].

As Case 2 illustrates, young people who experience complex trauma may feel unsupported by adults from multiple sectors. As a result, young people may develop a pervasive sense of mistrust and suspiciousness of authority figures, including health providers – an example of extreme attachment dysfunction [17]. Michael's issues with attachment are illustrated by his abusive relationships and his struggles with assertiveness and interpersonal boundaries. To address effectively both his eating disorder and his traumatic experiences while being trafficked, caregivers and health practitioners must understand that problems with attachment can lead to significant barriers in establishing trust with adolescents who experience complex trauma and should therefore act in a trauma-sensitive manner when providing care [17]. Similarly, youth like Michael are frequently testing boundaries and limits to determine if the adults in their lives will "give up on them" or let them down: this may manifest as difficulties with emotional regulation leading to frequent angry outbursts or periods of self-harm, and struggles in regulating basic bodily functions such as sleep and eating [17]. In addition, people with eating disorders who have experienced trauma engage in re-enactment patterns frequently through food, which can be overtly or covertly symbolic [23]. These re-enactments can be engaged through metaphorical, dissociative, and/or depersonalized means [24]. In this case, Michael's self-destructive behaviors involved a plethora of difficulties – impulsively wanting to run away with his exploiters after having a period of safety, self-destructive overdosing, engaging in re-enactments through punishing himself with exercise and verbally abusive relationships, and restricting during the day and binge-eating in the evening and at night.

Adverse Childhood Experiences in Human Trafficking and Eating Disorders

Adverse childhood experiences (ACEs) are exposures to abuse and family dysfunction during childhood and adolescence that can lead to long-term health consequences and well-being in adulthood [25]. These health consequences include, but are not limited to, cardiac disease, obesity, diabetes, substance use, high-risk sexual activity, stroke, cancer, and early death. Individuals who have more ACEs are at higher risk for the development of such health consequences in the future [25]. Although a history of being trafficked has not been examined as a separate ACE, a Florida study conducted among juvenile youth demonstrated that children with a sexual abuse history and a higher ACE score were significantly more predisposed to sexual exploitation [26]. Similarly, history of child sexual abuse is a known risk factor for binge eating disorder (BED). [27] BED is defined as eating large quantities of food in a short amount of time, having a feeling of loss of control in eating, and feeling of guilt and shame after eating, but not using unhealthy compensatory measures after these eating events such as purging [27]. Given that human trafficking survivors may have pre-existing experience with several ACEs, including child sexual abuse, it is important to consider that such individuals are at significant risk for BED, and the subsequent long-term health consequences of BED including obesity, diabetes, and hypertension as well as several other related chronic health conditions. It is imperative for healthcare professionals to recognize the risks of those who have been trafficked in developing an eating disorder in the short term (including restrictive or BED) as well as to be aware of the development of unhealthy eating behaviors in the long term, particularly for those with high ACEs, to prevent and manage these possible chronic health consequences.

Treatment and Management of Human Trafficking Survivors with Eating Disorders

The approach to mental and long-term medical healthcare for youth experiencing complex trauma requires a consistent team of health providers who are able to engage with youth both in formal settings and community-based settings where youth spend their time [16, 21]. This coordination of care should ideally be integrated with the education and physical healthcare settings so that youth are not left to navigate complex social structures on their own [16, 21]. Ideally all services would be located in one setting with providers meeting as a team frequently in order to support one another and ensure that consistent messages are being provided to youth [16, 21]. Care of these youth requires not only diagnostic assessment, case management, and medical management, but also psychosocial approaches borrowing from the principles of trauma treatment and dialectical behavior therapy [17, 21, 28]. Recovery plans should reconnect youth to appropriate social supports and to age-appropriate recreational activities, as these are important components of building a sense of competence and resiliency [16, 17]. In addition, it may take years, not weeks or months, to see improvement in the lives of such young people, and funding strategies should take into consideration that this type of approach is more successful than multiple short acute-care admissions.

References

1. Baldwin SB, Eisenman DP, Sayles JN, Ryan G, Chuang KS. Identification of human trafficking victims in health care settings. Health Hum Rights. 2011;13:E36–49.
2. Department of U.S. Immigration and customs enforcement. Human Trafficking and smuggling [Internet]. 2013 [cited 2019 Sep 24]. Available from: https://www.ice.gov/factsheets/human-trafficking.
3. Väyrynen R. Illegal immigration, human trafficking and organized crime. In: Borjas GJ, Crisp J, editors. Poverty, international migration and asylum. London: Palgrave Macmillan UK; 2005. p. 143–70.
4. Mostajabian S, Santa Maria D, Wiemann C, Newlin E, Bocchini C. Identifying sexual and labor exploitation among sheltered youth experiencing homelessness: a comparison of screening methods. Int J Environ Res Public Health. 2019;16.
5. Institute of Medicine (U.S.) Committee on the Commercial Sexual Exploitation and Sex Trafficking of Minors in the United States., Clayton EW, Krugman RD, Simon P, Institute of Medicine (U.S.), National Research Council (U.S.). Confronting commercial sexual exploitation and sex trafficking of minors in the United States. Washington, D.C.: National Academies Press; 2013.
6. U.S. Department of Health and Human Services, Administration for Children, Youth, and Families. Guidance to states and services on addressing human trafficking of children and youth in the United States [Internet]. 2014 [cited 2019 Sep 25]. Available from: http://www.acf.hhs.gov/sites/default/files/cb/acyf_human_trafficking_guidance.pdf.
7. United Nations Office on Drugs and Crime. Global Report on Trafficking in Persons, 2018 [Internet]. United Nations; 2018. Available from: https://www.unodc.org/documents/data-and-analysis/glotip/2018/GLOTiP_2018_BOOK_web_small.pdf.
8. Oram S, Ostrovschi NV, Gorceag VI, Hotineanu MA, Gorceag L, Trigub C, et al. Physical health symptoms reported by trafficked women receiving post-trafficking support in Moldova: prevalence, severity and associated factors. BMC Womens Health. 2012;12:20.
9. Ottisova L, Hemmings S, Howard LM, Zimmerman C, Oram S. Prevalence and risk of violence and the mental, physical and sexual health problems associated with human trafficking: an updated systematic review. Epidemiol Psychiatr Sci. 2016;25:317–41.
10. Fisher M. Treatment of eating disorders in children, adolescents, and young adults. Pediatr Rev. 2006;27:5–16.

11. American Psychiatric Association. Anxiety disorders. Diagnostic and statistical manual of mental disorders. Am Psychiat Ass; 2013.
12. Moskowitz L, Weiselberg E. Anorexia nervosa/atypical anorexia nervosa. Curr Probl Pediatr Adolesc Health Care. 2017;47:70–84.
13. Zimmerman J, Fisher M. Avoidant/restrictive food intake disorder (ARFID). Curr Probl Pediatr Adolesc Health Care. 2017;47:95–103.
14. Westwood J, Howard LM, Stanley N, Zimmerman C, Gerada C, Oram S. Access to, and experiences of, healthcare services by trafficked people: findings from a mixed-methods study in England. Br J Gen Pract. 2016;66:e794–801.
15. English A. Mandatory reporting of human trafficking: potential benefits and risks of harm. AMA J Ethics. 2017;19:54–62.
16. George JS, Malik S, Symes S, Caralis P, Newport DJ, Godur A, et al. Trafficking healthcare resources and intra-disciplinary victim services and education (THRIVE) clinic: a multidisciplinary one-stop shop model of healthcare for survivors of human trafficking. J Hum Traffick. 2018:1–11.
17. Cook A, Spinazzola J, Ford J, Lanktree C, Blaustein M, Cloitre M, et al. Complex trauma in children and adolescents. Psychiatr Ann. 2005;35:390–8.
18. Campbell K, Peebles R. Eating disorders in children and adolescents: state of the art review. Pediatrics. 2014;134:582–92.
19. McClain Z, Peebles R. Body image and eating disorders among lesbian, gay, bisexual, and transgender youth. Pediatr Clin N Am. 2016;63:1079–90.
20. Golden NH, Katzman DK, Sawyer SM, Ornstein RM, Rome ES, Society for Adolescent Health and Medicine, et al. Position Paper of the Society for Adolescent Health and Medicine: medical management of restrictive eating disorders in adolescents and young adults. J Adolesc Health. 2015;56:121–5.
21. Williamson E, Dutch NM, Clawson HJ. Evidence-based mental health treatment for victims of human trafficking. US Depart Health Hum Serv Off Ass Secret Plann Evaluat. 2010:1–13.
22. Tasca GA, Ritchie K, Balfour L. Implications of attachment theory and research for the assessment and treatment of eating disorders. Psychotherapy (Chic). 2011;48:249–59.
23. Farber SK. Self-medication, traumatic reenactment, and somatic expression in bulimic and self-mutilating behavior. Clin Soc Work J. 1997;25:87–106.
24. Farber SK. Dissociation, traumatic attachments, and self-harm: eating disorders and self-mutilation. Clin Soc Work J. 2008;36:63–72.
25. Felitti VJ, Anda RF, Nordenberg D, Williamson DF, Spitz AM, Edwards V, et al. Relationship of childhood abuse and household dysfunction to many of the leading causes of death in adults. The adverse childhood experiences (ACE) study. Am J Prev Med. 1998;14:245–58.
26. Reid JA, Baglivio MT, Piquero AR, Greenwald MA, Epps N. Human trafficking of minors and childhood adversity in Florida. Am J Public Health. 2017;107:306–11.
27. Palmisano GL, Innamorati M, Vanderlinden J. Life adverse experiences in relation with obesity and binge eating disorder: a systematic review. J Behav Addict. 2016;5:11–31.
28. Gordon M, Salami T, Coverdale J, Nguyen PT. Psychiatry's role in the management of human trafficking victims: an integrated care approach. J Psychiatr Pract. 2018;24:79–86.

Chapter 11
LGBTQIA+ Youth and Human Trafficking

Miriam Langer, Nat Paul, and Uri Belkind

Case Presentation
Name: Jesse
Pronouns: She/her/hers
Age: 24 years
Sex assigned at birth: Male
Gender: Transgender female
Cause of death: Multiple pulmonary emboli with pulmonary infarction, deep venous thrombosis of the legs

Introduction

Lesbian, gay, bisexual, transgender, genderqueer, questioning, intersex, and asexual (LGBTQIA) youth, by the very nature of their gender identity, gender expression, and/or sexual orientation, experience rejection and are victims of interpersonal and systemic discrimination [1–4]. The direct effects of this discrimination, as well as the effects of internalized homo/transphobia, lead to

M. Langer (✉)
Department of Pediatrics, Division of Adolescent Medicine Children's Hospital at Montefiore, Bronx, NY, USA

N. Paul
Bolivar, NY, USA

U. Belkind
Callen-Lorde Community Health Center, New York, NY, USA

K. E. Titchen, E. Miller (eds.), *Medical Perspectives on Human Trafficking in Adolescents*, https://doi.org/10.1007/978-3-030-43367-3_11

outcomes that place this population at high risk for being trafficked [5–9]. In fact, LGBTQIA youth are overrepresented among labor and sex trafficked youth [5, 8]. Avoidance or delay in seeking healthcare due to fear of discrimination, especially for those who have previously experienced discrimination in a healthcare setting, reduces opportunities for intervention [10]. Awareness of these risks and providing more comprehensive and inclusive care can lead to better health outcomes for these patients.

Creating a safe environment and strong rapport between medical professional and patient are important components in identifying youth who are being trafficked, as youth may distrust their clinician or the healthcare system at large [11]. This rapport building does not begin and end with the clinician but starts before the patient even sees a clinician. If clinics include welcoming and non-judgmental intake forms that have either more open-ended questions or more options with gender-inclusive language, trained front desk staff who do not assume that all patients are cisgender, and signs that promote inclusivity such as "all are welcome here" or a pride flag, LGBTQIA patients may feel more welcome and comfortable [12]. This may lead to a more productive encounter and increase the odds of disclosure [13].

We present the case of Jesse, who ultimately died of potentially avoidable medical complications after self-administering gender-affirming hormone therapy without access to adequate medical supervision. This case highlights the fact that there were many encounters between Jesse and medical professionals and yet, due to low suspicion, lack of knowledge in caring for transgender individuals, and failures in the health system, these all were missed opportunities to address potential human trafficking and safe, gender-affirming treatment.

Visit 1: Mobile Medical Unit

Information obtained from medical records:

Sixteen-year-old transgender female for sexually transmitted infection (STI) screening. Patient takes self-prescribed estrogen and spironolactone, otherwise healthy. Three sexual partners in the last 6 months (all assigned male at birth (AMAB)), receptive oral and anal intercourse with inconsistent condom use.

Plan: Gonorrhea/*Chlamydia trachomatis* (GC/CT) in urine, pharynx, and rectal swabs. Rapid HIV test: Non-reactive. Patient declined phlebotomy.

Referred for primary care; patient needs quadrivalent meningococcal (MenACWY) and human papillomavirus vaccines. Encouraged condom use.

Information not gathered during this visit:

Jesse lives with her mother and mother's boyfriend. She has a difficult relationship with her mother who is not supportive of Jesse's gender identity and continues referring to her as her "son," using male pronouns, and calling Jesse by her birth (dead) name. Despite this, Jesse has obtained estradiol tablets and spironolactone from the Internet which she buys with money given to her by her mother's boyfriend.

Jesse is sexually active with AMAB partners, and often she meets her partners online. She sometimes exchanges sex for money which she uses to buy estradiol shots from friends, as well as to buy clothes. Her mother will only buy her "masculine" clothes.

Epidemiology

Just over 10% of high school students identify with a sexual orientation other than heterosexual (8% bisexual, 2.4% gay or lesbian, etc.) [1]. That same nationally representative survey estimates 1.8% of high school students identify as transgender or gender nonconforming, although other studies put the number of adolescents and young adults as <0.7% of the population that age [2, 14].

Risks

Negative health outcomes such as higher rates of violence victimization, increased rates of depression and suicidality, high rates of substance use, and increased risk for STIs can be seen in LGBT youth [3]. A 2017 study of high school students shows double the prevalence of online bullying in LGB youth versus heterosexual youth, and almost one in three LGB youth are bullied on school property [1]. The same study showed higher prevalence of drinking, binge drinking, marijuana use, and other substance use among LGB compared to heterosexual high school students. Reisner (2015) actually links the bullying to the substance use showing that the increased bullying leads to the increased substance use [15]. One in five LGB high school students and almost one in four transgender high school students are forced to have sexual intercourse compared to one in 20 of their heterosexual peers. Almost two-thirds of LBG youth have been sad or hopeless with just under one-quarter having attempted suicide. A matched single-center cohort study of adolescents and young adults showed a two- to threefold increased risk of depression, anxiety disorder, suicidal ideation, suicide attempt, self-harm without lethal intent, and both inpatient and outpatient mental health treatment in transgender patients compared to cisgender patients [16].

That same 2017 nationally representative sample of high school students showed increased risky sexual behavior among transgender students than their cisgender peers [2]. Transgender students were more likely than cisgender students to have had coitarche prior to age 13 years, to have four or more lifetime partners, and to have used no birth control method at last sexual intercourse. Transgender students were almost twice as likely than were cisgender females to have drunk alcohol or used drugs before their last sexual intercourse. Transgender students were also almost twice more likely than cisgender males to report no condom use during their last sexual intercourse.

Protective Factors

A few factors have been identified as being protective against the negative risks associated with LGBTQIA youth. Family support is shown to be a key protective factor against some of the negative health outcomes seen in LGBTQIA youth such as depression, substance abuse, and suicidal ideation and attempts [17–19]. A child's positive school environment and supportive adults within that environment can also be protective against high-risk behaviors [20, 21]. Transgender adults name peer support as protective [22].

For transgender youth, social transitioning seems to be a protective factor too. One study showed that after socially transitioning, rates of depression in transgender youth were similar to those seen in cisgender youth and rates of anxiety dropped significantly, remaining only slightly higher than cisgender youth [23]. Another study showed that rates of suicide fall after having personal identification with the appropriate gender marker and also after medical transition [19].

In Jesse's case, the medical professional could have taken time to learn more about Jesse's life: without knowing much about Jesse's life, it was hard to tailor safety and anticipatory guidance. The psychosocial history is an important component of routine adolescent and young adult care. If performed effectively, it would have provided insight into Jesse's challenges and may have provided an opportunity to direct Jesse to available community support resources.

Questions that could have improved this medical encounter: **Good morning. What name do you like to be called? What pronouns do you use?**

A comprehensive psychosocial assessment is recommended by the American Academy of Pediatrics at all primary care visits [24]. Since adolescents often present for complaints and not for primary care, many recommend doing an assessment at every visit. The adolescent psychosocial "HEADSS" assessment or "SSHADESS" assessments are brief tools recommended by the AAP (Table 11.1) [25, 26] (For the similar SHEEADSSS assessment, see Chap. 4, Table 4.2). Psychosocial assessments result in higher disclosure of high-risk situations and behaviors [27]. A significant barrier to using these assessment tools is that disclosure generally is higher among adolescents with self-administered questionnaires, whereas these questions are asked by the clinician. Another barrier is that clinicians need to follow-up with patients based on affirmative answers to screening questions of high-risk behaviors; some clinicians may not feel equipped to respond. Provider training and clinic-level changes in practices and protocols are needed to improve care for LGBTQIA youth more broadly as well as for adolescents at risk for trafficking.

Using sexuality and gender-inclusive language while doing the psychosocial assessment is imperative to building rapport and trust with all teenage patients, especially LGBTQIA youth [28]. Using gender-neutral language such as "Have you had sex before? With girls, boys, or both?" instead of asking "Do you have a boyfriend?" avoids presumptions of the gender of sex partners and allows space for the patient to discuss their partners without having to correct the clinician and "out" themselves in an obvious way. The openness of the question helps to normalize the behavior and avoid judgment or the mere perception of judgment.

Table 11.1 Two examples of commonly used adolescent psychosocial assessments

HEADSS		SSHADESS	
Home	Who do you live with? Where do you live? Any recent changes to your home situation (new people, recent moves)? What are your relationships like with the people in your house? What do the adults in your house do for a living? Were you ever institutionalized/ incarcerated? Have you ever run away?	**S**trengths	What do you like doing? Tell me what you're most proud of about yourself? How would your best friends describe you?
Education and **e**mployment	What grade are you in? How are you doing in school? Has this changed since last year? What are your favorite subjects? Worst subjects? Any failed classes? Any suspensions or dropping out? What are your future plans for school or work? How are your relationships with your teachers/bosses? Do you have friends in school?	**S**chool	What do you like most/least about school? How many days have you missed or had to leave early or arrive late? How are your grades? Are they different than last year? Do you feel you are doing your best at school? Do you feel safe on your way to and from school and at school? What do you want to do when you get older?
Activities	Do you have friends out of school? What do you like to do after school? Do you do it alone or with friends? Do you exercise or do sports? Are you part of any religious groups or other clubs? Do you read for fun? How much TV do you watch? What's your favorite music? Any history of arrests?	**Home/a**ctivities	Who do you live with? Any changes in your family? Can you talk to your family if you're stressed? Who would you talk to? Do your friends treat you well? Do you have a best friend or trusted adult outside of your family? Are you involved in the same activities this year compared to last year? What do you do for fun? Are you spending the same amount of time with your friends as you used to?
Drugs	Do any of your friends or do you use drugs? … drink alcohol? … smoke cigarettes or Juul? Do any of your family members? How often? Do you get in a car when you use or in a car with a driver who has used? How do you pay for it/ where do you get it from?	**D**rugs/substance use	Do any of your friends talk about smoking cigarettes or tobacco products like e-cigarettes, taking drugs or drinking alcohol? Do you smoke cigarettes or Juul? Drink alcohol? Have you tried sniffing glue, smoking weed, or using pills or other drugs? If you do, how does it make you feel?

(continued)

Table 11.1 (continued)

HEADSS		SSHADESS	
Suicide/ depression	How well do you sleep? Any changes in your eating habits recently? Have you felt extra bored? How is your mood? Have you ever had any thoughts of hurting yourself or killing yourself? Are you thinking about hurting yourself or killing yourself today?	**E**motions/**e**ating/ depression	Have you been feeling stressed? Are you feeling more bored or annoyed than usual? Do you feel nervous a lot? Have you had trouble sleeping lately? Have you been trying to lose or gain weight? Have you been feeling down, sad, or depressed? Have you thought about hurting yourself or someone else? Have you ever tried to hurt yourself?
Sexuality	Do you know if you are sexually or romantically interested in girls, boys, or both? Have you ever had sex willingly before? If yes, with a girl, boy, or both? How many partners have you had? Has anyone tried to make you do something sexually that you did not want to do? Do you masturbate? Any history of pregnancy or sexually transmitted infections? What do you do to protect yourself against that? Do you get pleasure from sexual activity?	**S**exuality	Are you attracted to anyone? Tell me about that person. Are you comfortable with your sexual feelings? Are you attracted to guys, girls, or both? What kinds of things have you done sexually? Kissing? Touching? Oral sex? Have you ever had sexual intercourse? Have you enjoyed it? What steps do you take to protect yourself against pregnancy or sexually transmitted infections? Have you ever been pregnant or had a sexually transmitted infection? Have you ever been worried you were pregnant or had a sexually transmitted infection?
		Safety	Do you feel safe at school? Is there bullying? Have you been bullied? Do you carry weapons? What kinds of things make you mad enough to fight? Has anyone ever touched you physically or sexually when you didn't want them to? Does your partner get jealous? Do you ever get into fights with your partner? Physical fights? Have you seen people in your family hurt each other either with their words or physically?

Adapted from Cohen et al. [25] and Ginsburg [26]

Visits 2 and 3: Drop-in Clinic
Information obtained from medical records:

Eighteen-year-old transgender (TG) female, uninsured, c/o rectal pain, bloody stools, thinks it's a hemorrhoid.

PMHx: Takes estrogen and spironolactone, gets them from a friend, occasionally Depo-Provera injection when she can find it. Status post (s/p) breast augmentation 6 months ago in Florida (can't remember the surgeon's name).

PE: Thin male, well-appearing. Pertinent positives: +inguinal lymph nodes, normal genitals. Rectal exam: No external hemorrhoids; patient does not tolerate digital rectal exam and anoscope insertion. Rectal swab for GC/CT obtained.

Rapid HIV test: Reactive.

Assessment: Reactive rapid HIV test, anal fissure.

Plan: 1. Confirmatory HIV test. 2. Syphilis screening via RPR, hepatitis panel, or anal/oral/urine GC/CT. 3. Sitz baths. 4. Return to clinic (RTC) in 1 week for confirmatory test result.

Follow-up:

Eighteen-year-old TG female for confirmatory HIV results, persistent rectal pain.

HIV-1 antigen and antibody positive by fourth-generation immunoassay, confirmed by nucleic acid amplification test (NAAT). Viral load (VL) 130 K. CD4 count 435.

+Rectal chlamydia.

Assessment: 1. HIV, new diagnosis. 2. Rectal pain, +chlamydia, will treat for lymphogranuloma venereum (LGV) proctitis.

Plan: 1. Referral to infectious disease (ID) clinic. 2. Doxycycline 100 mg PO BID x 21 days.

Information not obtained from medical records/not gathered during this visit:

Jesse was kicked out of her house when she turned 18.

She was initially sleeping in friends' houses (couch surfing) and sometimes in the subway or on the street.

Mr. X approached Jesse her second night on the street when he offered her a place to sleep in exchange for sex. After a week, Mr. X offered to pay for Jesse's breast augmentation surgery in Florida in exchange for having sex with his friends.

LGBTQIA, Homelessness, and HIV

Of the estimated 1.6 million homeless American youth, between 20 and 40% are lesbian, gay, bisexual, or transgender [29]. As this subset of youth comprise <15% of the youth population, LGBTQIA youth are overrepresented among homeless youth. A 2015 survey of transgender people 18 years and older indicated that, of those "out" to their family, one in 10 ran away from home and one in 12 were kicked out of their house [30]. Acceptable shelter options are in particularly short supply for individuals who may face additional discrimination, such as LGBTQIA youth, especially those not eligible for women's shelters, e.g., transgender youth and gay and bisexual boys [31]. Transgender youth may not be given the gender-specific housing with which they identify or may be forced to disclose their transgender identity in order to obtain appropriate gender-specific housing, potentially exposing them to violence and/or discrimination [32] (More information on this can be found in Chap. 12).

Rates of HIV infection are five times higher in the population of homeless LGBT youth than the national rates (1.4% v 0.3%), with additional risk factors including homelessness, identification as transgender, and race. One study showed a sixfold higher risk of HIV infection when comparing high-risk adolescents who were homeless to high-risk teens living with their families, implying that homelessness could be a major contributor to this increased risk.

HIV rates among transgender women are higher than those even of homeless LGBT, at 3.4%. Specifically, transgender black women have a high risk, with nearly one in five (19%) black transgender women living with HIV [30, 33].

One 2017 national study of high school students found that transgender students were more likely than cisgender students to have ever been tested for HIV, perhaps implying that while they are not presenting routinely for care, they are presenting for testing [2].

Questions that could have improved this encounter: **What body parts do you use to have sex? Do you use toys? Do you share toys?**

Information about what body parts people use when they have sex and if they use toys are important pieces of the sexual history, as they inform screening. STI screening can be done orally, rectally, via urine, or via vaginal/urethral swab [34]. Patients can be instructed on how to use swabs to self-collect rectal and vaginal samples, if they find this acceptable and more comfortable.

HIV

HIV Screening

The AAP, CDC, and USPSTF recommend HIV screening at least once for everyone 13–64 years regardless of risk factors [35–37]. Given the higher incidence in males who have sex with males (MSM) and sex workers, this population should be screened at least annually. Additionally, the CDC recommends people being evaluated and treated for other STIs be screened at that time [37].

All sexually active adolescent and young adult females under 25 should be screened annually for gonorrhea and chlamydia. There are no recommended guidelines for STI screening in adolescent and young adult males who have sex with females; many follow the guidelines for girls under 25. MSM should also have at least annual gonorrhea and chlamydia screening, more frequently if at greater risk, as well as annual syphilis screening [35]. While there are no guidelines for transgender individuals, screening should be considered for those at risk. The guidelines recommend trichomonas screening annually in females who are HIV positive and should be considered in high-risk populations like females with multiple sexual partners and females who exchange sex for money, such as sex trafficking victims [35]. Similarly, this can be considered for transgender males and gender non-binary individuals assigned female at birth, at high risk, who have receptive vaginal intercourse. Cervical cancer screening with a Pap smear is recommended for all people with cervices every 3 years from ages 21 to 29 with cytology. Cervical cancer screening for people who are pregnant is the same. Cervical cancer screening for people living with HIV should start at coitarche or initial HIV diagnosis and then 6 months later [35].

Comment and question that could have improved this encounter: **Excellent job using condoms. It's the best way to protect yourself from sexually transmitted infections and prevent transmission of HIV. Do you know if any of your partners are taking pre-exposure prophylaxis (PrEP)?**

Sexual behaviors often change after an HIV diagnosis, for many reasons including fear of stigma after disclosure and concern for infecting a future partner [38]. Empowering patients to keep themselves and their partners safe through discussing the state law and medical recommendations can help patients with HIV continue to live romantically and sexually fulfilling lives. Some states have laws that people living with HIV must disclose their status to their partners, and others have laws that they must disclose to people with whom they share needles [39]. It is important to discuss these laws with patients so they do not inadvertently break the law. Knowing ways their partners can protect themselves, namely, condom use and PrEP, can allow patients to disclose and continue the relationship with their partner(s) more safely and, by alleviating secrecy and promoting healthy choices, can lead to a healthier and more stable relationship, if that is what is desired.

HIV Pre-exposure Prophylaxis (PrEP)

PrEP, comprised of once-daily, fixed-dose tenofovir (TDF) and emtricitabine (FTC), has been approved for use in adults and adolescents over 35 kg [40]. Indications for PrEP include all HIV-negative adults who have a partner who is HIV positive, MSM or people who have opposite sex partners who have multiple sex partners, and MSM or people who have opposite sex partners who have had a recent STI [41] (Table 11.2). (The guidelines say heterosexual people, but since many adolescents have sexual experiences that do not match their self-identified sexuality, it is important for clinicians caring for teenagers and young adults to consider the gender of the sexual partners and not exclusively the patient's sexuality.)

There is debate over whether PrEP interferes with female-affirming hormones as only one study of PrEP has been done in transgender women, with the majority of

Table 11.2 Summary of guidance for PrEP use

	Men who have sex with men	Heterosexual women and men	Persons who inject drugs
Detecting substantial risk of acquiring HIV infection	HIV-positive sexual partner, recent bacterial STI,* high number of sex partners, history of inconsistent or no condom use, commercial sex work	HIV-positive sexual partner, recent bacterial STI,^ high number of sex partners, history of inconsistent or no condom use, commercial sex work in high HIV prevalence area or network	HIV-positive injecting partner, sharing injection equipment
Clinically eligible	Documented negative HIV test result before prescribing PrEP, no signs/symptoms of acute HIV infection, normal renal function, no contraindicated medications, documented hepatitis B virus infection and vaccination status		
Prescription	Daily, continuing, oral doses of TDF/FTC (Truvada), ≤90-day supply		
Other services	Follow-up visits at least every 3 months to provide the following: HIV test, medication adherence counseling, behavioral risk reduction support, side effect assessment, STI symptom assessment at 3 months and every 6 months thereafter, assessment of renal function every 3–6 months, testing for bacterial STIs		
	Do oral/rectal STI testing	For women, assess pregnancy intent; perform pregnancy test every 3 months	Access to clean needles/syringes and drug treatment services

*Gonorrhea, chlamydia, and syphilis for MSM including those who inject drugs. ^Gonorrhea and syphilis for heterosexual women and men including those who inject drugs

Source: US Public Health Service. Preexposure prophylaxis for the prevention of HIV infection in the United States – 2017: Updated clinical practice guideline [42]

the studies done on MSM. Theoretically there should not be a drug interaction based on the metabolic pathway of tenofovir and feminizing hormones [43]. The iFACT study found that tenofovir did not lower levels of feminizing hormones in 20 transfemales; however, the levels of tenofovir were significantly lower, though still above the therapeutic level [44]. This study is reassuring to providers and should be discussed with transgender females who are starting on PrEP to increase adherence and dispel misinformation or prior suspicions.

Visits 4 and 5: Street HIV Clinic #1

Information obtained from medical records:

Nineteen-year-old male (MtF), HIV+ (diagnosed last year as per external medical records), lost to care. Patient is interested in starting antiretrovirals (ARVs), but is concerned that they will interfere with hormone replacement therapy.

Psychosocial history: Patient lives with roommates, has minimal contact with family, engages in sex work, and uses condoms always. Smokes cigarettes (1/2 pack per day). Alcohol on weekends, marijuana daily, no other drugs.

Assessment: HIV+.

Plan: HIV initial labs, STI screening, return to clinic (RTC) in 3 weeks to discuss results and medication options.

Follow-up:

Nineteen-year-old male-to-female for results.

*VL 55 K, CD4 385. Neg HLA-B*5701, no resistance.*

Rectal GC/CT.

Plan: 1. Start ARVs specifically TDF/FTC + darunavir/ritonavir (DVR/r). 2. Ceftriaxone and azithromycin. 3. RTC in 3 months.

Information not obtained from medical records/not gathered during this visit:

Jesse has continued working for Mr. X since she is indebted to him for her top surgery and needs money to pay for her hormones. Jesse gets her hormones online or from a friend. When she cannot access clean needles, Jesse will share needles in order to continue regular hormone injections. She feels even one missed dose of her hormones makes her feel masculine and dysphoric, and if she has to miss any injections she will double or triple the dose to "catch up." She has read the warnings online about doubling up but she can't keep a consistent dose, so she does the best she can to make herself feel as good as possible. Jesse's access to hormones is often limited by the fact that Mr. X will keep her hormones and use them as a bargaining chip in exchange for "good behavior."

Overrepresentation

LGBTQIA youth are overrepresented among victims of human trafficking. One multicenter study showed that transgender youth are four times more likely than cisgender females to engage in exchange sex, which is having sex or performing sexual acts in exchange for something they need, be it money, drugs, a place to live, employment, etc. [5]. They are more likely to have run away from home or used community housing services in the past year, engaged in poly-substance use including injectable drugs, had anal intercourse, experienced sexual coercion, reported depression, and had an STI/HIV diagnosis, all predictive factors for exchange sex [5–7]. LGBTQIA youth are at risk for homelessness, and among homeless youth, risk factors for exchange sex include history of family dysfunction and mental health problems, commonly experienced by LGBTQIA youth [8, 9]. In fact, homeless youth who were commercially sexually exploited were five times more likely to identify as LGBTQIA.

Transgender youth get involved in trafficking for many alluring reasons. Some transgender youth find sex work to be a means for expressing their gender identity. It allowed them to "date" in accordance with their gender identity. While some of these youth eventually worked without a trafficker or "pimp," many had previously been trafficked [45].

Some transgender youth are lured by the promise of money for hormones and gender-affirming surgeries, since they distrust and avoid traditional medical care.

Human Rights Watch interviews from 2017 to 2018 of many transgender individuals highlight the common use of hormones bought on the street [4]. Transgender youth who were interviewed stated that they engaged in sex work to earn money to buy these medications [45]. Many describe negative outcomes when using substances not prescribed, which are often unidentified and unregulated, or undergoing procedures by people not licensed or properly trained.

This offers an excellent opportunity for clinicians to engage with patients around risk behaviors, needle exchange and other harm-reduction interventions, and exploring other barriers to care.

Questions that could have been asked: **Are your hormones prescribed by a medical professional? If not, how and from whom do you get your hormones and other supplies?**

DIY (do-it-yourself) transitioning is not uncommon among transgender youth. Dangers of DIY transitioning include taking medications that are associated with greater likelihood of adverse events (e.g., conjugated estrogens vs. 17ß-estradiol), taking unknown doses, and not having a trusted clinician to ask medical questions. Jesse's disclosure of using self-prescribed hormones provides an opportunity for the clinician to ask follow-up questions and provide referrals to a clinic that can provide gender-affirming therapy. While Jesse may or may not choose to access these resources, her clinician would convey concern and care by providing them. This would also afford Jesse an opportunity to build her knowledge of available options and would leave open the possibility of her choosing to access them at a future date.

Questions that could have been asked: **What do you do to make money to buy your hormones? Have you ever exchanged sex for money, food, drugs, clothes, a place to sleep, transportation, or medication?**

Like other substance use, disclosure of buying medication on the street can prompt follow-up questions about the patient's sources of income. These questions can help open the door to exploring unsafe working environments and possible exchange sex. Understanding the risks patients face is key to providing the best care.

It is important to keep in mind that a patient may not be ready to change their life the day they are in the office, and in fact disclosure may not occur at all. A risk reduction model should be the goal, helping the patient to take steps to keep themselves safer and avoid some of the risks associated with their situation. Even a suspicion of exchange sex, with or without disclosure, can open a discussion of job training programs, and healthcare professionals can present resources such as the National Human Trafficking Hotline (888-3737-888) and programs to help youth change their life if and when they are ready [46]. Clinicians can show that they have resources available and can work toward building a trusting relationship with patients without providing printed pamphlets and handouts that a trafficker might find.

Visit 6: Street HIV Clinic #2

Twenty-one-year-old transgender woman, HIV+, here with boyfriend. Previously on PI-based antiretroviral therapy (ART), off meds for 1+ year.

No physical complaints.

Current medications: Estrogen, spironolactone.

Sex worker, uses condoms.

PE (pertinent findings): Thin, +diffuse lymphadenopathy, multiple tattoos, declines genital exam.

A/P: HIV+.HIV labs, switch to TDF/FTC/EFV daily. RTC in 3 months.

NOTE: Patient's boyfriend refused to leave room.

Information not obtained from medical records/not gathered during this visit:

"Boyfriend" was Mr. X. who forced patient to come to clinic by threatening to stop paying for gender-affirming hormones. Mr. X wanted patient back on ART due to concern for his reputation if his clients contracted HIV.

Patient had stopped taking ART because of fear that it would interfere with gender-affirming hormone therapy. During the time the patient was previously on both, patient had been able to acquire more estrogen "to overcome" the effect of ART but was not able to consistently buy both estrogen and the ART so she stopped the ART and went back to the original "dose" of estrogen. Patient had read online that there was no interaction but could not help thinking there must be.

Some of the tattoos were forced on patient by Mr. X as a marker that she was one of his girls.

Barriers to Care

There are many barriers to appropriate and timely care for LGBTQIA youth, especially those involved in sex work. One study found 8% of LGBTQIA adult respondents had delayed or avoided medical care because of concerns for discrimination [47]. Eight percent of lesbian, gay, and bisexual respondents and 29% of transgender respondents reported that a healthcare provider had refused to see them because of their sexual orientation or gender identity in the past year. Those who had previously experienced discrimination were particularly likely to avoid seeking care at all.

One theme that emerged in multiple qualitative studies was lack of trust of medical professionals and the concern of those involved in sex work about exposing their lifestyle to others [47]. While nondisclosure is an option for LGB patients, for many transgender patients, this is not an option because of their stage of transition, name or gender marker on their identification, or information listed in the chart or medication history. Only about half of LGBTQIA patients disclose their gender or sexual identity to their provider [48].

For transgender patients, the length of the medical process associated with gender-affirming care in traditional medical facilities was also a barrier to care [45].

Effects of avoiding medical care are numerous especially given the high rates of STIs and HIV. While more than half of LGBTQIA youth report having sex, less than half report ever having been tested [48].

Questions the provider could have asked: **Do you feel safe with your partner? Why do you think your partner might not have wanted to leave the room? Does it cause more trouble for you that your partner is not in the room right now?**

Confidentiality and Autonomy

The American College of Gynecology and the American Academy of Pediatrics recommend interviewing adolescents alone and confidentially. Having a clinic-wide policy in place that ensures that patients are seen alone at some point during the clinical encounter can assist the provider in ensuring that this recommendation is followed, even if a companion or patient is resistant to the confidential interview.

The partner might not want to leave the room because they are afraid the patient might disclose abuse. Other behaviors that an abusive or controlling companion might exhibit include answering questions directed to the patient and becoming increasingly more impatient and agitated during the visit [49].

It is also possible that the patient is hesitant to allow the partner to leave the room, fearing that this might arise suspicion of disclosure in their absence, which could lead to grave consequences. Sometimes this fear will come out through questioning and sometimes it will not, depending on the patient. It is unlikely that a patient will disclose on an initial encounter with a new clinician, and this highlights the importance of continuity and building strong rapport.

Reassuring comments that could have been made: **We can discuss more next time, or we don't have to talk about it at all. While I recognize I don't leave the office with you, I want to use our time together to help keep your mind and body safe.**

In recognition of patient autonomy, the goal when assessing safety should *not* be disclosure. The clinician must assess the patient's safety to the best of their ability. If the clinician *suspects* the patient might be in danger, they should offer a safety plan, for example, asking the patient to memorize the trafficking hotline number (or putting the number in their phone under a fictional name), scheduling a follow-up for a medical reason, and laying the groundwork for future conversations. However, if disclosure does occur, it is important to have identified resources for local programs aimed at helping victims of sex trafficking.

Probing questions that could have proved helpful: **Why did you stop the ARV treatment? Did you have physical side effects? Did you have difficulty getting the medication? Do you have a concern I could help with?**

Restarting a medication provides a unique opportunity to discuss previous medication side effects and complaints. It also may help identify a patient's specific barriers to treatment, be they physical, financial, or personal. Restarting a drug without exploring the previous barriers to care may not lead to the intended treatment plan, especially in teenagers and young adults who are concrete thinkers and need to understand the importance of something and the reasoning behind it before they will follow an adult's directive.

Visit 7: ER

Twenty-four-year-old MtF, HIV+, chest pain and severe shortness of breath. Cardiac arrest during transport to CT scan.

Summary

Jesse's experiences in late adolescence and young adulthood are not unique, especially among the overrepresented community of LGBTQIA homeless youth. While the experiences and risks do differ between the groups that comprise LGBTQIA youth, overall their risks for bullying, discrimination, and high-risk behaviors are higher than those of their cisgender heterosexual peers. LGBTQIA have low utilization of healthcare facilities due to mistrust of doctors and previous poor experiences in medical facilities.

Recognizing these facts is the first step toward better medical management of this population of patients. Starting with changing intake forms and educational materials in clinics to training personnel to ask more gender-inclusive questions to starting each encounter asking a patient for their preferred name and pronouns can change the rapport with LGBTQIA patients and welcome them before medical history-taking has begun.

Once the visit has begun, no matter the stated reason for the visit, it is important to perform a confidential comprehensive psychosocial history using open-ended and non-presumptive questions. Following up affirmative answers to screening questions for high-risk behaviors is crucial. In LGBTQIA youth specifically, asking about familial acceptance is important. Conversely, just because the question has been asked in an inclusive way does not mean the patient is ready to disclose, be it related to gender identity, sexual identity, or involvement in sex work or trafficking. In those situations, disclosure should *not* be the goal; rather, a risk reduction model should be explored, and the questions should be asked again at follow-up visits. Red flags for trafficking include use of self-prescribed hormones, a companion at medical visits who resists providing confidentiality to the patient, and patients carrying or wearing expensive things or with expensive drug habits or their own apartment but without a known source of income. All of these indicators should prompt further questioning in a trauma-sensitive manner.

A pitfall that clinicians must avoid is the well-intended but ill-informed desire to "save" the patient. Given time constraints and limitations of clinician knowledge and many patients' distrust of the medical system, the clinician must focus on risk reduction. Offering the patient the number to the trafficking hotline and ensuring that patients have a safe place to sleep, food to eat, and transportation to return for follow-up may be all that is possible. The medical professional likely will not be able to remove the patient from their trafficking situation but instead can use the visit to create a safe and affirming space, to screen for safety, and to provide excellent medical care that mitigates the risks faced by LGBTQIA youth who are trafficked. If disclosure does occur, it is important to have identified resources and safe places to refer patients.

References

1. Kann L, McManus T, Harris WA, Shanklin SL, Flint KH, Hawkins J, et al. Youth risk behavior surveillance - United States, 2015. MMWR SurveillSumm. 2016;65(6):1–174.
2. Johns MM, Lowry R, Andrzejewski J, Barrios LC, Demissie Z, McManus T, et al. Transgender identity and experiences of violence victimization, substance use, suicide risk, and sexual risk behaviors among high school students - 19 states and large Urban School districts, 2017. MMWR Morb Mortal Wkly Rep. 2019;68(3):67–71.
3. Herman JL, Flores AR, Brown TNT, Wilson BDM, Conron KJ. Age of Individuals who Identify as Transgender in the United States. UCLA Law Rev [Internet]. 2017 Jan [cited 2019 Oct 4]. Available from:https://williamsinstitute.law.ucla.edu/wp-content/uploads/TransAgeReport.pdf.
4. Thoreson R. "You Don't Want Second Best": Anti-LGBT Discrimination in US Health Care [Internet]. Human Rights Watch. 2018 [cited 2019 Oct 4]. Available from:https://www.hrw.org/report/2018/07/23/you-dont-want-second-best/anti-lgbt-discrimination-us-health-care.
5. Boyer CB, Greenberg L, Chutuape K, Walker B, Monte D, Kirk J, et al. Exchange of sex for drugs or money in adolescents and young adults: an examination of sociodemographic factors, HIV-related risk, and community context. J Community Health. 2017;42(1):90–100.
6. Edwards JM, Iritani BJ, Hallfors DD. Prevalence and correlates of exchanging sex for drugs or money among adolescents in the United States. Sex Transm Infect. 2006;82(5):354–8.
7. Kaestle CE. Selling and buying sex: a longitudinal study of risk and protective factors in adolescence. PrevSci. 2012;13(3):314–22.
8. Walls NE, Bell S. Correlates of engaging in survival sex among homeless youth and young adults. J Sex Res. 2011;48(5):423–36.
9. Patton RA, Cunningham RM, Blow FC, Zimmerman MA, Booth BM, Walton MA. Transactional sex involvement: exploring risk and promotivefactors among substance-using youth in an urban emergency department. J Stud Alcohol Drugs. 2014;75(4):573–9.
10. Singh S, Durso LE. Widespread Discrimination Continues to Shape LGBT People's Lives in Both Subtle and Significant Ways [Internet]. Center for American Progress. 2007 [cited 2019 Oct 4]. Available from:https://www.americanprogress.org/issues/lgbt/news/2017/05/02/429529/widespread-discrimination-continues-shape-lgbt-peoples-lives-subtle-significant-ways/.
11. National Research Council. Confronting commercial sexual exploitationand sex trafficking of minorsin the United States. Clayton EW, Krugman RD, Simon P, editors. Washington, D.C.: The National Academies Press; 2013.
12. Center of Excellence for Transgender Health: Department of Family & Community Medicine. Guidelines for the Primary and Gender-Affirming Care of Transgender and Gender Nonbinary People [Internet]. 2nd ed. Deutsch MB, editor. University of California, San Francisco: Center of Excellence for Transgender Health; 2016 [cited 2019 Oct 4]. Available from:https://transcare.ucsf.edu/sites/transcare.ucsf.edu/files/Transgender-PGACG-6-17-16.pdf.

13. Meckler GD, Elliott MN, Kanouse DE, Beals KP, Schuster MA. Nondisclosure of sexual orientation to a physician among a sample of gay, lesbian, and bisexual youth. Arch Pediatr Adolesc Med. 2006;160(12):1248–54.
14. Institute of Medicine (US).The health of lesbian, gay, bisexual, and transgender people: building a Foundation for Better Understanding. Washington, DC: The National Academies Press; 2011. 366 p.
15. Reisner SL, Greytak EA, Parsons JT, Ybarra ML. Gender minority social stress in adolescence: disparities in adolescent bullying and substance use by gender identity. J Sex Res. 2015;52:243–56.
16. Reisner SL, Vetters R, Leclerc M, Zaslow S, Wolfrum S, Shumer D, et al. Mental health of transgender youth in care at an adolescent urban community health center: a matched retrospective cohort study. J Adolesc Health. 2015;56:274–9.
17. Ryan C, Russell ST, Huebner D, Diaz R, Sanchez J. Family acceptance in adolescence and the health of LGBT young adults. J Child Adol Psych Nurs. 2010;23(4):205–13.
18. Ryan C, Huebner D, Diaz RM, Sanchez J. Family rejection as a predictor of negative health outcomes in white and Latino lesbian, gay, and bisexual young adults. Pediatrics. 2009;123(1):346–52.
19. Bauer GR, Scheim AI, Pyne J, Travers R, Hammond R. Intervenable factors associated with suicide risk in transgender persons: a respondent driven sampling study in Ontario, Canada. BMC Public Health. 2015;15(1):525.
20. De Pedro KT, Esqueda MC, Gilreath TD. School protective factors and substance use among lesbian, gay, and bisexual adolescents in California public schools. LGBT health. 2017;4(3):210–6.
21. Espelage DL, Aragon SR, Birkett M. Homophobic teasing, psychological outcomes, and sexual orientation among high school students: what influence do parents and schools have? School Psych Rev. 2008;37(2):202–16.
22. Bockting WO, Miner MH, Swinburne Romine RE, Hamilton A, Coleman E. Stigma, mental health, and resilience in an online sample of the US transgender population. Am J Public Health. 2013;103(5):943–51.
23. Olson KR, Durwood L, DeMeules M, McLaughlin KA. Mental health of transgender children who are supported in their identities. Pediatrics. 2016;137(3):1–8. https://doi.org/10.1542/peds.2015-3223.
24. HaganJF, ShawJS, DuncanPM. Bright futures: guidelines for health supervision of infants, children, and adolescents. American Academy of Pediatrics; 2007.
25. Cohen E, Mackenzie RG, Yates GL. HEADSS, a psychosocial risk assessment instrument: implications for designing effective intervention programs for runaway youth. J Adolesc Health. 1991;12(7):539–44.
26. Ginsburg KR. The SSHADESS screen: a strength-based psychosocial assessment. Reaching Teens Strength-Based Communication Strategies to Build Resilience and Support Healthy Adolescent Development. 2014:139–64.
27. Bradford S, Rickwood D. Psychosocial assessments for young people: asystematic review examining acceptability, disclosure and engagement, and predictive utility. Adolesc Health Med Therapeut. 2012;3:111.
28. Fuzzell L, Fedesco HN, Alexander SC, Fortenberry JD, Shields CG. "I just think that doctors need to ask more questions": sexual minority and majority adolescents' experiences talking about sexuality with healthcare providers. Patient EducCouns. 2016;99(9):1467–72.
29. RayN. An epidemic of homelessness. New York: National Gay and Lesbian Task Force Policy Institute and the National Coalition for the Homeless (US); 2006. p 192.
30. JamesS, HermanJ, RankinS, KeislingM, MottetL, AnafiMA. The report of the 2015 US transgender survey. National Center for Transgender Equality (US); 2016.
31. WatersE. Lesbian, Gay, Bisexual, Transgender, Queer, and HIV-affectedIntimate Partner Violence in 2015. New York, NY: National Coalition of Anti-Violence Programs (NCAVP); 2016. 84 p.

32. Institute of Medicine. The health of lesbian, gay, bisexual, and transgender people: building a foundation for better understanding. Washington, DC: The National Academies Press; 2011. http://www.ncbi.nlm.nih.gov/books/NBK64806.
33. Cohen E, Mackenzie RG, Yates GL. HEADSS, a psychosocial risk assessment instrument: implications for designing effective intervention programs for runaway youth. J Adolesc Health. 1991;12(7):539–44.
34. U.S. Food and Drug Administration. FDA clears first diagnostic tests for extragenital testing for chlamydia and gonorrhea [Internet]. U.S Food and Drug Administration; May 23, 2019 [cited 28 June 2019]. Availablefrom:https://www.fda.gov/news-events/press-announcements/fda-clears-first-diagnostic-tests-extragenital-testing-chlamydia-and-gonorrhea.
35. Adolescent Sexual Health [Internet]. US: American Academy of Pediatrics;2019. STI Screening Guidelines; 2019 [cited 2019 May 18]; [about 1 screen]. Available from:https://www.aap.org/en-us/advocacy-and-policy/aap-health-initiatives/adolescent-sexual-health/Pages/STI-Screening-Guidelines.aspx.
36. BransonBM, HandsfieldHH, LampeMA, JanssenRS, TaylorAW, LyssSB, ClarkJE. Revised Recommendations for HIV Testing of Adults, Adolescents, and Pregnant Women in Health-Care Settings. Atlanta, GA: CDC (US); 2006. Report No.:2.
37. Moyer VA. Screening for HIV: US preventive services task force recommendation statement. Ann Intern Med. 2013;159(1):51–60.
38. GreenG.Positive sex: sexual relationships following an HIV positive diagnosis. In: Aggleton P, Davies PM, Hart G, editors. AIDS: foundations for the future [internet]. Bristol, PA: Taylor & Francis; 1994. Chapter 10. Available from:https://books.google.com/books?hl=en&lr=&id=fxDMytljQ10C&oi=fnd&pg=PA136&dq=hiv+guilt+partner&ots=6OqcQLKci7&sig=_MT9FBWvJod9xuE9ruMlVKTMVEE#v=onepage&q=hiv%20guilt%20partner&f=false.
39. Centers for Disease Control and Prevention [Internet]. Atlanta, GA: US Department of Health and Human Services;2018 Nov 30. HIV and STD Criminal Law; 2018 Nov 30 [Cited 2019 Jun 28]. Available from:https://www.cdc.gov/hiv/policies/law/states/exposure.html.
40. Centers for Disease Control and Prevention (US). Sexually Transmitted Diseases Treatment Guidelines, 2015. MMWR Recomm Rep; 2015. 137p.
41. HIV/AIDS [Internet]. Atlanta, GA (US): Center of Disease Control, Dept of Health and Human Services; Dec 26, 2018. Preventing New HIV Infections; [cited May 19, 2019]; [about 2 screens]. Available from:https://www.cdc.gov/hiv/guidelines/preventing.html.
42. Centers for Disease Control and Prevention: US Public Health Service: Preexposure prophylaxis for the prevention of HIV infection in the United States—2017 Update: a clinical practice guideline. https://www.cdc.gov/hiv/pdf/risk/prep/cdc-hiv-prep-guidelines-2017.pdf. Published March 2018.
43. Anderson PL, Reirden D, Castillo-Mancilla J. Pharmacologic considerations for preexposure prophylaxis in transgender women. JAcquirImmune DeficSyndr (1999). 2016;72(Suppl 3):S230.
44. Hiransuthikul A, Himmad K, Kerr S, Thammajaruk N, Pankam T, Janamnuaysook R, et al. Drug-drug interactions between the use of feminizing hormone therapy and pre-exposure prophylaxis among transgender women: the iFACT study. J Inter AIDS Soc. 2018;21:170–1.
45. Hampton MD, Lieggi M. Commercial sexual exploitation of youth in the United States: a qualitative systematic review. Trauma Violence Abuse. 2017;1524838017742168
46. National Human Trafficking Hotline [Internet]. Washington, DC: Polaris; 2019 [cited Aug 27, 2019]. Available from: https://humantraffickinghotline.org/.
47. MirzaSA, RooneyC. Discrimination prevents LGBTQ people from accessing health care. Center for American Progress, January18, 2018. Available at:https://www.americanprogress.org/issues/lgbt/news/2018/01/18/445130/discrimination-prevents-lgbtq-people-accessing-health-care. Accessed May 24, 2019.
48. McRee AL, Gower AL, Reiter PL. Preventive healthcare services use among transgender young adults. Int J Transgenderism. 2018;19(4):417–23.
49. RobitzR, GajariaA, StoklosaH, JonesE, BaldwinSB. A youth transgender woman with fatigue, malnutrition and a previous suicide attempt. Psych Annals.2018; 48(3).

Chapter 12
Homelessness, Unstable Housing, and the Adolescent Patient

Nkemakolem Osian and Elizabeth Miller

Case Presentation

Tornia is a 17-year-old brought to the emergency room by ambulance following a syncopal episode at a local fast food restaurant. She states she had not eaten for a day and just passed out. In the emergency room, she was found to be slightly tachycardic with a blood pressure of 100/65. She states that she had just not been eating that day and that she is otherwise healthy. She says she is a junior in high school and lives with her mom and two younger siblings. She denies any substance use. She usually uses condoms when she is having sex with men. She thinks she's up to date on her shots. Her labs were all normal except for a slight microcytic anemia. Her EKG was normal. She received fluids, was able to eat a sandwich in the emergency room without difficulty, and was told to follow-up with her primary care clinician. A social worker came by to see her and offer food resources in case she and her family were food insecure. As she was a minor, the emergency room coordinator asked for a phone number of an adult caregiver to come pick her up. Eventually, an adult man stating he is her uncle came to the emergency room to sign her out and take her home.

Discussion Questions

(a) What are the important clinical "red flags" in this case? (Things to consider: not eating as a sign of food insecurity, unaccompanied in the emergency department, having a microcytic anemia (possibly malnutrition), and picked up from emergency department by an "uncle")
(b) How does housing insecurity impact health and well-being of young people?
(c) How does housing insecurity increase vulnerability for being trafficked?

N. Osian (✉)
HIV/AIDS Bureau, Division of Community HIV/AIDS Programs, Health Resources and Services Administration, Rockville, MD, USA

E. Miller
Division of Adolescent and Young Adult Medicine, UPMC Children's Hospital of Pittsburgh, University of Pittsburgh, Pittsburgh, PA, USA

K. E. Titchen, E. Miller (eds.), *Medical Perspectives on Human Trafficking in Adolescents*, https://doi.org/10.1007/978-3-030-43367-3_12

Youth Homelessness in the United States: At a Glance

Homeless youth are an invisible population, hidden in the shadows and undercounted. Part of this challenge stems from the fact that homeless youth have been extremely difficult to track as they generally are not seen on the streets (such as in parks or under bridges where adults who are chronically homeless may be). Homeless youth tend to experience unstable housing [1]. For example, unaccompanied youth might shelter at a friend's home for a night or two and then move on to other places, commonly referred to as "couch surfing." The lack of a standard definition for youth homelessness across federal agencies compounds the challenges that exist in tracking this population [2].

Despite these challenges, research suggests that the rate of homelessness among youth in the United States is on the rise. There are approximately four million youth and young adults (13–25 years) including about 700,000 unaccompanied youth ages 13–17 in the United States who experience homelessness in a single year. Based on a 2017 Point-in-Time (PIT) count, about 41,000 unaccompanied youth were identified as experiencing unsheltered or sheltered homelessness on any given night. Of these unaccompanied youth, about 88% were between the ages of 18 and 25 and 12% were under the age of 18. This PIT count also revealed an estimated 9400 parenting youth (under age 25) and their roughly 12,150 children experiencing homelessness in January 2017 [2].

Factors that Contribute to Youth Homelessness in the United States

Reasons for the rise in youth homelessness are vast and complex. Some factors that contribute to homelessness among youth include family dysfunctions that include child abuse and neglect, family conflict, parental substance abuse, sexual abuse, and domestic violence. Family conflict also may stem from intolerance of adult caregivers with the sexual orientation of youth. Lesbian, gay, bisexual, transgender, and questioning (LGBTQ) youth are often kicked out of the home by parents who cannot accept their lifestyle [3]. In one study with LGBT youth, one quarter reported that family rejection was the overarching cause of their homelessness. As a result, LGBTQ individuals make up a disproportionate number of those experiencing homelessness. Several studies have found that an estimated 40% of homeless youth are LGBTQ. According to the United States Interagency Council on Homelessness, LGBTQ youth are 120% more likely to report homelessness at some time during the year than their peers who identify as heterosexual and cisgender. National survey data also reveal that youth who are black and LGBT, specifically young men, report the highest rate of homelessness. Overall, the comparative risk of homelessness is 83% higher among African-American youth relative to youth of other racial/ethnic backgrounds [2].

Youth who are involved in the child welfare system are also more likely to become homeless. A good number of youth run away from their foster care families due to conflict, abuse, and/or rejection. About 12–36% of youth who age out (emancipate) from foster care become homeless. Relative to youth in the general population, youth who age out of foster care are less likely to finish high school or attend college. These youth also lack strong foundational support to help them gain financial stability and upward mobility. Collectively, these factors lead to restricted employment opportunities. As a result, these youth are more likely to experience economic hardship, become unemployed, and ultimately end up homeless [4].

In addition, justice-involved youth are at an increased risk of becoming homeless. The correlation between youth homelessness and the justice system is bidirectional. Youth involved in the justice system are more vulnerable to experiencing homelessness. A significant number of youth who are released from the justice system were previously a part of the child welfare system. Youth who are juvenile-justice involved (especially those with recurrent incarceration) often do not have the necessary skills to integrate back into society and either end up re-incarcerated or homeless [5]. Further, approximately 20–30% of homeless youth report frequent encounters with the justice system. Youth experiencing homelessness often find themselves engaging in illegal activities such as loitering and panhandling as a way to attain food and shelter and are frequently criminalized as a result. Homeless youth are also more vulnerable to becoming victims of commercial sexual exploitation and labor trafficking which puts them at a higher risk for ending up in the juvenile-justice system. The interconnection between youth homelessness and risk for becoming victims of trafficking is explored further in the next section [2].

The Intersection Between Youth Homelessness and Trafficking

Human trafficking and youth homelessness in the United States are both pressing and intersecting concerns. Many youth who experience homelessness report that they do not feel safe. Youth homelessness creates a pathway and a web of increased risk for both labor and sex trafficking [3].

Several studies reveal that the threat of sex trafficking is at a peak when both individual risk factors and environmental challenges intersect in the lives of youth including poverty, homelessness, sexual orientation, a history of maltreatment, and trauma, among many other underlying factors. One study found that LGBT youth and former foster care youth reported higher rates of victimization by trafficking compared to other youth. Runaway youth may be escaping abuse and violence in their home only to be further victimized when they end up on the streets [4]. As noted above, as youth experiencing homelessness lack basic needs such as food, shelter, and clothing, they are in survival mode. Traffickers exploit the unmet needs of homeless youth to lure them into forced labor or sex trafficking. According to one study, about 28% of homeless youth and 10% of those in shelter engage in survival sex in exchange for food, shelter, or money [6]. Furthermore, youth with a history of trauma are even more likely to engage in survival sex [2]. Another study conducted with 601 homeless youth who were seeking services in three US cities found that about 13% of the study participants reported engaging in sex trade to generate some form of income while homeless [7]. Similarly, a study with a sample of homeless youth who were receiving services from professionals in New York City showed that 34% of the study sample reported trading sex for money, drugs, food, or shelter [8].

While sex trafficking is more often identified, homeless youth also get caught up in labor trafficking. Similar to sex trafficking, homeless youth are lured into labor trafficking with the false promises of a "better life," a life that will provide them with all of the daily necessities that they are lacking. A survey conducted by the Alliance to End Slavery and Trafficking (ATEST) found that among programs serving homeless youth that screened for child labor trafficking, each program had identified at least one young person who had been trafficked for labor [9].

The largest-ever groundbreaking study in this area, with findings released in 2017, was conducted by Covenant House – a privately funded agency that provides shelter, food, and services to homeless and runaway youth — in collaboration with researchers from the Field Center for Children's Policy, Practice and Research at the University of Pennsylvania and Loyola University Modern Slavery Research Project in New Orleans. This study (conducted from 2014 to 2017) estimated the prevalence of and mechanisms for sex trafficking among homeless youth by interviewing close to 1000 youth experiencing homelessness (ages 17–25) in 13 cities. Debra Schilling Wolfe, the executive director of the Field Center, described that the goal of the study was to identify factors that could predict who is most at risk for sex trafficking: "This work can help shape national policy and create effective interventions, thereby stemming pipeline to predators and ultimately reducing the number of victims" [10].

Key findings from this study are:

- 19.4% of the 911 homeless youth who were interviewed were victims of human trafficking, with 15% sex trafficked (21.4% of young women and 10% of young men), 7.4% labor trafficked, and 3% trafficked for both.
- Similar to previous studies, this study found that LGBTQ youth were disproportionately affected. Even though the study sample was 19.2% LGBTQ, this population accounted for 33.8% of sex trafficking victims and 31.8% of those who engaged in sex trade. Transgender youth had the highest prevalence for experiences of trafficking.
- 68% of youth who were involved in commercial sex trade were homeless while doing so.
- 95% of youth who were sex trafficked reported a history of child maltreatment, with 49% reporting a history of childhood sexual abuse.
- 67% of homeless females reported being offered money for sex.

The stark findings from this study and previous studies emphasize the important role that addressing youth homelessness plays in curbing human trafficking among this population. Youth homelessness and human trafficking are intertwined and it would be ineffective to address child sex – as well as labor – trafficking without examining the underlying factors such as homelessness that increase vulnerability [11].

The Role of the Healthcare Professional

Addressing Gaps in Care

There are several service systems that youth trafficking victims encounter including law enforcement and the healthcare system. Healthcare professionals are on the frontlines and have the unique opportunity to identify, advocate for, and provide or refer victims of human trafficking to essential services. Youth who have been trafficked frequently interface with healthcare professionals while being trafficked but are often not identified as victims [12]. One study found that 43% of adolescents who were victims of trafficking had seen a healthcare professional in the previous 2 months. Another study found that 88% of trafficking victims encountered at least one healthcare professional at some point during captivity; however, none were identified as victims. As a result, none were offered assistance or essential services that could help them escape. This happens far too frequently, and these are missed opportunities for reducing youth isolation and increasing options for safety.

Several barriers to victim identification exist for both healthcare professionals and patients. Clinician barriers may include limited to no knowledge of human trafficking, failure to implement a trauma-informed approach to care, low rates of inquiry regarding trafficking, and preconceived notions (and biases) about the victims. Some of the barriers related to the patient include fear and stigma and not self-identifying as a victim resulting in low disclosure rates. It is critical for healthcare facilities to create policies and protocols that take into consideration these barriers to effectively serve victims of human trafficking [13].

To help address these gaps, there have been several promising assessment tools that have been developed to identify victims of trafficking among homeless youth in the healthcare setting. Some of these tools include the Commercial Sexual Exploitation – Identification Tool (CSE-IT), Trafficking Victim Identification Tool (TVIT), Human Trafficking Screening Tool (HTST), and the Child Sex Trafficking Tool (CST).

The CSE-IT was developed by the WestCoast Children's Clinic in 2014 with the contribution of over 100 survivors and service professionals. The validity of this tool was determined during a 15-month period of pilot testing in juvenile-justice, community-based organizations and child welfare organizations to ensure that the tool accurately identifies youth who have clear indicators of exploitation. In 2017, WestCoast Children's Clinic trained 4000 service professionals to recognize the signs of exploitation. CSE-IT has been introduced in five states and, as of January 2018, it has been used to screen over 20,000 youth.

The Trafficking Victim Identification Tool (TVIT) was developed by the Vera Institute of Justice and was tested for use with adults and youth to identify either sex or labor trafficking in community-based settings. The TVIT is distinct because it has been interpreted and validated for use in several languages. The TVIT is a 30-topic questionnaire that was tested by service professionals across the United States. This tool gives legal, healthcare, and social service professionals, law enforcement, and other professionals the ability to better recognize people who are being trafficked and offer supports that may help improve their legal, social, and health outcomes.

The Human Trafficking Screening Tool (HTST) was developed by the Urban Institute to help identify victims of trafficking involved in the child welfare and runaway and homeless youth systems. Research conducted on the tool found that it is accessible to youth and easy to administer. In addition, both versions of the tool (full and short lengths) are effective in identifying youth in the child welfare and runaway homeless systems who are being trafficked.

The Child Sex Trafficking Tool (CST) developed by Greenbaum et al. was created and tested specifically for the healthcare setting – in emergency departments, child advocacy centers, and adolescent clinics [14]. The six-item short form showed relatively good sensitivity and moderate specificity, such that the tool may help identify youth who are being trafficked as well as youth at elevated risk for becoming trafficked.

CSE-IT, TVIT, HTST, and CST may be useful tools for implementation within agencies serving youth who are involved in the child welfare, juvenile-justice, and homeless shelter systems. Integrating such assessment and routine inquiry into agencies serving youth at elevated risk, these tools may serve as an important opportunity for educating both staff and youth about the realities of trafficking as well as the available resources and can be a step forward in ensuring that homeless and unstably housed youth who are victims of trafficking are recognized and offered essential services [12]. Youth should always receive resources and information about trafficking regardless of disclosure to these assessment tools. (See Sect. 4.13 for additional considerations regarding trauma-sensitive implementation of any assessments and rationale for universal education approach.) Such assessment tools alone, however, will not curb trafficking and homelessness among youth. Systemic policy changes are needed.

A Call for Housing and Policy Changes

Ending youth homelessness is integral to the fight against human trafficking. In this effort, youth experiencing homelessness and youth who have been trafficked cannot be viewed as distinct populations. In many circumstances, they are the same youth and taking steps toward curbing exploitation must take into account the factors that make them vulnerable to such exploitation.

To effectively address youth homelessness requires collective effort across multiple sectors of society from the housing and homeless agencies serving young people to the child welfare system. For example, housing and homelessness agencies play a critical role in decreasing youth susceptibility to trafficking. These entities are in a unique position to respond quickly to a young person's homelessness because they provide a variety of options that are intended to fulfill the needs of youth and young adults in diverse situations [9]. Overall the services that these agencies provide include street outreach, emergency shelter, drop-in centers, education and employment supports, family intervention services, transitional housing, and independent housing options. Instead of expelling young people for behavioral challenges, it is important that transitional and other housing programs and services supported by public agencies (including health professionals) provide incentives as a way to retain and serve this population appropriately.

In several communities across the United States, partnerships have already developed between service professionals helping youth experiencing homelessness and victims of trafficking. Professionals serving youth experiencing homelessness are beginning to realize that many they serve have been victims of trafficking. Therefore, it is imperative to formalize and sustain these collaborations to effectively address these intersecting issues. It is also crucial for everyone who works with youth who are experiencing homelessness to be educated, trained, and well-informed about the interconnection between homelessness and trafficking.

The child welfare system also plays an integral role in closing the housing gaps that exist for homeless and trafficked youth. Child welfare agencies should provide services for youth who lack safe and stable housing and create safe pathways for reunification between youth and their families whenever possible. Child welfare agencies are also in a unique position to help significantly reduce the risks that make youth who are homeless more susceptible to trafficking. One approach is to develop a plan that helps youth transition once they age out of the system to become independent and self-sufficient. These agencies should provide these youth with opportunities to access education, job skills training, financial support, life skills, independent living, and important social supports. All of these factors work collectively to help reduce the trafficking risk for youth who age out of the child welfare system. The diagram below (Fig. 12.1), from a report by the National Network for Youth, highlights the key factors that can help decrease youth vulnerability to trafficking [4]. (See Chap. 8 for more information on human trafficking and intersections with foster care.)

Finally, while a focus on affordable housing and policy changes that support the needs of vulnerable youth are critical, additional considerations to assist LGBTQ youth are needed. As the homeless youth population is comprised of about 40% LGBTQ identified youth, they are at an increased risk for remaining homeless for extended periods of time compared to non-LGBTQ homeless youth. In addition, LGBTQ youth experiencing homelessness are more likely to endure discrimination and sexual abuse, to have mental health and substance abuse problems, and to have encounters with law enforcement, all of which further exacerbate both the

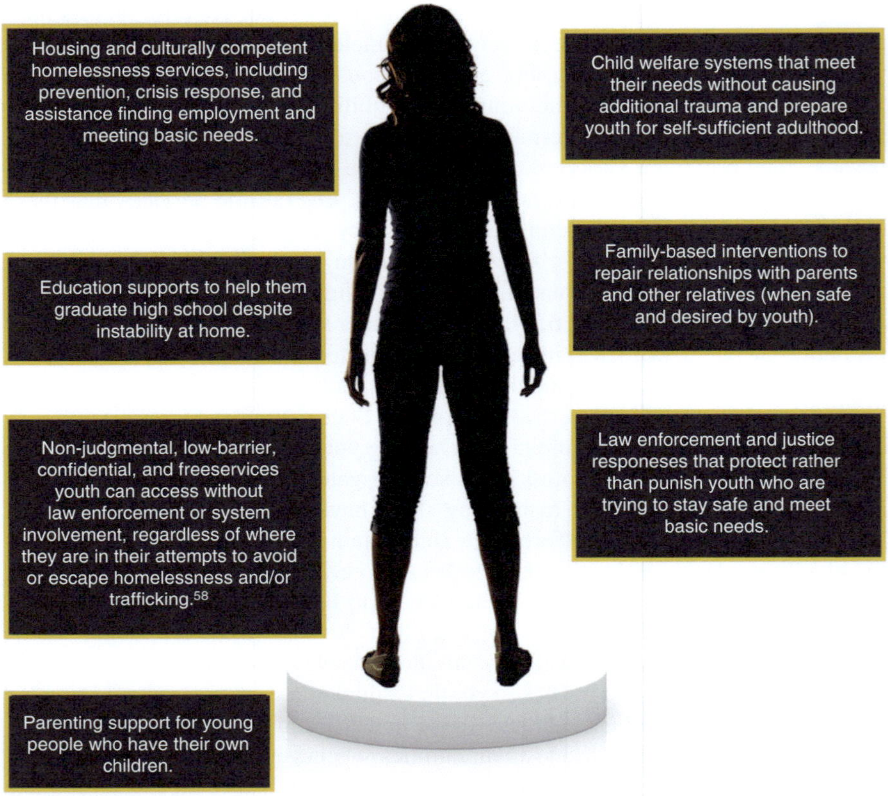

Fig. 12.1 Supportive and protective factors that reduce vulnerability for trafficking (*figure reproduced with permission from the National Network for Youth*)

likelihood of being unstably housed and being identified by traffickers as an easy target [15]. This reality becomes even more staggering when talking about LGBTQ youth of color. LGBTQ youth of color are at a heightened risk of becoming homeless and remaining in those circumstances compared to their white counterparts. This is due largely to the structural, social, and emotional barriers such as homophobia, racism, and conflicts even within their own communities which creates a culture of fear and isolation. More resources and funding are needed for housing programs that address the unique needs of LGBTQ homeless youth. Social services geared to this population should include comprehensive health services (including HIV testing as well as mental health and substance abuse treatment). Service professionals should also be appropriately trained to understand how best to support youth of diverse sexual and gender identities. This includes advocating for gender-neutral bathrooms as well as preferred gender pronouns and name in the electronic health record [16]. (See Chap. 11 for more information on LGBTQIA+ youth and human trafficking.)

Returning then to the case, given what is known about the intersections of housing insecurity, food insecurity, and risks for trafficking, the healthcare professionals in the emergency department missed an opportunity to connect with Tornia and offer her services and supports. An unaccompanied minor in the emergency department who has not eaten (including in this case some evidence of possible malnutrition) should not only prompt considerations for eating disorders and dehydration but also the possibility of social factors such as housing instability and trafficking that are contributing to her presentation. This young person was lost to follow-up without resources or connections that may have helped address any of her myriad immediate needs and build trust. It is also notable that a policy that is intended to keep children safe by requiring an adult be present at time of discharge (for non-confidential services) may have also resulted in her returning to the trafficker. A confidential conversation with Tornia about her social circumstances, an offer of information about trafficking and additional supports available to young people, and a system with careful check of identification of any adult arriving to "pick up" the child from a clinical setting may have resulted in a different story for this young person.

Although there is no one-size-fits-all approach to eradicating youth homelessness, there are steps that can be taken to decrease the number of homeless youth and to reduce risk for being trafficked. Human trafficking and youth homelessness are inextricably linked and it would be virtually impossible and ineffective to address trafficking without addressing one of the most prominent factors that make youth more susceptible to traffickers. From healthcare professionals to housing and homeless agencies, combating trafficking and homelessness among youth will necessarily take the collective effort of all sectors in society.

References

1. Fernandes-Alcantara AL. Runaway and homeless youth: demographics and programs. Washington, D.C.: Congressional Research Service; 2018.
2. United States Interagency Council on Homelessness. Homelessness in America: focus on youth. Washington, D.C.: United States Interagency Council on Homelessness; 2018.
3. The National Network for Youth. Human trafficking and the runaway and homeless youth population. Washington, D.C.: The National Network for Youth; 2014.
4. Pilnik L. Responding to youth homelessness, a key strategy for preventing human trafficking. Washington, D.C.: The National Network for Youth; 2018.
5. Morton MH, Dworsky A, Matjasko JL, Curry SR, Schlueter D, Chávez R, et al. Prevalence and correlates of youth homelessness in the United States. J Adolesc Health. 2018;62:14–21.
6. Greene JM, Ennett ST, Ringwalt CL. Prevalence and correlates of survival sex among runaway and homeless youth. Am J Public Health. 1999;89:1406–9.
7. Bender K, Yang J, Ferguson K, Thompson S. Experiences and needs of homeless youth with a history of foster care. Child Youth Serv Rev. 2015;55:222–31.
8. NetWork LW. Meeting the service needs of human trafficking survivors in the New York City metropolitan area: assessment and recommendations. lifewaynetwork.org.
9. Henry M, Mahathey A, Morrill T, Robinson A, Shivji A, Watt R, et al. The 2018 Annual Homeless Assessment Report (AHAR) to Congress. The U.S. Department of Housing and Urban Development; 2018.

10. Wolfe DS, Greeson JKP, Wasch S, Treglia D. Human trafficking prevalence and child welfare risk factors among homeless youth: a multi-city study. The Field Center for Children's Policy, Practice & Research at the University of Pennsylvania; 2018. Available at https://fieldcenteratpenn.org/wp-content/uploads/2013/05/6230-R10-Field-Center-Full-Report-Web.pdf. Accessed on June 21, 2020.
11. Murphy L. Labor and sex trafficking among homeless youth: a ten city study (executive summary). 2017.
12. Mostajabian S, Santa Maria D, Wiemann C, Newlin E, Bocchini C. Identifying sexual and labor exploitation among sheltered youth experiencing homelessness: a comparison of screening methods. Int J Environ Res Public Health. 2019;16(3):363.
13. Rollins R, Gribble A, Barrett SE, Powell C. Who is in your waiting room? Health care professionals as culturally responsive and trauma-informed first responders to human trafficking. AMA J Ethics. 2017;19:63–71.
14. Greenbaum VJ, Livings MS, Lai BS, Edinburgh L, Baikie P, Grant SR, et al. Evaluation of a tool to identify child sex trafficking victims in multiple healthcare settings. J Adolesc Health. 2018;63:745–52.
15. Choi SK, Wilson BDM, Shelton J, Gates G. Serving our youth 2015: The needs and experiences of lesbian, gay, bisexual, transgender, and questioning youth experiencing homelessness. Los Angeles: The Williams Institute With True Colors Fund. 2015.
16. Page M. Forgotten youth: homeless LGBT youth of color and the runaway and homeless youth act. Northwest J Law SocPolicy. 2017;12(2):17.

Chapter 13
The Patient with Substance Use

Elizabeth S. Barnert, Mikaela A. Kelly, Alexandra G. Shumyatsky, and Marti MacGibbon

Case Presentation

Jessica is a 16-year-old girl presenting to a community clinic for a sick visit with the chief complaint of, "It hurts to pee." You are the clinician, and this is the first time you are meeting Jessica. She is accompanied by a staff member from her group home, who is asked to wait in the clinic lobby. As you enter the examination room, you notice that Jessica appears visibly tense, anxious, and withdrawn, as evidenced by her physical posture and facial expression. You smile and introduce yourself before taking a seat across from her. When you ask Jessica about her symptoms, she states that she began experiencing pain while urinating 3 days ago. She also has noticed increased urinary frequency and urgency. She has not noticed abnormal vaginal discharge, odor, or pruritis; and she reports no hematuria, abnormal bleeding, fever, nausea, vomiting, abdominal pain, back pain, diarrhea, or constipation. She denies recent unprotected sex and history of sexually transmitted infections. You ask if you may perform a physical exam, and she agrees. During the exam you observe the name "Anthony" tattooed on her lower abdomen, which causes her to become very tense and quickly cover the tattoo with her clothing. Otherwise, the physical exam is unremarkable. She does not have signs of acute or chronic illness. She appears well-nourished and has good hygiene, good dentition, and no track marks or scars. Her point-of-care urinalysis is positive for leukocytes and leukocyte esterase. The urine pregnancy test in clinic is negative. You also order gonorrhea, chlamydia, and syphilis testing, and she consents to HIV testing. You send a urine culture to the lab. Jessica is prescribed nitrofurantoin for possible urinary tract infection and is taken back to the group home.

Several days later, you receive results showing that Jessica's urine sample is positive for gonorrhea and request that Jessica return to the clinic. When she returns later that day, you

E. S. Barnert (✉) · M. A. Kelly
Department of Pediatrics, David Geffen School of Medicine at UCLA, Los Angeles, CA, USA

A. G. Shumyatsky
Department of Cell Biology and Neuroscience, Rutgers University, Piscataway, NJ, USA

M. MacGibbon
Office for Victims of Crime (Expert Consultant), Sacramento, CA, USA

K. E. Titchen, E. Miller (eds.), *Medical Perspectives on Human Trafficking in Adolescents*, https://doi.org/10.1007/978-3-030-43367-3_13

again notice her anxious behavior. You tell her that she should stop the nitrofurantoin because her urine culture was negative. You inform Jessica of the positive gonorrhea test and tell her that it was good that she experienced symptoms, as most cases are asymptomatic. To treat her gonorrhea infection, you prescribe a single dose of intramuscular ceftriaxone and a single dose of oral azithromycin. You advise that Jessica avoid having sex until after her symptoms have completely resolved. To prevent further spread of the infection, you counsel about the importance of condoms and advise that Jessica and her sexual partners avoid sexual activity until at least 7 days after treatment.

You encourage Jessica to notify her current and recent sexual partners so that they are able to obtain appropriate treatment. At this suggestion, Jessica becomes visibly upset and withdrawn. You ask her if she is okay. She says that she has not had unprotected sex recently. She does not know where her past partners are. You decide to take more time to do a full adolescent psychosocial assessment (see Chap. 4 for a more detailed description of the SHEADSSS approach), assuring Jessica about her right to doctor-patient confidentiality, with explanation of mandated reporting considerations. When you ask Jessica sensitively about sexual risk factors, violence, abuse, and substance use, she reveals a history of human trafficking, which began after running away from her foster home at the age of 12. She states that this is in the past, and this information is known to her group home, where she was placed after an arrest for drug possession. In response to your nonjudgmental questioning, she divulges that although she has used methamphetamine and heroin in the past, she is in recovery and "only" uses marijuana now. When you ask her why she uses marijuana, she says that marijuana helps her "stay calm" and helps her sleep. She tells you that she often does not sleep at night and, when she does, she has nightmares.

The nurse knocks on the door to inform you that the ceftriaxone shot has been drawn up and that your next patient is waiting.

Background on Substance Use Among Youth with Histories of CSE

Jessica is a composite character based on our clinical experience as well as research interviews, conducted by two of the chapter authors (EB, MK), with youth impacted by commercial sexual exploitation (CSE) on their health needs and experiences with healthcare. As highlighted in other chapters in this handbook, several aspects of Jessica's presentation are risk factors for CSE, such as her prior involvement in foster care. In this chapter, we will focus on the aspects of Jessica's story relevant to the intersection of CSE and substance use.

Definition of Addiction/Substance Use Disorder (SUD)

The connection between addiction and commercial sexual exploitation is recognized by the federal criminal justice system [1, 2]. Service providers can benefit from understanding the American Society of Addiction Medicine's definition of substance abuse/addiction [3]:

> "Addiction is a primary, chronic disease of brain reward, motivation, memory and related circuitry. Dysfunction in these circuits leads to characteristic biological, psychological, social and spiritual manifestations. This is reflected in an individual pathologically pursuing reward and/or relief by substance use and other behaviors."

As further described by the American Society of Addiction Medicine, addiction is characterized by inability to abstain from the substance, lack of control over one's behavior, and a dysfunctional emotional response. Untreated, addiction is progressive and can result in death [3]. Survivors of CSE with substance use challenges often face double societal stigma, receiving judgment and condemnation for both their exploitation and their addiction.

Substance use disorder (SUD), or addiction, is a primary, chronic disease that is characterized by lack of choice [4–6]. In many situations, the judgment and condemnation directed toward individuals with SUD is based on a mistaken belief that the "addict" persists in making a series of "bad choices" and that shaming or punishing them will make them change their "bad" behavior. In fact, the link between shame and addiction is recognized by the addiction treatment profession and the broader behavioral health treatment community. Shame and fear can also exacerbate the cycle of trauma and substance use. Societal stigma and self-stigma may cause patients to minimize their substance use and misuse and/or under-report it. Denial and option reduction increase as SUD progresses. Option reduction can impair the SUD sufferer's ability to see all the available choices in a given situation. In active, ongoing SUD, denial and option reduction occur as a result of neurological changes in the brain that increase as the SUD progresses and impair the individual's ability to recognize the harmful effects of their own compulsive use. Recovery reverses the process as the brain and body heal from the negative effects of the disease. In active recovery, the patient learns how to make healthy choices again. When a patient has been trafficked/exploited, they've already been robbed of choice, and in active SUD, the substances make choices for the patient. Sometimes, circumstances or drug-using associates will act as default decision-makers. When mental health disorders co-occur with addiction disorders, healthcare providers must take care to connect patients with appropriate treatment resources. Adolescents with CSE history and substance use issues will benefit from playing an active role in their own treatment plans; the process of choosing interventions and setting goals is intrinsically healing for the recovering brain and is an exercise in discovering and building self-empowerment, dignity, and self-esteem.

Substance Use Prevalence Among Youth with Histories of CSE

Available literature suggests that rates of substance use among youth with histories of CSE are high [7, 8]. The authors (EB, MK) studied a sample of 364 youth with histories of CSE supervised in a specialty juvenile delinquency court in Los Angeles, and they found that 90% reported ever having used at least one illicit substance. The most common substances used were marijuana (87%), followed by alcohol (54%) and amphetamines (33%). Further, polysubstance use was common. While nearly half (46%) of the youth reported use of one or two substances, more than one-third (35%) reported having used three to four substances, and 8% reported using five or more substances [9]. The average age at first use for marijuana was 12.8 years, alcohol was 13.5 years, and methamphetamine was 13.6 years. Similarly, a

New York-based cross-sectional study of 237 youth with histories of CSE found that over half (54%) reported using marijuana on a regular basis. Other commonly used substances included cocaine (26%), alcohol (25%), and heroin (14%) [8]. Similar rates of substance use were seen between girls and boys; however, a higher proportion of girls used "crack" or prescription pain killers, while a higher proportion of boys abused heroin and methamphetamine [8].

Within the general adolescent population, substance use of all types has decreased in the past decade, with the exception of marijuana use [10]. Additionally, alcohol use among teens has been lower in recent years [10]. However, among adolescents impacted by CSE, substance use remains high and is often severe [8]. Further, substance use among youth with histories of CSE often begins at younger ages compared to adolescent peers without histories of CSE, which is notable as younger age at first use strongly predicts later life SUD [11].

Intersection of Risks

Adolescents with SUD/addiction problems have an increased likelihood of having a trauma history [7]. The extreme and often complex trauma endured by many youth with histories of CSE makes them highly vulnerable to addiction [7]. Likewise, addiction makes youth vulnerable to CSE [12]. Thus, adolescents impacted by CSE often have histories of substance use that precede or interact with their exploitation, in addition to their mental health and trauma histories [7]. Furthermore, adolescents impacted by CSE have high rates of post-traumatic stress, which can potentiate addiction risk [10, 13].

Specifically, chaotic or dysfunctional childhood home environments can directly contribute to CSE risk and adolescent substance use [14]. Many youth with histories of CSE have experienced childhood physical, sexual, and emotional abuse or neglect [14]. Additionally, histories of parental drug use or parental incarceration are common for youth with histories of CSE, which can also contribute to adolescent substance use [14, 15]. Mechanisms for this link may include increased exposure and access to drugs, normalization of drug use, and deterioration of youths' mental health. Additionally, unstable home environments can lead youth to run away from home and/or become involved in the child welfare or juvenile justice systems [16]. This instability is a well-documented risk for CSE and can perpetuate substance use [14, 17].

Substance Use and CSE

Adolescents with histories of CSE may suffer from co-occurring mental health conditions that may be linked to their exploitation [13]. Common mental health conditions among CSE youth include depression, anxiety, suicidality, and post-traumatic stress disorder (PTSD) [10, 13]. Youth with histories of CSE may rely on drugs or alcohol to reduce their mental health symptoms that develop or become exacerbated due to sexual exploitation [13]. Thus, substance use can be seen as a coping mechanism for unmet mental health need. Empirical evidence collected in the authors' (EB, MK) study of judicially involved youth with histories of CSE demonstrated a strong link between substance use and mental health conditions [9]. Among a sample of 364 youth with histories of CSE, the odds of using two or more substances for those with a mental health challenge was 8.5 times the odds of using two or more substances for those without a mental health challenge. Additionally, the odds of using methamphetamine for those with a mental health condition was 4.4 times the odds of using methamphetamine for those without a mental health condition [9].

Some traffickers subject CSE youth to drug or alcohol use to create physiological dependence as a form of control [18]. Exploiters may recruit youth with promises of drugs and then intentionally foster chemical dependence so that youth remain exploited. One study of youth with histories of justice involvement and CSE found that use of substances in 1 year predicted subsequent CSE in the following year [19]. Youth who have exited CSE may relapse because of their physiological and psychological dependence on drugs, including alcohol, as exploitation can often be seen as a means to access drugs [18]. CSE youth may also be forced to transport or sell drugs, creating an under-discussed intersection between labor and sex trafficking [20]. (See Chap. 5 for further discussion of this intersection around forced criminality.)

In addition, the trauma from being trafficked may increase the risk of relapse for youth who have achieved abstinence from substances and have begun the process of recovery from SUD. PTSD is among the most common co-occurring disorders found in individuals in treatment for substance misuse or disorders [13]. Clinicians need to understand and inform patients that becoming abstinent from substances does not resolve trauma, and in some cases abstinence can exacerbate certain trauma symptoms. Both disorders must be addressed in treatment [21].

Many youth with histories of CSE may not view alcohol or drug use as a problem [5]. Some youth may view their drug use as beneficial, or may want to quit but may feel so overwhelmed with their life circumstances that they remain entrapped in cycles of substance use and CSE. Given the high rates and severity of substance use seen among youth with histories of CSE, substance use treatment is an important aspect to consider in the care of youth with histories of CSE [22].

Jessica, in this case study, self-reports that marijuana helps her "stay calm" and helps her sleep. This is a possible example of self-medicating in an attempt to manage trauma. And it could be a red flag for dependence, or risk of developing dependence, on marijuana or other substances. In the case presentation, Jessica self-reports she has used methamphetamine and heroin in the past, but is in recovery now and "only" uses marijuana. Marijuana and alcohol are addictive substances, but they are perceived to be safe by young people because they are more socially acceptable. Societal stigma toward those who use alcohol and marijuana is less severe than the stigma toward "hard" drugs like methamphetamine, heroin, cocaine, etc. Addiction is a disease, and the physiological and neurological effects of the disease are equally serious regardless of which substance(s) the patient may be dependent upon. (See Chap. 17 for more on cardiovascular effects of substance use). In the case study, Jessica does not present with the stigmata of recent intravenous drug use, but she would benefit from non-judgmental patient education about drug use and chemical dependency [23].

In summary, the case presentation illustrates several aspects that youth may experience while being trafficked. As the literature illustrates, and as personified by Jessica, youth may feel that marijuana use is not a problem but rather a helpful coping mechanism for underlying depression and anxiety. The literature also shows that dependence on harder drugs, including use against one's will, can entrap youth in cycles of exploitation. Youth may not feel an allegiance with their clinicians, and their clinicians may not feel available or know how to direct youth to needed substance use treatment. While Jessica's case is not representative of all youth, the case narrative serves as an example to summarize salient points relevant to factors influencing substance use among trafficked persons. Understanding these factors can help yield a more effective approach to treatment – both of substance use and related health conditions.

Opportunities

Youth Impacted by CSE Do Present for Healthcare

Given the prevalence of substance use in this population, a number of opportunities exist for intervention. Current research, while limited, suggests that youth with histories of CSE do present for healthcare both during and after exploitation [23, 24]. One retrospective study involving youth who raised high suspicion for CSE ($N = 63$) found that 83% had received medical care within the past year [23]. Another study of youth impacted by CSE similarly found that a clinician had seen 81% of their participants within the past year [24]. Additionally, in a separate study of youth presenting to an emergency department who screened positive for commercial sexual exploitation, 35% had seen a healthcare professional within the previous 2 months [25]. Involvement with the healthcare system presents an opportunity for both substance use assessment and potential treatment. Research by EB and MK explored the interactions of adolescent girls impacted by CSE with various types of healthcare, utilizing mixed methods [16]: reproductive healthcare was generally actively sought, while behavioral healthcare (i.e., mental health and substance use treatment) was typically mandated after youth became involved in "the system" (i.e., juvenile justice system, child welfare system). In addition, reproductive healthcare facilities, such as Planned Parenthood, presented an opportunity to connect with youth impacted by CSE about their substance use treatment needs [16]. This care opportunity is consistent with our case example of Jessica, who presented for reproductive healthcare and subsequently revealed a history of CSE and associated substance use. However, clinicians need to be attuned that youth often deny the extent of addiction and also often do not view their exploitation as abuse, or their drug use as problematic. Some youth may be more ready for help than others – however, all should be offered help regardless of disclosure.

Systems Involvement

A unique opportunity exists to engage youth who are systems-involved (i.e., juvenile justice system, foster care system), as youth impacted by CSE often are referred or mandated to mental health and substance use treatment services [13]. Identifying the best means to achieve treatment engagement is key. Exploration of youths' "buy-in" or engagement in substance use treatment [12] revealed that engagement in behavioral healthcare hinged upon whether or not the adolescent girls had access to trusted clinicians. Clinician relationships that fostered autonomy and no judgment were the most impactful. These aspects were embedded within the context of their CSE histories, where youth experienced severe trauma, danger, and disappointment. Additionally, youth involved in a variety of systems often experienced fragmented care – where they may have had at least one clinician in juvenile detention, another in a group home, and another once at home with their parents. Consistency in care provided the optimal environment for youth to meaningfully engage in treatment [25].

Challenges

Context of CSE

Efforts to provide treatment and care for CSE youth with substance use pose a number of challenges. Within the context of CSE, youth may prioritize their survival needs rather than engaging in available treatment options [26]. Additionally, youth may be under the control of their trafficker, who may encourage or force substance use [18]. Furthermore, youth may have extensive difficulties coping with their unique trauma histories without the substances they have grown accustomed to using [27].

Healthcare-Related Challenges

With regard to specific treatment and healthcare, continuity of care can be a challenge for this often-transient population [28]. Clinicians need to understand that traffickers not only target youth but also people who are using substances. Some traffickers directly recruit people coming out of detox/rehab and SUD treatment facilities [29]. Traffickers know that people exiting detox or SUD treatment facilities have built-in vulnerabilities and will be "low-hanging fruit" – also they are easy to recognize; this is similar to the way that traffickers target group homes and foster homes and children aging out of foster care. Referral of any trafficking victim or survivor to SUD treatment must be well-researched, well-thought out, and trauma-informed to protect the patient.

Additionally, providers should be attuned to avoiding stigmatizing language, either with regard to exploitation history or substance use. Language should be (1) person-first, (2) focused on medical aspects of care, (3) strengths-based and recovery promoting, and (4) without slang or idioms that promote negative stereotypes or perpetuate stigma [23, 30]. (See Chap. 19 Survivor Insights for more on the importance of language.)

Some commercially sexually exploited adolescents with SUD may not identify openly about their gender identity and may not identify as being trafficked. LGBTQIA+ youth (lesbian, gay, bisexual, transgender, genderqueer, questioning, intersex, and asexual) are highly vulnerable to substance use issues and to being trafficked. (See Chap. 11 for more in-depth information.) Healthcare professionals can create a safe space for LGBTQIA+ patients in the clinical setting. In LGBTQIA+ culture, substance use settings are an integral part of connecting with others, and 12-step meetings generally don't list meetings that are LGBTQIA+; patients find out about them through word of mouth in areas that are not major urban centers. Establishing contact with local LGBT centers to find practitioners who are culturally competent and representing a truly LGBTQIA+ safe space with an equality flag (equal sign on blue background), rainbow flag, or a doormat/sign that says "All Are Welcome Here," will make patients feel more comfortable. (For more about LGBTQIA youth and trafficking, see Chap. 11.)

Moreover, clinical settings for addiction treatment vary and include acute rehab/detox, one-on-one counseling sessions, group counseling sessions, inpatient rehab, outpatient rehab, and transitional housing. Inpatient, outpatient, and transitional housing treatment settings generally include process group sessions, one-on-one counseling sessions, and educational group sessions. The best facilities are licensed and accredited, adhere to evidence-based and trauma-informed practices, and offer access to medication-assisted treatment (MAT) for patients with opioid and benzodiazepine dependence. There are many psychosocial approaches to treatment. Cognitive behavioral therapy (CBT) is a psychotherapeutic intervention that helps patients understand why they adopted addictive behaviors and thought processes. This approach helps patients learn how to "successfully modify addictive behaviors…and make such changes durable" [31]. Motivational interviewing (MI) and motivational enhancement therapy (MET) focus on enhancing the patient's desire for positive change.

Patients, including adolescent and young adult patients, with opioid use, misuse, or disorder need MAT to safely recover, and MAT is recommended for longer than a 28-day treatment interval. "Cold-turkey" withdrawal from opioids, especially opioids in combination with benzodiazepines and alcohol, is dangerous and can be fatal. Youth may present for care in one setting, such as in a group home, and subsequently be transitioned from placement to the care of their parents, disconnecting them from the treatment setting. Attempts to provide adequate care and support necessitate continuity and consistency [28]. Courts, families, and organizations often look to recovery support groups, the most well-known of which is Twelve Steps, as a means of continuity of care for youth and adults with substance use concerns [30]. This is understandable, as these programs are no cost or low cost and ubiquitous in our society. Healthcare professionals and other service providers need to understand the possible benefits, risks, and complications of participation in Twelve-Step programs.

Twelve-Step Programs – A Word of Caution

Twelve-Step meetings, such as Alcoholics Anonymous (AA) or Narcotics Anonymous (NA), are not supervised group sessions, rely on anonymity, lack formal research of their effectiveness, and are not equivalent to clinical mental health treatment. As a result, Twelve-Step meetings and events should be offered cautiously to young people who are connected to treatment and are interested in exploring peer support to enhance their treatment plan and/or to connect with others who are like-minded to build a positive social support network. The Twelve-Step programs focus on admitting that we are "powerless" over addiction; but focusing on powerlessness can be counterproductive for someone dealing with trauma, or for someone who has been sexually assaulted, abused, or commercially sexually exploited.

*While Twelve-Step programs have helped thousands of people to recover, the Twelve-Step program is not a trauma-sensitive program. In fact, the meetings may be a risky environment for newly exited survivors of commercial sexual exploitation, sex trafficking, or labor trafficking who may be re-traumatized as they mingle with members of the group – a group which could include (anonymous) sex offenders and violent offenders mandated to Twelve-Step meetings by the court system. Lay press articles have chronicled "Thirteenth-Stepping" within the culture of the meetings – a slang term within the Twelve-Step community that describes a harmful pattern of behavior where someone at a meeting will exploit the vulnerabilities of the newcomer for sex. *The potential risk goes beyond Thirteenth-Stepping – there is a possibility of sexual harassment, sexual assault, and sexual exploitation within the Twelve-Step setting. If a patient who is a survivor is court-mandated by a judge to attend Twelve-Step meetings, the healthcare professional should educate the patient/survivor about self-protective behaviors and strategies to use while in the Twelve-Step community such as feeling empowered to refuse hugs from people at meetings and to refuse answering personal questions. Advocates can also attend meetings with survivors, and youth survivors with substance use issues may indeed find support and success within those programs.*

Narcotics Anonymous and Alcoholics Anonymous have events for youth and adolescent survivors with substance use issues may find support and success within those programs. Some youth may prefer to attend meetings of

Marijuana Anonymous (MA), Cocaine Anonymous (CA), Crystal Meth Anonymous (CMA), or Heroin Anonymous (HA) because they may identify better with a group recognizing recovering from a specific substance dependence. Urban areas offer a panoply of choices in Twelve-Step model support groups, while rural areas may only have one or two AA meetings.

*Cunha D. "I was fresh meat": how AA meetings push some women into harmful dating; 2015 Sep The Guardian [Internet]. London (UK): Available from: https://www.theguardian.com/society/2015/sep/22/alcoholics-anonymous-aa-women-dating-addition-rehab

In sum, as previously mentioned, addiction is a devastating condition [3], and even under the most ideal circumstances, with ample support, recovery is difficult [32]. This aligns with the narrative surrounding CSE. CSE is often a cyclical process, where youth may be commercially sexually exploited, disengage, and subsequently return under a variety of circumstances [33]. Addiction often follows a similar process; and the forces that draw youth back into CSE and substance use often interrelate and self-perpetuate each other [25].

Conclusions

Clinicians and service providers can avoid re-traumatizing young people impacted by CSE and substance use by employing patient-centered best practices for trauma-informed care. Education about substance use/addiction for both service provider and patient is recommended because the double societal stigma is pervasive and can affect how provider and patient view the approach to treatment. Trauma-sensitive care delivered through a harm-reduction lens in settings that are flexible and accessible to youth is most likely to be effective. Substance use is intertwined with CSE and disentangling them requires compassionate, dedicated care to overcome the neuro-bio-behavioral patterns of substance use and to promote successful, long-lasting healing.

Discussion Questions

1. Why does Jessica appear so uncomfortable in the healthcare setting? What can you change about the way you interact with young people who are being commercially sexually exploited to appear more trustworthy? How can the clinic setting be more inviting?

2. How can you best meet Jessica's substance use treatment needs? How can you optimally help her while not over-stepping, re-traumatizing her, creating more care fragmentation, or falling behind at your busy clinic?
3. How can you ensure that Jessica is improving and receiving the right treatment?

Resources

1. *Polaris Project Referral Directory* provides addiction treatment services by location on their website. Go to https://humantraffickinghotline.org/training-resources/referral-directory, click "Services," and then select "Addiction Treatment/Services."
2. Healthcare professionals need to understand the importance of evidence-based recommendations for treatment of SUD and trauma. *Seeking Safety* is an evidence-based program for treatment of substance use issues and trauma: https://www.treatment-innovations.org/seeking-safety.html. *Seeking Safety* is for adolescents and adults and is free or low cost. Clinics with mental health practitioners working alongside medical practitioners can consider training mental health staff using *Seeking Safety*.
3. Treatment facilities can be found on this free tip sheet from the *Substance Abuse and Mental Health Services Administration (SAMHSA)*: https://store.samhsa.gov/product/Finding-Quality-Treatment-for-Substance-Use-Disorders/PEP18-TREATMENT-LOC.
4. Board-certified addiction medicine physicians can be located via the website of the *American Board of Addiction Medicine*: http://www.abam.net/.
5. *SMART Recovery (Self-Management and Recovery Training)* is a network of support groups based on cognitive behavioral therapy that is an alternative to Twelve-Step programs. Another alternative is LifeRing, a strength-based network of support groups that works on positive reinforcement of the qualities one already possesses, rather than the Twelve-Step practice of focusing on "admitting you are powerless" over the substance use issue.
6. If a patient presents with tracks or scars that indicate intravenous drug use, the patient will benefit from information/education about *harm reduction resources* like clean needle exchanges to protect individual and public health, Narcan (naloxone) kits to prevent overdose death, and safe injection sites for public health and the safety of individuals. Urban areas are more likely to provide one or all of these options, but smaller cities and rural areas have built harm reduction resources within their communities in response to the opioid crisis. A staff member at your clinic can become trained in administering naloxone and can train others. Learn more at https://harmreduction.org/issues/overdose-prevention/tools-best-practices/od-kit-materials/.

References

1. The United States Department of Justice. Massachusetts man sentenced to 17 years for sex trafficking women by exploiting their opioid addictions [Internet]. 2018 [cited2019 Sep 27]. Available from: https://www.justice.gov/opa/pr/massachusetts-man-sentenced-17-years-sex-trafficking-women-exploiting-their-opioid-addictions.
2. Stoklosa H, MacGibbon M, Stoklosa J. Human trafficking, mental illness, and addiction: avoiding diagnostic overshadowing. AMA J Ethics. 2017;19:23–34.
3. ASAM Definition of Addiction [Internet]. [cited 2019Oct 1]. Available from: https://www.asam.org/resources/definition-of-addiction.
4. Miller M, Gorski TT, Miller DK. Learning to live again: a guide for recovery from chemical dependency. REV 92. Independence: Herald House/Independence Press; 1992.
5. Matthews S, Dwyer R, Snoek A. Stigma and self-stigma in addiction. J Bioeth Inq. 2017;14:275–86.
6. Rinn W, Desai N, Rosenblatt H, Gastfriend DR. Addiction denial and cognitive dysfunction: a preliminary investigation. J Neuropsychiatry Clin Neurosci. 2002;14:52–7.
7. Barnert E, Iqbal Z, Bruce J, Anoshiravani A, Kolhatkar G, Greenbaum J. Commercial sexual exploitation and sex trafficking of children and adolescents: a narrative review. Acad Pediatr. 2017;17:825–9.
8. Curtis R, Terry K, Dank M, Dombrowski K, Khan B. Commercial sexual exploitation of children in New York City, volume one: the CSEC population in New York City: size, characteristics, and needs. New York: The John Jay College of Criminal Justice; 2008.
9. Barnert ES, Ports K, Mondol S, Thompson L, Kelly M, Godoy S. Mental health profiles of judicially-involved commercially sexually exploited youth. Toronto: Pediatric Academic Societies Annual Meeting; 2018.
10. Teen substance use shows promising decline [Internet]. [cited 2019 Oct 1]. Available from: https://www.drugabuse.gov/news-events/news-releases/2016/12/teen-substance-use-shows-promising-decline.
11. Goldman B. The neuroscience of need: understanding the addicted mind. Menlo Park: Stanford School of Medicine; 2012.
12. Barnert E, Kelly M, Godoy S, Abrams LS, Bath E. Behavioral health treatment "Buy-in" among adolescent females with histories of commercial sexual exploitation. Child Abuse Negl. 2019;100:104042.
13. Ijadi-Maghsoodi R, Cook M, Barnert ES, Gaboian S, Bath E. Understanding and responding to the needs of commercially sexually exploited youth: recommendations for the mental health provider. Child Adolesc Psychiatr Clin N Am. 2016;25:107–22.
14. Greenbaum VJ. Commercial sexual exploitation and sex trafficking of children in the United States. Curr Probl Pediatr Adolesc Health Care. 2014;44:245–69.
15. National Research Council. Confronting commercial sexual exploitation and sex trafficking of minors in the United States. Washington, D.C.: National Academies Press; 2013.
16. Barnert E, Kelly M, Godoy S, Abrams LS, Rasch M, Bath E. Understanding commercially sexually exploited young women's access to, utilization of, and engagement in health care: "work around what I need". Womens Health Issues. 2019;29:315–24.
17. What are the common risk factors for adolescent addiction? [Internet]. [cited 2019 Oct 1]. Available from:https://www.projectknow.com/parents-guide/common-risk-factors/.
18. Reid JA. Entrapment and enmeshment schemes used by sex traffickers. Sex Abus. 2016;28:491–511.
19. Reid JA, Piquero AR. On the relationships between commercial sexual exploitation/prostitution, substance dependency, and delinquency in youthful offenders. Child Maltreat. 2014;19:247–60.
20. Chisolm-Straker M, Einbond J, Sze J, White J. Recognizing human trafficking among homeless youth. Covenant House New Jersey: Newark; 2017.

21. Center for Substance Abuse Treatment. Understanding the impact of trauma. In: Trauma-informed care in behavioral health services : a treatment improvement protocol. Rockville: U.S. Department of Health and Human Services, Substance Abuse and Mental Health Services Administration, Center for Substance Abuse Treatment; 2014.
22. Greenbaum J, Crawford-Jakubiak JE, Committee on Child Abuse and Neglect. Child sex trafficking and commercial sexual exploitation: health care needs of victims. Pediatrics. 2015;135:566–74.
23. Hadland SE. How clinicians caring for youth can address the opioid-related overdose crisis. J Adolesc Health. 2019;65:177–80.
24. Hornor G, Sherfield J. Commercial sexual exploitation of children: health care use and case characteristics. J Pediatr Health Care. 2018;32:250–62.
25. Goldberg AP, Moore JL, Houck C, Kaplan DM, Barron CE. Domestic minor sex trafficking patients: a retrospective analysis of medical presentation. J Pediatr Adolesc Gynecol. 2017;30:109–15.
26. Greenbaum VJ, Titchen K, Walker-Descartes I, Feifer A, Rood CJ, Fong H-F. Multi-level prevention of human trafficking: the role of health care professionals. Prev Med. 2018;114:164–7.
27. Ijadi-Maghsoodi R, Bath E, Cook M, Textor L, Barnert E. Commercially sexually exploited youths' health care experiences, barriers, and recommendations: a qualitative analysis. Child Abuse Negl. 2018;76:334–41.
28. Wills TA. Stress and coping in early adolescence: relationships to substance use in urban school samples. Health Psychol. 1986;5:503–29.
29. Powell C, Asbill M, Louis E, Stoklosa H. Identifying gaps in human trafficking mental health service provision. J Hum Traffick. 2017;4:1–14.
30. Broyles LM, Binswanger IA, Jenkins JA, Finnell DS, Faseru B, Cavaiola A, et al. Confronting inadvertent stigma and pejorative language in addiction scholarship: a recognition and response. Subst Abus. 2014;35:217–21.
31. Human trafficking and opioid abuse [Internet]. [cited 2019 Oct 1]. Available from:https://www.acf.hhs.gov/archive/blog/2016/05/human-trafficking-and-opioid-abuse.
32. Carroll KM, Kiluk BD. Cognitive behavioral interventions for alcohol and drug use disorders: through the stage model and back again. Psychol Addict Behav. 2017;31:847–61.
33. Mendola A, Gibson RL. Addiction, 12-step programs, and evidentiary standards for ethically and clinically sound treatment recommendations: what should clinicians do? AMA J Ethics. 2016;18:646–55.

Chapter 14
Human Trafficking in Suburban and Rural America

Sarah Chaffin, Sarah Hofer, Sawan Vaden, and Ronald Chambers

Case Presentation

A 15-year-old female, "Amanda," presents for evaluation of depression. She is accompanied by her mother after being referred to a rural family medicine clinic by Child Protective Services (CPS); there are concerns of ongoing human trafficking. Amanda states that she lives at home with her mother and two younger half-siblings in a small town (pop. 2,500); while she notes an overall positive relationship with her mother, she reports that she has never had a relationship with her biological father and that her mother's former partner (the father of her half-siblings) treated her like an "outsider in the home." At one point, when she was in the 7th grade, she considered committing suicide because she felt so worthless. She continued to struggle with these feelings until 1 year ago when she made a new male friend from another school; they began a romantic relationship and became sexually active, but in order to secure enough money to pay for dates, he convinced her to perform "small sex stuff" with "people on the Internet." She denies vaginal/anal intercourse with any "johns," but does report engaging in fetish fantasies and oral sex with advertisements on Backpage and other websites. She acknowledges that the men and women who engaged in her services would "drive in" from neighboring cities. Amanda's mother was unaware of this activity until the patient's "boyfriend" was incarcerated for sex trafficking and FBI/CPS became involved in her daughter's case. The patient denies that she is currently being trafficked or exploited though she understands that there are "illegal things" that are occurring given her minor status.

Despite her "boyfriend's" incarceration, Amanda maintains contact with him and his friends; she reports regularly going on "dates" arranged for her via Internet postings and performing sexual acts for money. She later turns over this cash to her "boyfriend" via his

S. Chaffin (✉) · R. Chambers
Department, Family Medicine, Dignity Health, Sacramento, CA, USA

S. Hofer
Aspirus Wausau Hospital, Wausau, WI, USA

S. Vaden
Community Against Sexual Harm (Program Administrator & Survivor Leader), Sacramento, CA, USA

K. E. Titchen, E. Miller (eds.), *Medical Perspectives on Human Trafficking in Adolescents*, https://doi.org/10.1007/978-3-030-43367-3_14

network of friends, who regularly communicate with him and monitor her while he is incarcerated. This persistent exploitation despite the trafficker's incarceration demonstrates both the network of individuals that may impede attempts to leave a trafficking situation and the effects of trauma-coerced attachment (or trauma bonding) that continue to bind an individual to their exploiter. Amanda's mother is distraught over this activity but is at a loss for what to do: she works full-time and cannot constantly monitor her daughter. Amanda admits to feeling overwhelmed by her multiple encounters with law enforcement; she feels isolated, unhappy, and alone at school. She further states that she "hates being at home" and wishes she could move out. She has contemplated running away and living with the people that arrange her "dates." Additionally, she has struggled with generalized fatigue, sadness, loss of appetite, unintentional weight loss, and insomnia. Her mother reports that Amanda is extremely irritable when they are together at home. During the clinical encounter Amanda states that she doesn't "know why [she's] here" or "what the fuss is about." Her mother states, "We need help and heard about this clinic that treats patients who have experienced trafficking. What else can I do?" Despite denying recent or planned vaginal intercourse, both Amanda and her mother request contraception in addition to addressing her depression.

During this initial visit, Amanda's clinician spent significant effort discussing the concept of human trafficking with her, including the manipulative and/or fraudulent methods by which a trafficker might entice a potential victim. Amanda demonstrated little insight regarding her own exploitation but was open to meeting with peer survivors through a local community agency. Amanda and her mother explored contraceptive options and proceeded with Nexplanon placement that same day. Amanda was started on an SSRI, and plans for close follow-up were established.

Over the course of 18 months, Amanda continued to follow-up with her clinician, who actively collaborated with community agencies to provide additional support. Her mother noted that Amanda was gradually becoming less irritable and more engaged with her family. Her sleep quality, fatigue, energy, and ability to concentrate on tasks improved; she expressed a desire to focus on a career in hairstyling and began applying herself more in her independent study program. With the above measures and medication management, she noted that improvement in her depression resulted in a significant "confidence boost." This, in addition to ongoing counseling from her clinician and support from local agencies, allowed her mindset to shift in regard to her relationship with her trafficker. Her clinician followed up regularly with Amanda and remained a consistent presence in her recovery during times of both success and setback. Her clinician assisted her along her nonlinear progression working with her through pre-contemplative to contemplative to active stages of change. Amanda eventually disclosed, "I just went along with doing [stuff] because of all the praise I got from [him and his friends] … The money was nice, but it was nicer to feel free without anyone telling me what to do. It got my attention." Presently, Amanda continues to be seen for follow-up management of her mental health and contraceptive needs; at her latest visits, she has solicited feedback, and her clinician has been reviewing her college applications.

Discussion Questions

1. Are there specific aspects to rural trafficking that present challenges to providers, patients, family and friends, and others? Consider long travel distances to care, boredom among rural youth, substance use, etc.
2. Are there specific aspects to suburban trafficking that present challenges to providers, patients, family, friends, and others? Consider beliefs and stereotypes about populations at risk for trafficking, etc.

3. Trauma-coerced attachment, or trauma bonding, occurs as the result of ongoing cycles of abuse in which intermittent reward and punishment creates powerful emotional bonds that are resistant to change. How does abuse or neglect at home influence a patient's susceptibility to trauma bonding? How does this influence the role a healthcare provider must play when working with a patient?

Background

Human trafficking studies produced by legal, governmental, and nonprofit organizations have focused largely on trafficking in highly populated, urban centers around the country. This may lead to the misconception that this is an issue specific to metropolitan areas when, in fact, human trafficking is increasingly recognized as a human rights and public health issue affecting both urban and rural/suburban communities worldwide. It occurs in every state in the United States and affects victims of all genders, ages, race/ethnicities, and socioeconomic backgrounds [1]. Case reports and studies have recorded the stories of human trafficking survivors from both suburban and rural areas, thus providing insight into the challenges specific to each environment [2, 3]. While the true number of human trafficking cases in both urban and rural/suburban areas remains unclear, healthcare professionals in all regions ought to be aware of the likelihood that they will encounter victims of human trafficking in their practice and thus be able to identify risk factors and indicators of trafficking in order to provide quality, trauma-informed care to survivors.

Risk Factors

While there is no single profile of a human trafficking victim, there are several risk factors for victimization, many of which apply to individuals in both urban and rural/suburban areas. Specifically within rural areas, individuals may be at increased risk for human trafficking due to poverty, limited resources, and/or minority status (especially Native American/Native Alaskan individuals) [2, 4]. In agricultural communities, there may be an elevated risk of labor trafficking among documented and undocumented immigrants [5] (see Chap. 5); sex trafficking is also observed frequently along rural interstate and highway routes at truck and rest stops [6]. As in our case study above, victims are often female minors in their early-to-mid-teen years; however, adults, males, and non-binary individuals are victimized as well, and LGBTQ individuals may be at enhanced risk of victimization [2] (see Chap. 15). Homeless and run-away youths are at increased risk of trafficking (see Chap. 12), and research has shown that contact with child welfare; economic insecurity; prior physical, verbal, emotional, and/or sexual abuse; drug and substance abuse and addiction; and social isolation are also indicators of elevated risk [2, 7, 8]. These topics are addressed in depth in Chaps. 7, 8, and 13 of this textbook.

Challenges and Limitations

Confronting rural and suburban human trafficking presents specific challenges. Particularly in rural communities, resources such as law enforcement, healthcare facilities, and nonprofit organizations receive less funding and have fewer areas of specialization when compared to their metropolitan counterparts; providers often receive less training on human trafficking and have less knowledge around relevant legislature [2, 9]. Consequently, individuals may have to travel long distances in order to access resources and obtain necessary healthcare.

In rural settings, trafficking is often conducted remotely using the Internet or social media, as was the case with Amanda. Traffickers may use websites such as Backpage (now defunct), Eros Guide, P411, Skip the Games, AdultLook, Private Delights, and others to sell their victims frequently and undercover with limited repercussions, accessing a wider span than would have been possible otherwise [10, 11] (see Chap. 6). Youth in rural/suburban settings, especially those who may have limited parental or guardian supervision, may also be influenced by boredom and social pressures which can increase the likelihood of behaviors such as drinking, substance abuse, and unprotected sexual activity. In fact, when compared to their urban counterparts, non-metro areas had the highest rate of tobacco use and underage alcohol abuse [12]. This is especially concerning in light of the link between substance abuse and human trafficking; a 2014 study shows that approximately 85% of trafficking victims reported some type of substance abuse [13] and the link between opioid use and intimate partner violence is well documented across the literature [14]. While victims may use substances to cope with the trauma of being trafficked, traffickers often exploit already present addictions in order to coerce individuals into trafficking. A recent letter to the *American Journal of Public Health* cites a report that 66% of clients indicated that substance abuse led to their trafficking, while only 4.5% said their abuse was the result of being trafficked [15]. There is a need for additional research on the role that substance abuse plays in facilitating and maintaining human trafficking victimization, as well as the effects of the opioid epidemic on trafficking in rural areas [16]. (See Chap. 17 for more on substance use and cardiovascular effects.)

Misconceptions About Rural Trafficking

Perhaps the greatest threat to the rural/suburban fight against human trafficking is the misperceptions of trafficking, traffickers, and their victims. Unfortunately stigmatization has the potential to undermine a victim's attempts to access resources and implement lasting change, as it is often difficult to maintain privacy in a small town and victims may be shunned and/or mistreated by their peers [6]. Similarly, the assumption that human trafficking doesn't happen in wealthy suburban neighborhoods to "good" families or "good" kids [9, 17] allows traffickers to hide in plain sight, among unassuming parents, residents, and officials [18]. This lack of awareness of trafficking within rural/suburban areas is a significant obstacle to the development and funding of necessary resources. The authors of this chapter have treated trafficked minors from suburban areas who reported understanding what they were "getting into," but described a lack of resources and parental guidance, as well as normalization by peers at school as they entered "the life." Finally, it is important to remember that the demand for purchased sex crosses suburban, rural, and urban lines and ultimately propagates exploitation.

Identification of Trafficking Victims in the Rural/ Suburban Clinic

Healthcare providers are often the first line of care for victims of human trafficking in all communities and regions, with research estimating that up to 88% of trafficked individuals interact with healthcare at some point during their exploitation [13]. It is the responsibility of healthcare professionals to recognize indicators of human trafficking in order to appropriately respond and care for these patients. (See Chap. 17 for more on medical subspecialties and trafficking). The red flags of human trafficking are as varied as the risk factors, with each patient presenting differently. However, as our case study demonstrates, there are several common indicators that help to identify victims of trafficking in the clinic. These include depression and suicidality, feelings of isolation and "outsiderness," fatigue, loss of appetite, weight loss, insomnia, and irritability. Additionally, the patient's reports of family and home-life instability, wanting to run away from home, the presence of a manipulative romantic partner, and coercion to perform sexual acts for money (which is illegal sex trafficking despite the patient's claims to abstain from intercourse) are all indicators that the patient is likely being trafficked. Other common indicators may include the presence of physical wounds and bruising, sexually transmitted infections and diseases, lack of immunizations and other routine preventative healthcare, substance use, and severe mental and psychological illness. It is important to keep in mind that these signs may be much more subtle than expected, especially with young victims still living at home or having only been recently trafficked. These patients may also lack insight into their exploitation, having a sense of normalization if these experiences are commonplace in their peer group, community, or schools. Also of note, when providing longitudinal care, the authors have witnessed the devastating effects of trauma bonding (trauma-coerced attachment) as individuals often attempt to dissociate from their trafficker but relapse to "the life." In these situations, it is important to rely on the expertise of law enforcement and community agencies to help in the identification of victims and the administration of comprehensive care. There are a growing number of screening tools available to help with the identification of victims, and continued research and education on this topic is imperative as the culture continues to evolve (see Additional Resources).

Trauma-Informed Care

As with all victims of human trafficking and other forms of violence and trauma, a longitudinal, trauma-informed, victim-centered, comprehensive model of care is required to ensure the best course of action for recovery. Practices must be built and implemented with survivor input (see Dignity Health Medical Safe Haven – "Survivor-Informed Checklist and Scoring System"). Trafficked persons often experience complex recurring traumas which may require a coordinated care effort that includes the primary care physician, psychiatric or psychological counseling, support groups, law enforcement, and providers of additional services for victims including housing, transportation, legal assistance, food assistance, financial and career training, and family counseling. This comprehensive, longitudinal approach is especially important as a history of victimization increases risk of future victimization for survivors. In the case of suburban and rural victims, some or all of these resources may be limited [6, 9], making clinical partnerships with community agencies even more essential to comprehensive longitudinal care. Internet resources including screening tools, online support groups, and government services may be more accessible than local resources and are able to provide additional information for both healthcare providers and victims themselves (see Additional Resources). It is important to keep in mind that victims may not self-identify as victims, perhaps because they have maintained belief in their own autonomy and ability to decide their own fate, as was the case for Amanda in the case report. Some may be aware of the risks, but choosing the lesser of two evils, for example, deciding between staying with a sexually abusive and neglectful parent and a "romantic" interest offering an opportunity to make money. For healthcare professionals, using language that mirrors that of the victim and their guardians is a crucial step in developing trust and rapport (see Chap. 19).

Another complicating aspect may be that the victim is a child with parents or guardians who are unaware that trafficking has occurred. Similarly, minors may also still be attending school and with peers who are also at risk or may be a component of the patient's initial victimization. In these situations, involvement of school officials, law enforcement, and social services are often essential to helping victims and preventing further victimization. As presented by our case report, comprehensive trauma-informed care means a whole-patient approach involving both preventive and curative care. This may include contraceptive and sexual healthcare (STI/STD treatments and immunizations), mental healthcare (SSRI), counseling and therapy, and support to help the patient recover and reintegrate into society, such as career or educational support services and peer support groups. In rural areas, accessing resources may be more of a challenge and providers may need to investigate alternative options such as telehealth, videoconferencing, use of local transportation services (e.g., Uber Health), hospital-based indigent care services, and others. Support groups and survivor groups, which can often be accessed through anti-human trafficking and domestic violence organizations or their online services, offer an additional network to support victims throughout their recovery. One way that this can be accomplished is through coordination with advocacy services across neighboring towns; for example, if an individual has to travel to a hospital for a sexual abuse case, organizations can coordinate to provide an advocate that is local to the patient's place of residence, thus easing the transition of services and care. Additionally, these organizations are also able to design programs specific to community needs, whether through partnering with neighboring nonprofits to provide emergency transportation, coordinating with organizations like Wheels to Work where public transportation is not available, or providing education for local organizations and raising community awareness. This latter is something that nonprofits such as Truckers Against Trafficking and others are doing. A few resources can be found at the end of this chapter.

For patients like Amanda, involving family and parental support is extremely important in aiding recovery and preventing recidivism. Amanda felt safe and supported in her clinical visits and learned to trust her care providers over an extended period of time, eventually opening up and even asking for feedback on her college admissions efforts. While there are many challenges faced by those supporting victims of human trafficking in rural and suburban areas, resources are available and continue to grow, expanding the access of care to victims in communities everywhere.

Additional Resources

1. National Human Trafficking Resource Center (resources for service providers) – https://humantraffickinghotline.org/audience/service-providers.
2. Rural Behavioral Health (List of resources on human trafficking) – https://ruralbehavioralhealth.org/resources/resources-2018-rural-behavioral-health-webinar-series-webinar-1-human-trafficking-rural.
3. Rural Health Information Hub (Violence and Abuse in Rural America resources – https://www.ruralhealthinfo.org/topics/violence-and-abuse/resources.
4. Dignity Health Medical Safe Haven program – https://www.dignityhealth.org/msh.
5. Physicians Against the Trafficking of Humans (PATH) – https://www.doc-path.org/.
6. HEAL Trafficking – https://healtrafficking.org/.
7. US Department of Homeland Security Blue Campaign (resources) –https://www.dhs.gov/blue-campaign/share-resources.
8. Uber Health – https://www.uberhealth.com/.
9. Truckers Against Trafficking – https://truckersagainsttrafficking.org/.

References

1. National Human Trafficking Hotline. Hotline Statistics [Internet]. Polaris. 2018 [cited 2019 Mar 30]. Available from: https://humantraffickinghotline.org/states.
2. Bowers P. Sex trafficking and rural communities: areview of the literature. Contemp Rural Soc Work J. 2017;9(1):13.
3. Talbot EP, Suzuki YE, LaPlante K, Omanson S. Human trafficking in Small Urban & Rural Communities. Annapolis: NACSW Convention; 2014.
4. Greer BT. Hiding behind Tribal Sovereignty: rooting out human trafficking in Indian country. J Gender Race Just. 2013;16:453–82.
5. Fyksen J. Human trafficking lurks in rural areas [Internet]. [cited 2019 Mar 30]. Available from: https://www.agupdate.com/agriview/news/crop/human-trafficking-lurks-in-rural-areas/article_5a28676d-d2ea-5bf9-9e8d-fc98f5626bd3.html.
6. Occhiboi A. Trafficking in rural America [Internet]. Love146. [cited 2019 Mar 30]. Available from: https://love146.org/trafficking-in-rural-america/.
7. National Human Trafficking Hotline. The victims [Internet]. Polaris. [cited 2019 Oct 2]. Available from: https://humantraffickinghotline.org/what-human-trafficking/human-trafficking/victims.
8. Davis L. Human trafficking in rural America and the rural health system response. 2018. [Internet]. [cited 4/22/20]. Available from: https://nosorh.org/wp-content/uploads/2018/10/We-Have-that-Here-Human-Trafficking-in-Rural-America-and-Rural-Helath-System-Response-Lisa-Davis-1.pdf.
9. Cole J, Sprang G. Sex trafficking of minors in metropolitan, micropolitan, and rural communities. Child Abuse Negl. 2015;40:113–23.
10. US Department of Justice. Child Sex Trafficking [Internet]. [cited 2019 Mar 30]. Available from: https://www.justice.gov/criminal-ceos/child-sex-trafficking.
11. Cooney V. Sex trafficking in the suburbs [Internet]. SWNewsMedia. [cited 2019 Mar 30]. Available from: https://www.swnewsmedia.com/sex-trafficking-in-the-suburbs/article_9e6581a7-df56-5b32-9626-26485134b0f7.html.
12. Rural Health Information Hub. Substance abuse in rural areas introduction [Internet]. [cited 2019 Mar 30]. Available from: https://www.ruralhealthinfo.org/topics/substance-abuse.
13. Lederer LJ, Wetzel CA. The health consequences of sex trafficking and their implications for identifying victims in healthcare facilities. Ann Health Law. 2014;23:61.
14. Stone R, Rothman EF. Opioid use and intimate partner violence: a systematic review. Curr Epidemiol Rep. 2019;6:215–30.
15. Haney KN. Increasing public health awareness of the intersection between human trafficking and the opioid epidemic. Am J Public Health. 2019;109:e3.
16. Concepcion-Zayas MT, Ayling R. The intersection between the opioid epidemic and child trafficking: viewpoints from a rural state. J Am Acad Child Adolesc Psychiatry. 2018;57:S106.
17. Rogers A. Human sex trafficking is now affecting America's elite communities [Internet]. Business Insider. 2012 [cited 2019 Mar 30]. Available from: https://www.businessinsider.com/human-trafficking-in-the-suburbs-2012-9.
18. Landesman P. The girls next door [Internet]. The New York Times. 2004 [cited 2019 Mar 30]. Available from: https://www.nytimes.com/2004/01/25/magazine/the-girls-next-door.html.

Chapter 15
Boys Are Trafficked Too?

Sarah Chaffin, Ronald Chambers, and Erik Gray

Case Report

A 20-year-old man, "Adam," with a past medical history significant for attention-deficit/hyperactivity disorder (ADHD) presents to your clinic to establish care and discuss possible medication refills. You are the physician evaluating Adam for the first time. Adam states that he was first diagnosed with ADHD at the age of 14 when one of his teachers recommended that he be evaluated for the condition. When you ask about previous medication regimens, Adam notes that he has been managed on "Vyvanse, Adderall, Seroquel, Prozac, and Effexor to name a few" but states that he has never been able to achieve "stability in [his] life" on any mono- or combination therapy. When you ask him to clarify this statement, Adam alludes to a history of depression, suicidality, and substance use all stemming from a "weird" home situation.

Discussion Question

What is your next step? How do you gauge whether or not Adam would like to discuss this "weird" home situation in more detail?

At this initial visit, you prescribe Adam a stimulant for his ADHD, test him (and subsequently treat him) for sexually transmitted infections, start a "catch-up" schedule for immunizations which he never received in childhood, treat his musculoskeletal complaints from old injuries, and connect him with a psychiatrist and therapist. You are able to accomplish all this in part due to the training implemented for all clinic staff on human trafficking (using the Assessment Tool for Health Care Provider Human Trafficking Training, a guide to identifying areas for improvement and to ensuring comprehensive training in human trafficking) and in part due to the victim centered, trauma-informed principles that were

S. Chaffin (✉) · R. Chambers
Department, Family Medicine, Dignity Health, Sacramento, CA, USA

E. Gray
Innovations Human Trafficking Collaborative, Olympia, WA, USA

K. E. Titchen, E. Miller (eds.), *Medical Perspectives on Human Trafficking in Adolescents*, https://doi.org/10.1007/978-3-030-43367-3_15

employed in the clinic setting that actively incorporated survivor-informed best practices [2, 3].

Adam states that he was born in the Midwest and that his family situation was not necessarily supportive; he notes a significant family history of depression and suspects that he himself has struggled with depression since the age of 12. Adam offers that he turned to substances such as alcohol, opiates, benzodiazepines, and LSD in an attempt to cope with his hopelessness but felt himself becoming more and more isolated from his peers and family, which ultimately worsened his depressive symptoms. He did make several attempts at the age of 15 to seek psychiatric help and was at one point hospitalized for being a danger to himself, but he cannot recall if he was subsequently connected within the healthcare system for additional support. With worsening social isolation, Adam turned to the Internet to "distract [himself] from overwhelming thoughts"; ultimately, he became quite enmeshed in certain interactive threads on websites such as Reddit.

He notes in particular developing a close relationship with a married couple who lived out-of-state. His relationship with them had become so close that, in an effort to leave behind a difficult home life, the patient accepted their offer to move in with them when he turned 16. The patient reports conflicted feelings about his time with this couple, as they had "treated me like I was their son." While living in a seemingly supportive environment was a welcome change, Adam notes that he began to struggle with having firm boundaries with the people he felt he owed so much to; shortly after moving into their home, Adam recalls being "guilted into" engaging in sexual acts with them. This behavior later escalated into non-consensual sexual acts consisting mostly of receptive and insertive oral sex. After some time, the patient stated that the couple suggested he trade sex for money on the street as he had no other way to help offset the cost of housing him. In the face of rent, groceries, utilities, and other bills, the patient felt he had to "sell himself" for sexual acts or face abandonment by the couple. Adam states that, more than homelessness, the possible lack of a support system "terrified" him.

While he became involved in commercial sex, Adam states that the couple actually helped him to establish care with a primary doctor and always accompanied him to his appointments; because of this, he is not sure if the medications he was prescribed or the diagnoses he was given are actually accurate. He admits that his recollection of events is hazy and that all attempts at trying to piece together chronology end in frustration. The patient reports feelings of deep shame and confusion regarding his sexuality, shame regarding physiologic responses such as erection and orgasm; these feelings actually hindered him from leaving this "arrangement" for years and kept him from establishing care with a new healthcare professional until he was able to seek help from a community agency about 1 year ago. He had "convinced" himself that he was ultimately to blame for what he now understands to have been an abusive and exploitative situation; he had felt that he was "undeserving" of help.

With the continued support and assistance of local outreach workers, Adam was able to find gainful employment and achieve financial independence, giving him the power to end his relationship with his traffickers. He had just started classes at the local community college and realized that without significant help his "mental health" would continue to be an insurmountable challenge. Over the course of 9 months, you follow Adam closely and are gratified that he is able to adhere to therapy and reach a stable dose of medication which allows him to complete his first year of college. He continues to follow-up at your clinic for healthcare.

Discussion Questions

How is the care you offer Adam changed by his history of trafficking?

Does Adam need/want legal counseling? What other services might benefit Adam?

Background on Human Trafficking of Male Victims

There is increasing understanding among the academic, legal, and healthcare communities about human trafficking and its victims; however, many of the studies and policies have focused on female victims of sex trafficking. While females and especially female minors are at particularly high risk of victimization and indeed the majority (approximately 75%) of documented and predicted human trafficking victims are female [4], men and boys can be victims of both forced labor and commercial sex trafficking as well. The International Labour Organization, using 54 surveys of over 71,000 respondents across 48 countries in combination with international migration databases, estimated in 2017 that up to 99% of victims of commercial sex trafficking globally were women and girls, while they represent 58% of human trafficking victims in other exploitation sectors such as labor trafficking [4]. While women and girls may be particularly vulnerable to trafficking victimization, it is important for healthcare professionals to be aware that male victims of both sex and labor trafficking do exist and that healthcare professionals may encounter male victims in their practice. A recent telephone survey found that of 161 professionals in mostly rural Kentucky who worked with at-risk youth and at least one victim of child sex trafficking, 58% had worked with at least one male victim [1]. These providers identified many commonalities between the risk factors and care needs of male and female victims, but some differences along gender lines exist as well. Healthcare professionals should be aware of the special considerations, risk factors, healthcare needs, and resources available for male victims of human trafficking.

While every person's path to exploitation is different, there are several known risk factors that enhance vulnerability to victimization. As in the case of Adam in our case study, an unstable or unsupportive home situation and family life can be a major risk factor for victimization, especially if it results in homelessness or youth runaway status. Indeed, homeless and runaway youths are some of the most vulnerable populations to sex trafficking [5]. (See Chap. 12 for more on homelessness and trafficking.) LGBTQ status, especially when compounded with an unsupportive family or community which can lead to feelings of isolation or hopelessness, also greatly enhances the risk of victimization [6]. (See Chap. 11 for more on LGBTQ populations and trafficking.) Additionally, mental health issues and prior trauma including physical, sexual, and emotional abuse are risk factors for exploitation, especially if substance use and addiction are involved [5, 7]. (See Chap. 13 for more on mental health and trafficking.) As in Adam's case, poverty and financial instability are another risk factor that pulls some victims, both male and female, into the life of sex or labor trafficking. According to the Counter Trafficking Data Collaborative, the primary means used by traffickers to coerce male victims into trafficking situations and keep them there include false promises, withholding of earnings, psychological abuse, and excessive working hours [8], while women are coerced via similar means but often accompanied with threats and physical abuse.

An important challenge to identifying and treating male trafficking victims is the misconception that men are not generally vulnerable to human trafficking, especially sex trafficking. There are several possible reasons that male victims are often considered the "invisible" victims of human trafficking [9, 10]. Male victims of sex trafficking are particularly disregarded due to bias that men in the commercial sex trade are typically there by choice and not coercion [11, 12], likely compounded by the stereotype that men are not vulnerable to coercion or abuse. We also have a limited understanding of the true extent of human trafficking, especially in male victims. Methodological limitations and inconsistent definitions of sexual exploitation and abuse have made tracking youth male victims of trafficking difficult and unreliable [13]. Additionally, it is thought that frequently there is low self-reporting of male victims, likely due to the stigmatization that male victims are weak or less masculine [14]. Male victims also may be unaware of their own victimization, which may be reinforced by their own internalized societal expectations, traditional gender roles, and stereotypes [15]. Male victims when they do self-report are often met with disbelief from authorities including law enforcement, healthcare professionals, and even loved ones [14]. The biases that men and boys are not vulnerable or in need of assistance can lead to these victims being ignored and neglected. In many cases, male victims do not come forward because there are limited resources to help them if they do, including a lack of shelter beds, survivor groups, and anti-trafficking organizations dedicated to supporting male victims [9]. Male victims also are at greater risk of being penalized by fine or imprisonment for crimes committed as a result of their exploitation [15]. Despite these challenges and misconceptions, the number of male victims identified has grown in recent years, likely due to increased awareness of male victims by authorities and agencies that offer victim assistance [8]. (See Chap. 19 Survivor Insights for more.)

Identification of Male Trafficking Victims in the Clinic

Healthcare professionals often represent the first line of response for victims of human trafficking of all genders. The identification of patients as victims in the clinic is crucial to their ongoing care, as victims may have several physical and psychological needs that are informed by their experiences during exploitation. There are several red flags which can help healthcare professionals identify potential victims of human trafficking. Some of the red flags exhibited in the case study above include Adam's use of illicit and prescription drugs as a coping mechanism for the mental health issues he describes. Adam's history of learning deficits and mental illness including depression, suicidality, memory loss, and self-medication are all red flag indicators of possible exploitation. Adam describes his relationship with the couple who he began living with as a minor as controlling, restrictive, and psychologically manipulative. He states that he was financially dependent on them, and his conflicted and confused emotions toward his traffickers are indicative of trauma bonding. Controlling, dominating, one-sided relationships and especially the presence of someone who speaks for the patient and refuses to allow the patient privacy are strong indicators of an abusive or exploitative situation [16]. Other red flags of human trafficking and sex trafficking include physical signs of abuse and neglect such as bruising, burns, scars, unhealed or improperly treated wounds, chronic pain, neurological conditions, cardiovascular and respiratory conditions, sexually and non-sexually transmitted infections, and lack of routine preventative care including immunizations and dental care. Additional psychological indicators include fear, anxiety, self-harming behaviors, nightmares, flashbacks, PTSD, hypervigilance, hostility, dissociation disorders, and social/developmental issues such as impaired social skills, developmental delays, and increased risk-taking behaviors [16, 17]. (See Chap. 13) Assessment tools to aid healthcare professionals in the appropriate identification of human trafficking survivors are listed in the Additional Resources section at the end of this chapter.

Providing Care to Male Victims of Human Trafficking

Due to the chronic and recurring trauma that victims experience throughout their exploitation, victim-survivors of human trafficking have many health and other needs that must be addressed through coordinated, comprehensive, and trauma-informed care. The specific health issues of male victim-survivors of human trafficking remain understudied. There are many typical psychological needs of victim-survivors, so it is important to involve therapy and counseling, as well as to stabilize medication doses and schedules to address these needs and any underlying traumas from previous abuse (including childhood exposures) [18]. Many victim-survivors benefit from working with local agencies as well as survivor groups that can provide additional services such as group therapy. Coordinating care between primary healthcare professionals and other services including career counseling, legal counseling, food/shelter providers, and psychological therapy/counseling can help survivors on the path to recovery.

In addition to the psychological sequelae of human trafficking, the physical health consequences specifically from labor trafficking often include unhealed injuries and wounds resulting in chronic pain, asthma and breathing problems, infections, malnutrition, and dental diseases. Catch-up immunizations and treatments for chronic infections and diseases resulting from malnutrition and years of poor or absent healthcare may be required. Additionally, both sex trafficking victims and labor trafficking victims who have been sexually assaulted often present with STIs including HIV/AIDs.

Overall, male victims of human trafficking, and especially sex trafficking, remain poorly studied and underappreciated within the healthcare, legal, and service agency communities. Additional studies and resources are needed to bring male victims out of the shadows and ensure their equitable access to healthcare and victim-based services now and in the future.

Perspectives

By Erik Gray

Men are celebrated for feeling three emotions: anger, violence, and sexual arousal. Almost exclusively, men are limited to expressing these three emotions to be seen as "manly." This creates an environment where male survivors of human trafficking – who may inwardly feel submissive, fearful, and vulnerable – are demonized, not believed, and generally lack services.

My father molested me around the age of 5 years old. I didn't remember the trauma for some time, until I was in my 20s. I believe my father's molestation is the largest contributing risk factor to my own human trafficking. My father modeled for me that the love of a father comes with violation, hurt, and theft. He taught me that my body was for consumption and that I should silently give that up. He reinforced that no matter how much I cried or ran from him that no one would keep me safe. This created a huge gap in my sense of safety, security, and stability and made me to long for the love of a father, because I never received true fatherly love. When other men treated me similarly, not only was I familiar with the feeling: I felt like it was the piece of fatherly love that I had never received and so longed for. See, their abuse replicated the kind of love I received from my father. When I later opened up about the molestation, I wasn't supported or believed for a number of years. This caused further emotional damage and insecurities around safety, trust, and healing.

(For more of Erik's story and his insights about prevention, recovery, healing, and resilience, refer to Chap. 19)

Additional Resources

National Human Trafficking Resource Center (resources for service providers) – https://humantraffickinghotline.org/audience/service-providers.

Human Trafficking Task Force e-Guide (Male Victims) – https://www.ovcttac.gov/taskforceguide/eguide/4-supporting-victims/45-victim-populations/male-victims/.

Dignity Health Medical Safe Haven program – https://www.dignityhealth.org/msh.

Physicians Against the Trafficking of Humans (PATH) – https://www.docpath.org/.

HEAL Trafficking – https://healtrafficking.org/.

US Department of Homeland Security Blue Campaign (resources) – https://www.dhs.gov/blue-campaign/share-resources.

References

1. Cole J. Service providers' perspectives on sex trafficking of male minors: comparing background and trafficking situations of male and female victims. Child Adolesc Soc Work J. 2018;35:1–11.
2. Miller C, Greenbaum J, Napolitano K, Rajaram S, Cox J, Bachrach L, et al. Healthcare provider human trafficking education: assessment tool. Laboratory to Combat Human Trafficking and HEAL Trafficking; 2018. Available from: https://healtrafficking.org/assessmenttoolforhealthcareproviderhumantraffickingtraining/.
3. 2017 Human Trafficking Leadership Academy. Survivor-informed practice: definition, best practices, and recommendations [Internet]. Available from: https://www.acf.hhs.gov/sites/default/files/otip/definition_and_recommendations.pdf.
4. International Labour Organization (ILO). Forced labour, modern slavery and human trafficking [Internet]. International Labour Organization (ILO). 2017 [cited 2019 Oct 2]. Available from: http://www.ilo.org/global/topics/forced-labour/lang%2D%2Den/index.htm.
5. National Human Trafficking Hotline. The victims [Internet]. Polaris. [cited 2019 Oct 2]. Available from: https://humantraffickinghotline.org/what-human-trafficking/human-trafficking/victims.
6. Barron IM, Frost C. Men, boys, and LGBTQ: invisible victims of human trafficking. In: Walker L, Gaviria G, Gopal K, editors. Handbook of sex trafficking: feminist transnational perspectives. Cham: Springer; 2018. p. 73–84.
7. National Human Trafficking Hotline. Growing awareness. growing impact. 2017 Statistics from the National Human Trafficking Hotline and BeFree Textline [Internet]. PoLAR; 2017. Available from: https://humantraffickinghotline.org/sites/default/files/2017NHTHStats%20%281%29.pdf.
8. Counter Trafficking Data Collective. Human trafficking and gender: differences, similarities and trends [Internet]. International Organization for Migration (IOM). 2018 [cited 2019 Oct 2]. Available from: https://www.ctdatacollaborative.org/story/human-trafficking-and-gender-differences-similarities-and-trends.
9. Lillie M. Invisible men: male victims of sex trafficking [Internet]. Human Trafficking Search. 2014 [cited 2019 Oct 2]. Available from: https://humantraffickingsearch.org/invisible-men-male-victims-of-sex-trafficking/.
10. Greve A. Human trafficking: what about the men and boys? [Internet]. Human Trafficking Center. 2019 [cited 2019 Oct 2]. Available from: https://humantraffickingcenter.org/men-boys/.
11. Office for Victims of Crime Training and Technical Assistance Center. Male victims [Internet]. Office of Justice Programs. [cited 2019 Oct 2]. Available from: https://www.ovcttac.gov/taskforceguide/eguide/4-supporting-victims/45-victim-populations/male-victims/.
12. Dennis JP. Women are victims, men make choices: the invisibility of men and boys in the global sex trade. Gend Issues. 2008;25:11–25.

13. Mitchell K, Moynihan M, Pitcher C, Francis A, English A, Saewyc E. Rethinking research on sexual exploitation of boys: methodological challenges and recommendations to optimize future knowledge generation. Child Abuse Negl. 2017;66:142–51.
14. National Center on Sexual Exploitation. Bringing the sex trafficking of boys and men out of the shadows [Internet]. National Center on Sexual Exploitation. 2017 [cited 2019 Oct 2]. Available from: https://endsexualexploitation.org/articles/bringing-sexual-abuse-exploitation-boys-men-shadows/.
15. United States Department of State. Assisting male survivors of human trafficking [Internet]. United States Department of State. 2017 [cited 2019 Oct 2]. Available from: https://www.state.gov/assisting-male-survivors-of-human-trafficking/.
16. National Human Trafficking Resource Center. Identifying victims of human trafficking: what to look for in a healthcare setting [Internet]. Polaris. 2010 [cited 2019 Oct 2]. Available from: https://traffickingresourcecenter.org/sites/default/files/What%20to%20Look%20for%20during%20a%20Medical%20Exam%20-%20FINAL%20-%202-16-16.docx.pdf.
17. National Human Trafficking Hotline. Recognizing the signs [Internet]. Polaris. [cited 2019 Oct 2]. Available from: https://humantraffickinghotline.org/human-trafficking/recognizing-signs.
18. Ottisova L, Smith P, Shetty H, Stahl D, Downs J, Oram S. Psychological consequences of child trafficking: an historical cohort study of trafficked children in contact with secondary mental health services. PLoS One. 2018;13:e0192321.

Chapter 16
Surgery and ObGyn: Beyond the Chief Complaint

Elizabeth A. Berdan, Julia Geynisman-Tan, Deborah Ottenheimer, Miriam L. Tarrash, and Brittany A. Jackson

Introduction

When contemplating human trafficking, it is essential to consider it in the larger context of human rights abuse and violations. The acceptance of the buying and selling of human beings requires that an individual, or group of individuals, be considered less than human. As Brené Brown explains, the psychological process of dehumanization on the part of the persecutor – or trafficker – is necessary to overcome "our wiring as members of a social species to actually harm, kill, torture, or degrade other humans" [1].

E. A. Berdan (✉)
Pediatric Surgery, Mary Bridge Children's Hospital and Health Network, Tacoma, WA, USA

Department of Surgery, University of Washington School of Medicine, Tacoma, WA, USA

J. Geynisman-Tan
Female Pelvic Medicine and Reconstructive Surgery, Department of Obstetrics and Gynecology, Northwestern University, ERASE Trafficking Clinic, Chicago, IL, USA

D. Ottenheimer
Women's Holistic Health Initiative, Harlem United/URAM – The Nest Community Health Center, New York, NY, USA

M. L. Tarrash
Department of Obstetrics and Gynecology, Northwell Health at Long Island Jewish Medical Center and North Shore University Hospitals, Queens, NY, USA

B. A. Jackson
Obstetrics and Gynecology, Capital Women's Care- Division 37, Alexandria, VA, USA

K. E. Titchen, E. Miller (eds.), *Medical Perspectives on Human Trafficking in Adolescents*, https://doi.org/10.1007/978-3-030-43367-3_16

Groups or individuals who have been deemed less than human are often subjected to multiple types of violence and discrimination, as recognized in and delineated by the United Nations [2–4]. As clinicians, it is critical to remember that a patient who has been a victim of one human rights abuse has likely suffered others. For example, in a social setting in which certain types of people are considered to be commodities or property, trafficking is often accompanied by societal permissiveness for domestic violence, child marriage, and sexual abuse [5].

The cases in this chapter illustrate that broader and more complex diagnostic considerations, as seen through a human rights lens, must be used when treating a patient who has a constellation of symptoms that seem incongruous or conflicting. Rather than dismissing that patient as malingering, drug-seeking, or mentally impaired, it is incumbent upon us to consider that trafficking, along with other human rights abuses, may be the root cause of the presenting symptoms.

One of the greatest challenges to identifying patients who are trafficked is that, on the surface, some trafficking survivors can challenge our compassion or push our boundaries. Some survivors can act manipulative, belligerent, abusive, or ungrateful. Trafficking survivors may appear to be drug-seeking, threaten to leave against medical advice or else refuse to leave when discharged, use derogatory language toward staff, or show up frequently in the ER with the same complaint. They are often labeled "the difficult patient." We challenge you to recognize "difficult" as a coping mechanism for "loss of control" and to see this as a red flag for psychological trauma of any kind.

The first reaction often heard when discussing human trafficking with healthcare professionals (HCPs) is, "that's terrible… but…that doesn't happen here." In fact, it happens everywhere. Trafficked individuals can, and do, present for care to emergent, inpatient and outpatient health services [6]. They can be seen in every type of health system (public and private) and by every subspecialty (see Chap. 17). It is a common misconception among HCPs that, if they work in a private, heavily resourced clinical setting, they are unlikely to see trafficking victims. This is not the case for several reasons. First, trafficking victims, like all patients, want the best possible care for themselves and will travel to the best hospital in their area. Second, trafficking often happens in places where individuals with disposable income live and work. Your hospital or clinic may be in one of these affluent neighborhoods and could be the closest health center for a trafficked individual. Finally, traffickers may intentionally bring their victims to health systems that are less attuned to such social issues in order to avoid suspicion and detection (see Chap. 14).

Trafficked individuals use the healthcare system for a variety of reasons, including (but not limited to) acute traumatic injury, drug overdose, pregnancy, respiratory or pelvic infection, chest pain, abdominal pain, chronic fatigue, depression, or suicidal ideation. In their landmark report, *Stolen Smiles*, Cathy Zimmerman et al. detailed the health complaints of 207 trafficked individuals [7]. They found that 57% of the women interviewed reported suffering between 12 and 23 concurrent physical and/or mental health symptoms when they entered post-trafficking care. These findings are supported by a number of other studies, which repeatedly detail the physical and psychological consequences of trafficking [8, 9].

The experience of trauma also changes the individual's perception of pain over the long term [10]. Trauma, both physical and psychological, leads to heightened neuronal sensitivity and plasticity which results in the perception of pain from normally non-painful stimuli (allodynia) and greater pain than would be expected from painful stimuli (hyperalgesia). Survivors of trauma often carry diagnoses such as fibromyalgia, chronic fatigue, irritable bowel syndrome, chronic pelvic pain, and chronic daily headache [8]. Recent studies show these conditions are manifestations of an underlying syndrome known as *central sensitization* [9]. Unfortunately, healthcare biases about these syndromes, lack of awareness of trafficking victimization, and time constraints which limit comprehensive patient care make it difficult to recognize, let alone address, the underlying trauma of trafficking survivors.

Healthcare professionals often miss the signs of trafficking due to a lack of training, or because they are afraid to ask the difficult questions, or because of the biases they carry either consciously or unconsciously, including biases about race, gender, poverty, prostitution, and/or immigration [11]. Furthermore, our academic model of multiple providers (medical student, resident, attending) together conducting a history and physical exam may make any patient, especially a trafficked person, feel intimidated or humiliated. This in turn will inhibit revelations about his or her trafficked status.

Further, trafficked persons often do not want to be identified as a "victim": trauma bonding between the victim and abuser/perpetrator can be intense and lead many victims to believe they have chosen or are deserving of their abuse [12]. Traffickers often scare victims to ensure silence with threats and lies about the legal and social consequences of disclosure. Many traffickers come to healthcare visits or send a representative to ensure that a victim does not reveal the true nature of their situation.

In this chapter, you will read five real case presentations. These cases are meant to illustrate the multitude of ways in which a trafficking victim-survivor may present in the healthcare system. This short list of cases is by no means an exhaustive discussion of trafficked patients. After each case, there will be a series of questions that will touch on ethical, social, or medical considerations for further discussion and exploration. The short commentary following each question is meant to be a launching pad for further self-reflection and discussions with your colleagues.

A word of caution as you read this chapter: the practice of medicine encourages us to recover, to fix, and to heal. It is natural to read these stories – or hear of cases in your own healthcare setting – and to want to "rescue" the victim. Indeed, why do we have trainings and hospital protocols on trafficking if the goal is not to identify victims and to help our patients? This desire, while well intentioned, robs the patient of their own agency to choose how and when to leave their situation. Outside of mandatory reporting circumstances, our job is to ensure that the patient feels seen, heard, safe, and respected so they may return for services when they feel the time is right.

Emergency Department and Urgent Care Patient Presentations

Chief Complaint: Ankle Pain

"Allison" presents to an urgent care center with left ankle pain and swelling. She reports that she twisted her ankle and felt a "pop" while walking. She is a well-appearing 26-year-old woman with no significant prior medical or surgical history. The urgent care provider is too overwhelmed with patients that day to take a social or sexual history and stays focused on the primary presenting complaint. On physical exam, there is point tenderness of the left fifth metatarsal with associated swelling. The range of motion of her foot is limited secondary to pain, and she has normal sensation to light touch with 2+ distal pulses. An X-ray of the left ankle demonstrates a minimally displaced fracture involving the base of the fifth metatarsal with adjacent soft tissue swelling. The urgent care physician prescribes acetaminophen with codeine for 5 days. Allison is instructed to follow-up with an orthopedic surgeon in 2–3 days and is fitted for an ankle boot and crutches. As is typical of urgent care visits, she is given a referral to an orthopedic surgeon, but an appointment is not made on her behalf.

Six days later, Allison returns to the same urgent care clinic complaining of persistent left ankle pain and swelling and is seen by a second provider. Allison states that she could not get in to see the orthopedic surgeon and that she had used all of the pain medication that was prescribed to her. She had not worn the boot, nor had she used the crutches. The urgent care physician documents that the patient appears to be drug-seeking and is non-compliant with recommendations. Allison is given a prescription for ibuprofen and another referral for the orthopedic surgeon prior to being discharged. Again, no appointment with the surgeon is arranged.

Three days later, Allison is seen by you in your hospital's emergency department (ED). She presents with the same complaint of left ankle pain and swelling. This time, she reports that the fracture occurred when she fell at work and that she could not miss more work to go to an orthopedic surgery appointment. She requests more pain medication until she is able to get to an appointment. You order another X-ray, which confirms a displaced fracture of the left 5th metatarsal with associated soft tissue swelling. Allison reports her pain to be 8/10 and you give her IV morphine. You also conclude that the patient appears to be drug-seeking, and you refuse to prescribe more narcotic pain medication.

Approximately 3 weeks after her ED visit with you, Allison is arrested and charged with prostitution. She is referred to a human trafficking court where further investigation reveals that she had been coerced and deceived into providing commercial sex acts. Allison is brought for medical evaluation to yet another hospital ED. At *this* visit, she reports that the ankle fracture actually occurred when she was pushed down the stairs by her trafficker. She also reveals that she was forced to go on "dates" and was required to wear high heels, further aggravating her fracture. Her trafficker took away the ankle boot she was given because "it was not sexy" and took the narcotics she was prescribed for pain and sold them. Her trafficker threatened Allison, saying that if she saw an orthopedic surgeon, the surgeon would perform an emergency operation and that the trafficker would not pay her hospital bills. He told her that she would be obligated to pay back her "debt" by "working overtime."

In a review of the medical documentation preceding Allison's arrest, there was no documentation of a search of the prescribing database to investigate her prior narcotic use. Furthermore, there was no documentation of any social history, no work excuse letter was offered, and no social work consult placed. During her visit in your ED, Allison left "against medical advice" while awaiting final discharge planning for more than 2 hours. There is no documentation of an attempt to reach her for follow-up. Eventually, after her arrest and identification as a victim of trafficking by the judicial system, Allison is seen in a clinic specifically for the treatment and support for victims for sex trafficking.

The Social History

What is the appropriate social history to take at a new patient encounter, including in the ED and urgent care setting?

As medical students we are taught, through simulated patient encounters, how to take a complete social history. We are taught to ask about the patient's relationships, safety at home, occupation, sexual orientation, seatbelt use, stressors, and any barriers to healthcare. Unfortunately, on the wards, we are taught to adhere to the "focused history and exam" – essentially narrowing the evaluation to a series of pertinent questions and findings. In doing so, our social history is amputated to include only enough to satisfy billing requirements – does the patient use tobacco, alcohol, or drugs? In some cases, the record simply states "non-contributory," which is another way of saying "I didn't ask" or "it wouldn't be related to the diagnosis anyway." Some might argue that a social history is not relevant in an emergent or urgent care setting where the goal is stabilization. However, we would argue that following "stabilization," a patient's "disposition" from an acute care setting should be directly tied to whether, how, and when they can follow-up for the long-term care of their illness. It is not possible to plan an appropriate "disposition" without understanding the patient's social history. (See Chap. 20 for more on medical education.)

A Word on "Drug-Seeking Behavior"

What is drug-seeking behavior and the implications of assuming a patient is drug-seeking?

"Drug-seeking behavior" is a widely used, derogatory term that refers to demanding, manipulative, or dishonest behavior while trying to obtain an addictive medication. Patients who are "drug-seeking" employ multiple strategies: they may have an excuse for why other non-addictive medications don't work for their pain; they may "doctor-shop" or "pharmacy-shop" to fill multiple prescriptions; or they may return to the same doctor frequently, stating that they ran out of the prior prescription. Doctors who thoughtlessly prescribe opioids are considered outdated at best or complicit in the opioid epidemic at worst. In an effort to significantly reduce the availability of opioid medications, most urgent and emergent care settings have drastically curtailed opioid prescribing [13]. Unfortunately, for patients like the one described in this case, this meant that her pain was untreated for weeks and that she felt stigmatized and unwelcome in the healthcare setting. Could a search of the prescription monitoring program have helped? Could a social work or mental health consult have helped uncover the root of her apparent drug-seeking behavior and revealed her sexual exploitation?

Obligations for Follow-Up

What is an urgent care center's obligation for follow-up on a patient who has repeat admissions?

In a call-to-action article, Ayers describes the ethical and practical imperative of ensuring a patient can and does follow their discharge plan [14]. Before a patient leaves the center, Ayers writes, a knowledgeable and responsible provider should:

- Determine that the patient truly understands the clinical findings and the instructions for follow-up or self-care *and intends to follow them.*
- If the patient received a prescription, assess whether *he or she intends to get it filled and whether the cost of the drug is affordable.*
- Arrange for follow-up with a specialist or primary care provider if necessary, including forwarding the chart to the patient's personal physician.
- Detail where the patient should go if his or her condition worsens, with instructions on the criteria for returning to the urgent care center or going straight to the emergency department.

Furthermore, urgent care centers should have a clear protocol to telephone a day or two after the visit to determine whether or not all is going well with the therapeutic journey:

- The patient should be told that the center *will* call to follow-up.
- The patient should be asked *what number and what time* to call.
- The patient should never be asked *whether* the center should call.

A protocol like this may have helped this patient by determining that she could not fill her prescription, alerting the orthopedic surgeon that a patient had been referred who never called for an appointment, or following up by phone with the patient at a time when she may have been able to disclose her social situation.

Opioids and Human Trafficking

What is the relationship between the opioid epidemic and trafficking?

There are several ways in which the opioid epidemic intersects with human trafficking. (See Chap. 13 for further discussion of this nexus.) First, individuals who are already addicted to opioids are vulnerable to recruitment and exploitation by traffickers. Traffickers will often post themselves near methadone clinics, detox centers, and drug rehabilitation homes in the hopes of manipulating an individual during a vulnerable time in his or her life [15]. Since methadone use requires a person to present to the same location every day to get their pills, a trafficker is afforded the opportunity to slowly and deliberately groom and recruit someone over time. Secondly, traffickers may use opioids to control victims who did not previously have an addiction, using the drug to subdue their victims into compliance, or to mask pain that would otherwise require attention. For individuals who are addicted, traffickers can exploit the fear of withdrawal. Lastly, until we have better access to mental health services for survivors, opioids will be used by survivors to avoid, ward off, and cope with the flashbacks, nightmares, depression, and anger they often develop during their captivity. For more information, refer to Chap. 13, and view the webinar on the intersection of the opioid crisis with trafficking at https://www.acf.hhs.gov/otip/resource/nhttacopioidcrisis.

Red Flags for Trafficking

- Extremity fracture – for further reading, see George et al. [16].
- Multiple urgent care visits for the same complaint.
- Unable to follow through with recommended treatment.
- Left without disposition from the ED.

Chief Complaint: Vulvar Pain and Discharge

"Lourdes" presents to your outpatient gynecology clinic for an urgent appointment with the report of 4 days of vaginal pain and discharge. She is an 18-year-old adolescent with no previous health issues. Prior to this appointment, Lourdes was seen in a local ED, with the same symptoms. A review of the ED notes showed documentation of a pelvic exam with "no cervical discharge and no lesions appreciated." A point-of-care urinalysis was negative. Cervical chlamydia and gonorrhea swab testing were negative. Lourdes was diagnosed with a yeast infection, given a prescription for a topical antifungal treatment, and discharged home with no referral for follow-up.

Three days later, Lourdes returned to the same ED with persistent and worsening dysuria, so much so that she had begun to avoid toileting and had developed urinary retention. A bladder scan revealed distension with 800 mL of urine, for which she was straight catheterized. At the time of catheterization, she was noted to have multiple tender ulcers on her labia bilaterally. She was told that she likely had syphilis, and she was empirically treated with penicillin G. The patient refused a speculum exam at that visit secondary to pain. She was discharged home with lidocaine jelly for topical relief of her pain, told to void every 2 hours, and given a referral to a gynecologist (you). RPR and HIV testing from that ED visit were negative.

Lourdes presents to your outpatient gynecology office for follow-up subsequent to her recent ED visit. Her labia majora and minora are swollen and erythematous with a cluster of herpetic-appearing ulcerations on the posterior fourchette that are open and draining. The lesions are tender to the touch. A herpes simplex virus PCR sample is collected.

When you ask about her past medical and surgical history, Lourdes discloses two prior pregnancies; one in which she miscarried, with the other resulting in an elective termination of pregnancy. She has never had prior surgery. She reports that she is not currently using contraception because she hopes to get pregnant again; a urine pregnancy test is negative at this time.

When you inquire about her family history, she says she was adopted as a child through an open adoption. She communicates with her birth family as well as her adoptive family and her godmother. Throughout her childhood she moved from home to home frequently. Currently, Lourdes is going to an alternative school after a recent arrest for possession of a handgun, and she lives in a court-mandated group home. She states that she carried a handgun because she and her boyfriend sometimes need to rob people. Lourdes reports that she loves her boyfriend and feels safe and comfortable with him and that she would like to have a child with him.

When you counsel her about the diagnosis of herpes, she becomes tearful and angry. Lourdes says that she has never had a sexually transmitted infection (STI), and she thought her risk for STIs "was over now that she was out of the life." She discloses that when she was 14–16 years old, she was "working for a pimp" who would "trick her" into performing commercial sex acts. As a result of this previous relationship, she was arrested and incarcerated on charges of prostitution. Lourdes had thought that chapter of her life was over, but when she was in jail, she met a different man, "John," through Facebook. After her release from jail 2 weeks ago, she met up with "John" (10 days prior to her initial presentation to the ED) and reports that she was gang-raped by him and several of his friends. She thinks one of them had ulcers on his mouth.

Sexual Assault Exam

Given that the patient reports being gang-raped 10 days ago, is it appropriate to offer a sexual assault evidence collection kit? What information could be gained from this kit? What information could not be gained?

A sexual assault evidence collection kit involves a systematic standardized examination with a victim of sexual assault, which includes specific specimen collection and storage instructions. This examination includes but is not limited to examination and forensic sample collection from the mouth, vagina, and anus; photographic documentation of injuries; saliva, blood, and urine samples; STI testing; and hair sample collection. The standardized collection and secure storage of evidence increases the likelihood of prosecution and conviction of perpetrators of sexual violence. Even if an assailant is not prosecuted for one particular assault, entry of an individual's DNA profile into databases such as CODIS (Combined DNA Index System) may help to link the offender to past and future crimes. Victims do not bear the cost of the collection or processing of the kit, nor are victims obligated to pursue legal action after having completed the evidence collection process [17].

Patients who report a sexual assault should be counseled to seek medical attention immediately [18]. For optimal collection of evidence, especially that of DNA, the patient should avoid bathing, changing or washing clothing, urinating/defecating, cleaning fingernails, or washing the mouth. Smoking, eating, teeth brushing, or drinking should also be avoided. Time is of the essence for evidence collection: in many jurisdictions there is a 72-hour cut-off time for evidence collection, potentially extended to 1 week in specific cases [19]. Certain hospitals/institutions may have the benefit of having specially trained examiners known as Sexual Assault Nurse Examiners (SANE), who work with both adult and pediatric populations [20]. A lack of specially trained personnel at your institution should not preclude evidence collection; instead, this should prompt a rapid transfer to an appropriate facility. In some institutions, a consulting gynecologist or adolescent medicine specialist may be the best resource for completing the forensic examination and specimen collection. A sample protocol for the use of a sexual assault kit is available through the US Department of Justice's Office on Violence Against Women (https://www.forensicnurses.org/search/custom.asp?id=2093). Additional guidance is also available through the SAFE Technical Assistance program (https://www.safeta.org). It is critical that examiners follow local jurisdictional policies regarding the packaging and labeling of evidence. Time from collection to transport and storage should be minimized, and these transfers should only be undertaken by law enforcement or another authorized official. Evidence should be stored at an appropriate crime laboratory or law enforcement facility, and chain-of-custody information should be appropriately documented to ensure no loss or alteration of evidence which could affect its legal integrity [19].

For Lourdes, because 10 days have elapsed from the time of the assault, there has likely been a significant loss or degradation of collectable evidence due to changing of clothing, bathing, eating/drinking, and so forth. Nonetheless, a thorough exam should be performed as there may be physical evidence of violence that can still be documented, such as bruising or abrasions. An examination also would allow for appropriate STI screening, STI treatment, assessment of pregnancy, and consideration for emergency contraception. We would therefore suggest performing a full forensic evaluation of this patient. The pelvic exam should be performed in a trauma-sensitive manner, as outlined in Table 16.1.

At her first ED visit, Lourdes was tested for gonorrhea and chlamydia, which are two of the most common STIs reported by victims of sexual assault, as well as for HIV and syphilis. In your clinic, you should also consider screening for hepatitis B and C infections, as well as trichomonas. Although in this particular case the applicable time frame has been exceeded, it is important for providers caring for victims of sexual assault to consider HIV post-exposure prophylaxis, which should be administered as soon as possible and no later than 72 hours after a potential

Table 16.1 The pelvic exam should be conducted in a trauma-informed and sensitive manner

Trauma-informed gynecologic exam
Allow the patient *to keep on any clothing they want* – especially if its unrelated to your exam.
Do *NOT* force knees apart from the inside. Say, "relax your knees to the side as much as is comfortable."
Words matter! Footrests, not stirrups. Table, not bed. Drape, not sheet. The vagina looks healthy, not "it looks good." In general, avoid any statements evaluating her looks, even if they are compliments.
Communicate what you are going to do *BEFORE you do it, not as you are doing it.*
Is there anything I can do to make this exam more comfortable?
Make it clear that if something hurts or the patient says "stop," *you will immediately stop and the exam will be over.* Never say, "I'm almost done."
The *bimanual exam can be performed from the side of the patient* rather than from a standing position between her legs. The visual of you hovering over her is often traumatic.
The most traumatic part of speculum use is the insertion – *ask the patient if she would prefer to insert it herself, like a tampon.*
Use the smallest speculum possible and upsize only if necessary.
Once you know that the patient feels comfortable with your description, *perform the exam at your normal speed to adequately obtain the views or samples you need.* Don't rush and get an inadequate exam to "make it quicker for her." If you put her through an exam, the patient wants it to be useful to her health.

exposure, as well as emergency contraception for which there are options extending up to 120 hours after unprotected intercourse [19].

Lourdes had a negative urine pregnancy test at the time of the first emergency department evaluation; however, this would have been too early to detect a pregnancy on urine testing resulting from her assault. Serum testing of beta-HCG is significantly more sensitive in the first few weeks of gestation but is not recommended as a screening test unless the patient is having pain or bleeding. Given that she is not currently using contraception and is past the applicable time frame for emergency contraception, she should be counseled on the potential for resulting pregnancy and instructed to obtain a repeat pregnancy test in the instance of missed menses [17].

Herpes Simplex Virus and Syphilis

What were the classic signs of herpetic ulcers (rather than syphilitic ulcers) that could have led to an earlier diagnosis and treatment for this patient? What is the incidence of herpes compared to the incidence of syphilis in the United States?

There are several important differences between genital herpes infection (caused by herpes simplex virus (HSV) types 1 and 2) and syphilitic infection (caused by the spirochete *Treponema pallidum*) which could have avoided misdiagnosis and inaccurate treatment. These include differences in incidence/prevalence, presentation, and mode of diagnostic testing.

Of all genital ulcerative diseases, genital herpes is the most common and is one of the most prevalent of all STIs. Both HSV-1 and HSV-2 can lead to genital infection, with most genital infections in the United States resulting from HSV-2. Approximately 45 million adolescents and adults have been infected with HSV-2. In addition, while HSV-1 is more commonly contracted via orolabial transmission in childhood, the prevalence of genital HSV-1 infections among young adults (ages 14–19 years) appears to be rising [21]. In fact, up to 80% of new genital infections may be secondary to HSV-1 [22]. Overall, rates of genital HSV infections are likely to be significantly underestimated, due to mild or unrecognized infections, leading to inadvertent spread between sexual partners, as well as the fact that it is not a nationally reportable condition [21, 23]. Syphilis infection is notably less common, with just over 30,000 reported cases in 2017. However, after reaching a "historic low" in 2000, rates of syphilis infection have risen yearly, including a dramatic 10.5% increase from 2016 to 2017.

Genital herpes infections are characterized by recurrent and painful lesions, with primary infections (initial outbreak in setting of absent antibodies) generally being more severe. Prodromal symptoms prior to appearance of lesions occur in up to two-thirds of patients and can include vulvar burning or pruritus, which may lead to misdiagnosis of a urinary tract infection (UTI) or yeast infection. The subsequently developing vesicular lesions (often multiple) can be exquisitely tender to the touch, and may lead to significant dysuria when in contact with urine (as in this patient's case, which led to urinary retention). The characteristic lesion of a primary syphilitic infection is the chancre, which is typically isolated and described as having a crater-like appearance. In stark contrast to herpetic lesions, the chancre is classically *non*-tender [23]. Given the prevalence of herpes in the general population and its intersection with sexual violence, everyone caring for patients in the emergency department should familiarize themselves with the diagnosis and management of herpes lesions. If the diagnosis is uncertain, utilize the gynecologic or urologic consultants at your institution. It is also important to recognize that there are multiple atypical appearances of herpetic lesions, especially in varying stages of healing. These include but are not limited to, fissures, varying levels of erosion, and confluence of lesions. Thus, as a baseline recommendation, any new ulcerative lesion(s) of the vulva should prompt PCR testing for herpes by direct swab.

Contraception and Family Planning Counseling

How would you counsel this patient about contraception and family planning in light of her diagnosis and her desire for conception with her current boyfriend?

In the setting of an initial visit to an outpatient clinic, the primary goal is treating the patient's current outbreak for relief of her symptoms, followed closely by counseling her about prevention of transmission to her current partner. It is important to inform the patient that she should avoid sexual contact until the lesions have fully healed to avoid infecting her partner as a result of the active episode. Given the chronic nature of genital HSV and potential for recurrent outbreaks with viral shedding, this counseling must also include the prevention of transmission during future outbreaks [24]. It is critical for the patient to know that a history of genital herpes is important to relay to a future provider in a future pregnancy [22].

Who Is a Victim of Sex Trafficking?

Is this patient a survivor of human trafficking?

The patient's disclosed history of coercion into commercial sex acts as a minor means that she meets the definition of a victim of human sex trafficking, but the concept of survivorship is more complicated. Although she reports having exited "the life" at the age of 16, she remains vulnerable to exploitation. The events surrounding her recent assault are a direct result of her incarceration for prostitution and subsequent manipulation by the perpetrator online.

While she reports a good relationship and a desire to conceive with her "boyfriend," the exact nature of their relationship is suspicious in light of her admission that they engaged in armed robbery together. She clearly identifies her prior trafficker as a man who "tricked" her into sex work, but her "boyfriend" may also be exploiting her. There are many possible mechanisms of control or coercion, many of which may not be obvious to the victim. It is critical to consider that possessing a handgun and committing robbery may be the result of "pressure" from her "boyfriend" and that her complicity in armed robbery could be used to blackmail her into sex trafficking or other criminal activities.

Criminality

What is the relationship between incarceration and sex trafficking?

As described in a 2019 report on criminal record relief for victims of trafficking, often the first contact with law enforcement and the justice system is as an offender rather than a victim. While their illegal behavior is almost always a result of force or coercion on behalf of a pimp or trafficker, many victims will be arrested for crimes including prostitution, drug-related offenses, robbery, or theft. This report also cites the results of a 2016 survey by the National Survivor Network in which 91% of 130 trafficking victims reported having been arrested [25]. There are also incidents where victims commit crimes so as they will be sent to prison as an escape from their captor [26].

Incarceration itself may lead to an initial act of victimization or even re-victimization for women who have already been trafficked. Outside traffickers may prey on the insecurities of incarcerated women via written/online communication or via fellow female inmates currently under their influence. This can lead to the recruitment of imprisoned women, often through promises of food, shelter, relationship stability, or other basic needs upon release from prison [26]. A 2018 news article in *The Guardian* discusses the ways in which some traffickers use inmates under their control, corrupt bondsmen, and online information to identify women currently awaiting a court date. The trafficker then may communicate with these women, post their bond to free them from jail, and subsequently use this "incurred debt" as leverage to coerce them into criminal activity or commercial sex acts with the threat of rescinding their bond payment should they refuse or fail to comply with the trafficker's wishes [27].

Recidivism

What risk factors does she have for re-engaging in commercial sex work and being re-trafficked in her adult years?

The patient's history of incarceration itself generates significant risk of a return to "the life." This patient's specific experience of being contacted via social media while in jail, which resulted in her being lured into a premeditated gang rape, is quite similar to the baiting tactics used by traffickers as described above. It is critical to remember that a history of incarceration has long-lasting ramifications which increase the victim's vulnerability to traffickers, including limitations on future options for legal employment and/or the right to apply for public aid, with subsequent inability to afford safe housing and other basic necessities [25].

Red Flags for Sex Trafficking

- History of “working for a pimp” who would “trick her” into performing commercial sex acts
- Previous arrest and incarceration
- Victim of gang rape
- History of an unstable housing situation
- Participation in other illegal activities – armed robbery

Chief Complaint: Gunshot Wound

“Trudy” is a 14-year-old girl seen in the emergency department with a gunshot wound to the left upper extremity. She walks in unaided and alone. You are the pediatric trauma surgeon who has been consulted to assess the magnitude of Trudy’s injuries. When you ask Trudy what happened, she says she was on a date with an older man who beat her with the butt of a handgun. During the struggle, the weapon was discharged, and she sustained an injury to the left upper extremity.

On exam, Trudy is defiant, gives one-word responses to your questions, and is disheveled. Apart from soft tissue bruising of her face and the superficial gunshot wound to the lateral aspect of her proximal left arm, her exam is unremarkable. She has no significant past medical, surgical, or family history. Trudy says she lives with her mother. She does not use any drugs or alcohol. You did not obtain additional social history.

Because a gunshot wound raises significant concerns for her safety, you admit Trudy in an effort to provide protection and to connect her with potentially helpful resources. In a private conversation with Trudy, you discuss your concerns for her safety, disclose your mandatory reporting obligations, and attempt to establish a trusting relationship between her and the healthcare team. You discuss her case with your social work and child abuse team, concerned that Trudy may be involved in a gang, experiencing intimate partner violence or a victim of sex trafficking. The clinical team offers Trudy a host of services, you arrange for an outpatient adolescent medicine follow-up appointment, and you verbally provide her with the number to the National Human Trafficking Hotline (888-373-7888).

The following day, a man who is not Trudy’s guardian arrives at the hospital demanding that she be discharged since she has no injuries that require hospitalization. The bedside nurse and charge nurse are concerned for Trudy’s safety as they had overheard “heated discussions” between the man and Trudy. Because no legal guardian is present, Trudy is not discharged. Trudy’s mother comes to the hospital later that evening; Trudy is discharged home with her mother who is accompanied by the same man who is not her guardian.

Opportunity for Harm Reduction Intervention

The development of a trusting relationship between at-risk youth and safe adults is a critical part of harm reduction strategies and can offer potentially life-changing resources. Effective injury prevention and overall harm reduction have the ability to positively impact a vulnerable patient population [28, 29].

Gun Violence and Sex Trafficking

Patients who are at risk for sex trafficking often present with other "at-risk" behaviors that require harm reduction intervention, such as gun violence [30]. Gun violence in the context of an intimate relationship creates an environment that fosters coercive control facilitating chronic and escalating abuse [31]. Gun violence is known to be a serious concern for high-risk, socioeconomically disadvantaged patients [32]. Firearm fatalities were the second leading cause of death among children in 2013, and for over a decade, the United States has had the highest pediatric firearm fatality rate of all industrialized nations [32]. While there is a paucity of data on the use of gun violence in sex trafficking, we can extrapolate from data on gun use against an intimate partner which reveal that a staggering 4.5 million women have had an intimate partner threaten them with a gun, and one million have been shot or shot at by an intimate partner [29]. The identification of a patient who is high-risk for being trafficked presents an opportunity for engagement and to offer support with the overall intent of patient safety, injury prevention, and harm reduction. While protocols for screening are outside the scope of this chapter, gun violence can be an entry point of questioning for someone you suspect may be trafficked. Questions such as "Do you carry a weapon to protect yourself?" or "Who do you feel you need to protect yourself against?" or "Have you ever wished you had a weapon to protect yourself?" may be a way of initiating a conversation concerning violence and abuse.

Red Flags for Sex Trafficking
- Minor who reports dating a much older partner
- Minor who is present without a legal guardian
- Gun violence
- Dating violence
- An adult present who is not the legal guardian and appears to be verbally abusive toward a minor

Outpatient Presentations

Chief Complaint: Routine Prenatal Care

"Mariama" is a 15-year-old girl who presents for her first prenatal visit at a hospital-based women's health center. You are the pediatric and adolescent gynecologist on staff, and Mariama is a new patient on your clinic schedule. This is her first pregnancy, and she believes she is about 5 months pregnant. She has no complaints of bleeding, cramping, or rupture of membranes. There is no other past medical or surgical history. She reports that she arrived in the United States several months ago from her native West Africa and currently lives with her husband.

On exam, Mariama is well groomed, soft spoken, and fluent in English; but you notice she is not appropriately dressed for the cold weather. She makes poor eye contact during the visit. Her fundal height is 25 cm, and two fetal heart rates are detected. Ultrasound confirms a twin gestation. On genital exam, her labia minora, clitoris, and clitoral hood have been removed, consistent with Female Genital Mutilation/Cutting (FGM/C), Type IIb, which is practiced in her country of origin. When you ask about the cutting, Mariama discloses that she was cut at the age of 5 in her home country.

Mariama returns for each of her scheduled prenatal visits, and her pregnancy progresses normally. You notice that she becomes increasingly depressed with each passing week. When you ask her if she's okay, she reveals that her husband is verbally and physically abusive. He frequently hits her with his fists and a belt. He is particularly angry with her for carrying female twins. He wanted a son. He hits her most often when she asks to go to school.

At a later clinic visit, Mariama tells you that she was actually sold by her older sister and sent to the United States to be her husband's second wife. Upon her arrival, her travel documents and identification were taken from her, and she was never legally married. She lives with her "husband," who is in his 40s, and his first wife, who also is very abusive. She says that her "husband" told her she could never leave him as she had no legal immigration status and that he is in possession of all of her identification.

Mariama eventually delivers twin girls at 36 weeks' gestation via cesarean section.

Female Genital Mutilation/Cutting

What is the significance of her FGM/C?

Female genital mutilation/cutting affects an estimated 200 million women and girls [33]. FGM/C is practiced around the world, primarily in Africa, the Middle East, and Southeast Asia. The World Health Organization (WHO) has defined FGM/C as "all procedures that involve partial or total removal of the external female genitalia, or other injury to the female genital organs, for non-medical reasons" [33]. WHO has classified FGM/C into four fundamental types (with several sub-classifications added in 2016): (1) Type I, *clitoridectomy*, partial or total removal of the external clitoris; (2) Type II, *excision*, partial or total removal of the external clitoris and labia minora; (3) Type III, *infibulation*, cutting and repositioning the labia minora or labia majora to form a covering seal, narrowing the vaginal opening; and (4) type IV, all other harmful procedures to the female genitalia for non-medical purposes including, but not limited to, pricking, piercing, incising, scraping, and cauterizing the genital area [33].

Increasingly, due to migration, women and girls affected by FGM/C have become members of societies where the practice is not normative, including in the United States. Currently, more than an estimated 513,000 women and girls living in the United States have undergone FGM/C or are at risk of being cut [34]. Recognition of FGM/C in patients is essential to addressing their medical, gynecologic, and psychological symptoms. It is also imperative to recognize that affected women and girls are more likely to experience other forms of gender-based violence/human rights violations including intimate partner violence, sexual violence, child marriage, and forced marriage [35]. In our case, the patient has experienced all of these abuses.

Safety Planning

What steps should be taken in light of the revelation of domestic violence, particularly in pregnancy?

As with any patient experiencing intimate partner violence, the patient's immediate safety and risk of homicide must be assessed. If possible, a safety plan should be formulated with the expert guidance of a victim service advocate. Because Mariama is pregnant, fetal health is a significant concern. Involvement of social services, provision of hotline information, and detailed documentation of the violence and related medical sequelae are essential and may be used as evidence in the future should Mariama wish to pursue charges.

According to the American College of Obstetricians and Gynecologists (ACOG), approximately 324,000 pregnant women experience intimate partner violence (IPV) each year in the United States. IPV is associated with multiple complications in pregnancy and the severity of violence, including homicide, sometimes may escalate during pregnancy or the postpartum period [36].

This case is complicated by Mariama's age. As noted in the ACOG committee opinion, "Reporting of the abuse of children is mandatory; however, reporting IPV, particularly mandatory reporting, is controversial. Although the intent of mandatory reporting is to identify and protect individuals before the next act of violence, the individual's safety, in fact, may be jeopardized" [36, 37]. We recommend careful review of local and state laws as well as consultation with law enforcement and social work about mandatory reporting requirements in your region.

Depression

How should her depression be treated?

Depression is very common in women, especially in women of reproductive age. It is estimated that 14–23% of pregnant women experience depression during pregnancy and 5–25% experience depression postpartum [38]. In this case, our patient should be administered a validated questionnaire, such as the Patient Health Questionnaire (PHQ-9), and assessed for suicide risk [39]. She should be offered counseling services, as well as medication. It is important to remember that not all psychiatric medications are contraindicated in pregnancy.

Forced Marriage

In what ways is forced/child marriage a form of trafficking?

Forced marriage refers to situations where persons, regardless of their age, have been forced to marry without their consent. Forced marriage is prohibited through legislation regarding slavery and slavery-like practices, including servile marriage [40]. Child marriage is now recognized as a form of human trafficking. According to Girls Not Brides (www.girlsnotbrides.org), "Child marriage is any formal marriage or informal union where one or both of the parties are under 18 years of age." Child marriage is, de facto, forced marriage since a child cannot legally consent to the union. Each year, 15 million girls are married globally before the age of 18. The overwhelming majority of children wed were girls, though boys are also affected [41]. Child marriage fits most criteria for enslavement including forced work and serving others under the threat of mental or physical or mental punishment, dehumanization, treatment as property, forced sexual servitude, and severely restricted social interaction [42].

Red Flags for Human Trafficking
- Teen pregnancy.
- FGM/C is a possible marker for other forms of gender-based violence.
- The patient's admission that she is "married" at age 15.
- Undocumented immigration status/confiscated identity documents.

Chief Complaint: Abdominal Pain

"Vicky" is a 10-year-old girl, accompanied by her mother, who presents to the ED for evaluation of 3 days of abdominal pain. You are the pediatric surgeon on-call and you are asked to evaluate Vicky for possible acute appendicitis. Vicky reports nausea, but no emesis, no diarrhea, no recent travel, and no sick contacts. She reports no significant past medical, surgical, family, or social history.

As is your standard practice, you politely instruct Vicky's mother to leave the room at the conclusion of your physical exam in order to obtain a good social history in private. Vicky's mother refuses to leave. Rather than engage in a verbal altercation with Vicky's mother, you take Vicky to the radiology room for her ultrasound to speak with her alone. In private, Vicky reports no drug or alcohol use. When you ask about sexual activity, including intercourse, Vicky gives unusually long-winded, evasive responses and offers no specific information.

Vicky is a soft-spoken, well-groomed girl who is in obvious discomfort. At Vicky's request, you perform her physical assessment in her mother's presence. Her abdomen is soft, not distended, and tender to percussion throughout all quadrants. The urine pregnancy test is negative. Laboratory tests are significant for an elevated white blood cell count. An ultrasound of her abdomen reveals a normal appendix, fully visualized to the tip, with no fecalith. There is free fluid in the abdomen. A urine gonorrhea and chlamydia test is sent. Vicky and her mother both refuse a bimanual pelvic exam, and as a result, the gynecology service is not consulted.

Vicky is hospitalized on the inpatient pediatric service for observation, IV fluids, and serial abdominal exams with a diagnosis of possible acute appendicitis. On the day after admission, you take Vicky to the operating room for a diagnostic laparoscopy due to persistent peritonitis. During the laparoscopy, you diagnose pelvic inflammatory disease with significant adhesions within the pelvis, throughout the abdomen, and over the liver to the diaphragm (Fitz-Hugh-Curtis syndrome). Later that day, her urine gonorrhea test returns positive. You discuss your operative and lab findings with Vicky alone in the recovery room before allowing her mother to come into the recovery area.

Broad Differential Diagnoses: Abdominal Pain

What are the top considerations for abdominal pain in this patient?

In this age group, the most common causes of abdominal pain with no prior past medical or surgical history include appendicitis, gastroenteritis, and pyelonephritis. Appendicitis is less likely in this case in light of several days of abdominal pain without fever and an ultrasound that identifies a normal appendix. She does not have any findings consistent with gastroenteritis or pyelonephritis. Given the prevalence of child sexual abuse, it is critical not to neglect the possibility of sexually transmitted infections and pelvic inflammatory disease as the cause of her symptoms. Approximately 28.4% of child sex abuse victims are children between the ages of 4 and 7 years old, 25.5% between the ages of 8 and 11 years old, and 35.9% between the ages of 12 and 17 years old [43]. Furthermore, one must always rule out pregnancy, even if the patient denies heterosexual sexual activity.

When to Discuss Sex with the Pediatric Patient

In what situations do you include sexually transmitted infections and pelvic inflammatory disease on your differential and complete associated testing?

There is no standard guideline regarding the appropriate age at which to begin questioning patients about their sexual activity. Even when asked, many children do not disclose sexual abuse [44]. In this case, the patient's young age likely deterred the clinicians from initiating a conversation about sexual activity. Data show that even in outpatient settings, general practitioners are not regularly having these conversations with their patients. One study found that one-third of all adolescents had annual visits without any mention of sex. Of those conversations that did include sexual health and development, they lasted an average of 36 seconds [45]. Given this deficit of care, the American Academy of Pediatrics (AAP) recently published guidelines urging providers to engage in discussions of sex and sexuality at every visit along with education regarding puberty, birth control options, and protection against sexually transmitted infections [46]. As children and their families navigate through puberty during the teenage years, this early education may help them recognize warning signs of sexual abuse and trafficking in an effort to reduce the likelihood of becoming a victim.

One study of children who were victims of sexual abuse found that 67.5% of girls with a confirmed STI had normal or nonspecific physical exam findings [47]. Given the prevalence of childhood sexual abuse, STIs must be included in the differential. Interview questions should be asked in order to ascertain risk, and providers must perform the appropriate screening tests for these infections.

STIs and Sex Trafficking

Victims of sex trafficking are at an extremely high risk of contracting an STI for numerous reasons: condom use may be limited by their trafficker or the buyers, they have multiple sexual partners, and often they are unable to negotiate the terms of the sexual encounter [48–52]. Victims of sex trafficking often have a delayed presentation to healthcare providers resulting in delayed treatment. In this case the patient had evidence on laparoscopy of Fitz-Hugh-Curtis syndrome, which is a complication of PID causing inflammation of the liver capsule and typically presents with pain in the upper right quadrant.

Let's Talk About Sex Trafficking

How does a provider hold a conversation with a suspected sex trafficking victim?

This case highlights the importance of getting patients *alone and comfortable* to begin sensitive conversations, including taking a sexual history. Children who are sexually abused or victims of sex trafficking may present with their parents, other supervising adults, or other relatives. The person present with the child may not be aware of the abuse. Oftentimes, the accompanying adult will insist on being present for the evaluation; however, it is necessary to separate them to have a private conversation with the patient. After all non-HCPs have left the exam room, it is important to establish trust with the patient. We recommend that providers disclose their mandatory reporting obligations (refer to Chap. 18). Given that victims of exploitation and abuse are often led to believe they are to blame, we encourage providers to acknowledge the psychological coercion that exists in sexual abuse in an age-appropriate manner.

Suggestions for delicate conversations with children [53, 54]:

- See the patient alone, without guardians or other accompanying non-healthcare professionals.
- Disclose your mandatory reporting obligations.
- Put them in control and allow them to disclose information they are comfortable with discussing.
- Begin with open-ended questions such as:
  - Tell me about a time you were scared.
  - Who do you spend time with when you're not at home?
  - Who do you text or talk to online?

Use words the child is familiar with while being careful not to condescend the patient. It is critical to allow sufficient time for the child to respond fully.

Multidisciplinary communication with social workers, child abuse teams, nurses, and other professionals involved in this patient's care should be engaged to facilitate appropriate follow-up. While some patients have a primary care provider who can provide continuity of care, patients who do not have a medical "home" present an extra challenge. One solution is to take advantage of every point of patient contact for motivational interviewing and employ techniques of harm reduction. Counseling patients and their caretakers about sex education and the risk factors for sex trafficking may be a powerful way to increase awareness and prevention of further sexual exploitation [55].

It is vital to elicit a history of sexual abuse in pediatric patients *whenever* the suspicion arises. Victims of child sexual abuse are extremely vulnerable. Given our unique role as healthcare professionals, we have the opportunity to intervene and educate patients to empower themselves and possibly prevent future human trafficking [56]. By educating our patients, their parents, and our colleagues, we may recognize warning signs for the risks of human trafficking. Additional advice for strategies that parents can use to talk to their kids about sex and healthy relationships may be found at https://www.plannedparenthood.org/learn/parents/tips-talking and https://www.parents.culturereframed.org.

Red Flags for Sex Trafficking
- Sexual abuse
- Late presentation to care for an STI
- Evasive responses to straightforward questions about sexual activity

Conclusion

This chapter presents five ways in which victim-survivors of human trafficking may present to a healthcare setting. Our intention is not to provide an exhaustive description of patient presentations, but to illustrate the depth and nuance of examination skills and interview techniques required to reveal a situation involving trafficking. The most challenging patients – those whose symptoms do not seem to make sense, those who tend to be labeled as "drug-seeking" or "malingering," and those who seem to be "noncompliant" – are those who deserve our most diligent care. Adverse childhood events are known to have far-reaching effects. We must also bear in mind that an individual who presents with one type of abuse is at risk for others, as well. It is not sufficient to simply attend to a presenting complaint; rather, a holistic approach to every patient is critical to provide proper care and essential for the illumination of potentially abusive circumstances. This approach requires significant resources that are challenging to harness. It necessitates continued education and advocacy within our local healthcare communities, as well as acknowledgment of the greater risks to society at the national level.

Resources

1. https://healtrafficking.org/.
2. Alpert EJ, Ahn R, Albright E, Purcell G, Burke TF, Macias-Konstantopoulos WL. Human Trafficking: Guidebook on Identification, Assessment, and Response in the Health Care Setting. MGH Human Trafficking Initiative, Division of Global Health and Human Rights, Department of Emergency Medicine, Massachusetts General Hospital, Boston, MA and Committee on Violence Intervention and Prevention, Massachusetts Medical Society, Waltham, MA. September 2014.
3. Human Trafficking: ACOG Committee Opinion Number 507, September 2011.
4. Julia Geynisman, MD and Debra Taubel, MD. The Devil is in the Detail: Practical aspects of identifying and responding to sex trafficking. December 2, 2015. https://www.contemporaryobgyn.net/modern-medicine-news/devil-detail-practical-aspects-identifying-and-responding-sex-trafficking.

References

1. Brown B.Chapter 4, People are hard to hate close up. Move in. Braving the wilderness: the quest for true belonging and the courage to stand alone. New York: Random House; 2017. [cited 2019 Mar 25]; p. 63–88. Available from: https://www.brenebrown.com/articles/2018/05/17/dehumanizing-always-starts-with-language/.
2. United Nations of Human Rights. Convention on the rights of the child [Internet]. Switzerland. Office of the United Nations High Commissioner for Human Rights (OHCHR). [1989 Nov; cited 2019 May 5]. Available from: https://www.ohchr.org/EN/ProfessionalInterest/Pages/CRC.aspx.
3. United Nations General Assembly, Human Rights Council. Protection against violence and discrimination based on sexual orientation and gender identity [Internet]. Switzerland. Office of the United Nations High Commissioner for Human Rights (OHCHR). [2016 Jul; cited 2019 May 5]. Available from: https://www.un.org/en/ga/search/view_doc.asp?symbol=A/HRC/RES/32/2.
4. United Nations Entity for Gender Equality and the Empowerment of Women. Convention on the elimination of all forms of discrimination against women [Internet]. [1979 Dec; cited 2019 May 5]. Available from: https://www.ohchr.org/EN/ProfessionalInterest/Pages/CEDAW.aspx.
5. Hudson VM, Ballif-Spanvill B, Emmett CF. Sex and world peace. New York: Columbia University Press; 2012. p. 304.
6. Chisolm-Straker M, Baldwin S, Gaïgbé-Togbé B, Ndukwe N, Johnson PN, Richardson LD. Health care and human trafficking: we are seeing the unseen. J Health Care Poor Underserved [Internet]. 2016 cited [2019 May 05];27(3):1220–33. Available from: https://muse.jhu.edu/article/628131.https://doi.org/10.1353/hpu.2016.0131.
7. Zimmerman C, Hossain M, Yun K, Roche B, Morison L, Watts C. Stolen smiles: a summary report on the physical and psychological health consequences of women and adolescents trafficked in Europe [Internet]. London: The London School of Hygiene & Tropical Medicine. 2006 [cited 2019 Apr 12]. p. 27. Available from: https://www.icmec.org/wp-content/uploads/2015/10/Stolen-Smiles-Physical-and-Psych-Consequences-of-Traffic-Victims-in-Europe-Zimmerman.pdf.

8. Gupta MA. Review of somatic symptoms in post-traumatic stress disorder. Int Rev Psychiatry [Internet].2013 [cited 2019 May 19];25(1):86–99. Available from: https://doi.org/10.3109/09540261.2012.736367.
9. McKernan LC, Johnson BN, Crofford LJ, Lumley MA, Bruehl S, Cheavens JS. Posttraumatic stress symptoms mediate the effects of trauma exposure on clinical indicators of central sensitization in patients with chronic pain. Clin J Pain [Internet]. 2019 [cited 2019 May 05];35(5):385–93. Available from: https://journals.lww.com/clinicalpain/toc/2019/05000.https://doi.org/10.1097/AJP.0000000000000689.
10. Jenewein J, Erni J, Moergeli H, Grillon C, Schumacher S, Mueller-Pfeiffer C, et al. Altered pain perception and fear-learning deficits in subjects with posttraumatic stress disorder. J Pain [Internet]. 2016 [cited 2019 May 05];17(12):1325–33. Available from: https://doi.org/10.1016/j.jpain.2016.09.002
11. Fitzgerald C, Hurst S. Implicit bias in healthcare professionals: a systematic review. BMC Med Ethics. 2017 [cited 2019 May 05];18(1):1–18. Available from: https://doi.org/10.1186/s12910-017-0179-8.
12. Doychak K, Raghavan C. "No voice or vote:" trauma-coerced attachment in victims of sex trafficking. J Hum Traffick [Internet]. 2018 Oct [cited 2019 May 05];2332–705. Available from: https://doi.org/10.1080/23322705.2018.1518625.
13. Osborn SR, Yu J, Williams B, Vasilyadis M, Blackmore CC. Changes in provider prescribing patterns after implementation of an Emergency Department prescription opioid policy. J Emerg Med. 2017 [cited 2019 May 05];52(4):538–46. Available from: https://doi.org/10.1016/j.jemermed.2016.07.120.
14. Ayers AA. Post-visit follow-up calls: improving patient satisfaction, center profitability and clinical outcomes. JUCM [internet]. [cited 2019 May 05]. Available from:https://www.jucm.com/post-visit-follow-up-calls-improving-patient-satisfaction-center-profitability-and-clinical-outcomes-2/.
15. Chon K. US Department of Health and Human Services Office on Trafficking in Persons. Human trafficking and opioid abuse [Internet]. 2016 [2016 May; cited 2019 Aug 15]. Available from: http://www.acf.hhs.gov/blog/2016/05/human-trafficking-and-opioid-abuse.
16. George E, Phillips CH, Shah N, Lewis-O'Connor A, Rosner B, Stoklosa HM, et al. Radiologic findings in intimate partner violence. Radiology. 2019 [cited 2019 May 05];291(1):62–69. Available from: https://doi.org/10.1148/radiol.2019180801.
17. Rape, Abuse & Incest National Network (RAINN). What is a rape kit? [Internet]. [cited 2019 May 05]. Available from: https://rainn.org/articles/rape-kit.
18. Crawford-Jakubiak JE, Alderman EM, Leventhal JM. Care of the adolescent after an acute sexual assault. Pediatrics [Internet]. 2017. [cited 2019 May 05]; 2017;139(3):e2–e16. Available from: http://pediatrics.aappublications.org/lookup/doi/10.1542/peds.2016-4243. https://doi.org/10.1542/peds.2016-4243.
19. ACOG Committee Opinion: Committee on Health Care for Underserved Women. Sexual assault. ACOG Committee Opinion No. 777. Obstet Gynecol. 2019. [cited 2019 May 05];133(4):e296–302. Available from: https://insights.ovid.com/pubmed?pmid=30913202.https://doi.org/10.1097/AOG.0000000000003178.
20. International Association of Forensic Nurses. Sexual Assault Nurse Examiners [Internet]. Elkridge, MD; 2019. Available from: https://www.forensicnurses.org/page/AboutSANE.
21. Center for Disease Control and Prevention. Together for girls – Sexual Violence – Violence Prevention – Injury Center. 2011[cited 2019 May 05]. Available from: www.cdc.gov/ViolencePrevention/sexualviolence/together/index.html.
22. ACOG Committee on Practice Bulletins. Management of herpes in pregnancy. Practice Bulletin No. 82. Obstet Gynecol [Internet]. 2007. [cited 2019 May 05];109(6):1489–98. Available from: https://www.ncbi.nlm.nih.gov/pubmed/17569194. https://doi.org/10.1007/978-3-319-57675-6_9.
23. Hoffman BL, Schorge JO, Bradshaw KD, Halvorson M, Schaffer JI, Corton MM. Williams gynecology. 3rd ed. New York: McGraw-Hill Education; 2016. p. 55–60.

24. Sheth S, Keller JM. Infections of the genital tract. In: Johnson CT, Hallock JL, Bienstock JL, Fox HE, Wallach EE, editors. The Johns Hopkins manual of gynecology and obstetrics. 5th ed. Philadelphia: Wolters Kluwer; 2015. p. 356–78.
25. MohrG. The impact of human trafficking. Corrections Today [Internet]. 2017 [cited 2019 Apr 5];79(6):22–25. Available from: http://www.aca.org/ACA_Prod_IMIS/DOCS/Corrections%20Today/2017%20Articles/November%202017/CT-Nov-Dec%202017_Trafficking.pdf.
26. Kelly A, McNamara M. The guardian [Internet]. 2018. [cited 2019 Apr 5]. Available from: https://www.theguardian.com/global-development/2018/jun/29/americas-outcasts-women-trapped-in-cruel-cycle-of-exploitation.
27. Cunningham RM, Chermack ST, Zimmerman MA, Shope JT, Bingham CR, Blow FC, et al. Brief motivational interviewing intervention for peer violence and alcohol use in teens: one-year follow-up. Pediatrics. 2012. [cited 2019 May 05];129(6):1083–90. Available from: https://www.ncbi.nlm.nih.gov/pmc/articles/PMC4074654/.https://doi.org/10.1542/peds.2011-3419.
28. Cunningham R, Knox L, Fein J, Harrison S, Frisch K, Walton M, et al. Before and after the trauma bay: the prevention of violent injury among youth. Ann Emerg Med [Internet]. 2009. [cited 2019 May 05];53(4):490–500. Available from: https://doi.org/10.1016/j.annemergmed.2008.11.014.
29. Sorenson SB, Schut RA. Nonfatal gun use in intimate partner violence: a systematic review of the literature. Trauma Violence Abuse. 2018. [cited 2019 May 05];19(4):431–42. Available from: https://doi.org/10.1177/1524838016668589.
30. Ottisova L, Hemmings S, Howard L, et al. Prevalence and risk of violence and the mental, physical and sexual health problems associated with human trafficking: an updated systematic review. Epidemiol Psychiatr Sci. 2016. [cited 2019 May 05];25(4):317–341. Available from: https://doi.org/10.1017/S2045796016000135.
31. Carter PM, Cook LJ, Macy ML, Zonfrillo MR, Stanley RM, Chamberlain JM, et al. Individual and neighborhood characteristics of children seeking emergency department care for firearm injuries within the PECARN network. Acad Emerg Med [Internet].2017. [cited 2019 May 05];24(7):807–813. Available from: https://www.ncbi.nlm.nih.gov/pubmed/28423460. https://doi.org/10.1111/acem.13200.
32. CDC Web-based Injury Statistics Query and Reporting System (WISQARS). National Center for Injury Prevention and Control. [Internet]. 2019 [cited 2019 Apr 27]. Available from: http://www.cdc.gov/injury/wisqars/index.html.
33. World Health Organization. Care of women and girls living with female genital mutilation: a clinical handbook [Internet]. Geneva: World Health Organization; 2018. Report No. CC BY-NC-SA 3.0 IGO. Available at http://www.who.int/reproductivehealth/publications/health.
34. Goldberg H, Stupp P, Okoroh E, Besera G, Goodman D, Danel I. Female genital mutilation/cutting in the United States: updated estimates of women and girls at risk, 2012. Public Health Rep [Internet]. 2016. [cited 2019 May 05];131(2):340–7. Available from:https://www.ncbi.nlm.nih.gov/pmc/articles/PMC4765983/. https://doi.org/10.1177/003335491613100218.
35. Lever H, Ottenheimer D, Teysir J, Singer E, Atkinson HG. Depression, anxiety, post-traumatic stress disorder and a history of pervasive gender-based violence among women asylum seekers who have undergone female genital mutilation/cutting: a retrospective case review. J Immigr Minor Health [Internet]. 2019 [cited 2019 May 05];21(3). Available from: https://doi.org/10.1007/s10903-018-0782-x.
36. ACOG Committee Opinion: Committee on Health Care for Underserved Women. Intimate partner violence. ACOG Committee Opinion No. 518. Obstet Gynecol [Internet]. 2012. [cited 2019 May 05];110(385):1203–8. Available from: https://www.acog.org/-/media/Committee-Opinions/Committee-on-Health-Care-for-Underserved-Women/co518.pdf?dmc=1&ts=20190630T1642596467.
37. English A. Mandatory reporting of human trafficking: potential benefits and risks of harm. AMA J Ethics [Internet]. 2017 [cited 201915];19(1):54–62. Available from: https://journalofethics.ama-assn.org/article/mandatory-reporting-human-trafficking-potential-benefits-and-risks-harm/2017-01. https://doi.org/10.1001/journalofethics.2017.19.1.pfor1-1701.

38. ACOG Committee Opinion: Screening for perinatal depression. ACOG Committee Opinion No. 757. Obstet Gynecol [Internet]. 2018. [cited 2019 May 05];132(5):e208–12. Available from: https://www.acog.org/-/media/Committee-Opinions/Committee-on-Obstetric-Practice/co757.pdf?dmc=1&ts=20181024T2023437995. https://doi.org/10.1097/AOG.0000000000002927.
39. Kroenke K, Spitzer RL, Williams JB. The PHQ-9. J Gen Intern Med [Internet]. 2001 [cited 2019 Aug 15];16(9):606–13. Available from: https://www.ncbi.nlm.nih.gov/pubmed/11556941. https://doi.org/10.1046/j.1525-1497.2001.016009606.xr.
40. International Labour Organization and Walk Free Foundation. Global estimates of modern slavery: forced labour and forced marriage [Internet]. Geneva: International Labour Office (ILO); 2017 [cited 2019 May 05]; 68 p. Available from: https://www.ilo.org/wcmsp5/groups/public/%2D%2D-dgreports/%2D%2D-dcomm/documents/publication/wcms_575479.pdf.
41. United Nations Children's Fund (UNICEF). Child marriage [Internet]. 2018. [cited 2019 May 05]. Available from: https://data.unicef.org/topic/child-protection/child-marriage/.
42. United Nations: General Assembly. Preventing and eliminating child, early and forced marriage. Report No. A/HRC/26/22. 2014. [cited 2019 May 05]. p. 18. Available from: https://www.ohchr.org/EN/HRBodies/HRC/RegularSessions/Session26/Documents/A-HRC-26-22_en.doc.
43. Putnam FW. Ten-year research update review: child sexual abuse. J Am Acad Child Adolesc Psychiatry [Internet]. 2003. [cited 2019 May 05];42(3):269–278. Available from: https://doi.org/10.1097/00004583-200303000-00006.
44. Lahtinen HM, Laitila A, Korkman J, Ellonen N. Children's disclosures of sexual abuse in a population-based sample. Child Abuse and Negl [Internet]. 2018 [cited 2019 May 14];76:84–94. Available from: https://doi.org/10.1016/j.chiabu.2017.10.011.
45. Alexander SC, Fortenberry JD, Pollak KI, Bravender T, Davis JK, Ostbye T, et al. Sexuality talk during adolescent health maintenance visits. JAMA Pediatr [Internet]. 2014. [cited 2019 May 14];168(2):163–169. Available from: https://doi.org/10.1001/jamapediatrics.2013.4338.
46. BreunerCC, MattsonG. Sexuality education for children and adolescents. Pediatrics [Internet]. 2016[cited 2019 June 22];138(2):e1–e11. Available from: http://pediatrics.aappublications.org/content/138/2/e20161348Pediatrics.https://doi.org/10.1542/peds.2016-1348.
47. Girardet RG, Lahoti S, Howard LA, Fajman NN, Sawyer MK, Driebe EM, et al. Epidemiology of sexually transmitted infections in suspected child victims of sexual assault. Pediatrics [Internet]. 2009. [cited 2019 June 22];124(1):79–86. Available from:www.pediatrics.org/cgi/doi/10.1542/peds.2008-2947. https://doi.org/10.1111/j.1365-2214.2009.01023_5.x.
48. Wirtz AL, Schwartz S, Ketende S, Anato S, Nadedjo FD, Ouedraogo HG, et al. Sexual violence, condom negotiation, and condom use in the context of sex work. J Acquire Immune Defic Syndr [Internet]. 2015. [cited 2019 June 22];68(2):S171–S179. Available from:https://journals.lww.com/jaids/fulltext/2015/03011/Sexual_Violence,_Condom_Negotiation,_and_Condom.14.aspx. https://doi.org/10.1097/qai.0000000000000451.
49. Decker MR, Mack KP, Barrows JJ, Silverman JG. Sex trafficking, violence victimization, and condom use among prostituted women in Nicaragua. Int J Gynaecol Obstet [Internet]. 2009[cited 2019 June 22];107(2):151–2. Available from https://www.ncbi.nlm.nih.gov/pmc/articles/PMC3623281/. https://doi.org/10.1016/j.ijgo.2009.06.002.
50. Sarkar K, Bal B, Mukherjee R, et al. Sex-trafficking, violence, negotiating skill, and HIV infection in brothel-based sex workers of eastern India, adjoining Nepal, Bhutan, and Bangladesh. J Health Popul Nutr [Internet]. 2008. [cited 2019 June 22];26(2):223–231. Available from https://www.ncbi.nlm.nih.gov/pmc/articles/PMC2740670/.
51. Decker MR, McCauley HL, Phuengsamran D, Janyam S, Silverman JG. Sex trafficking, sexual risk, sexually transmitted infection and reproductive health among female sex workers in Thailand. J Epidemiol Community Health [Internet]. 2011. [cited 2019 June 22];65(4):334–9. Available from:https://www.ncbi.nlm.nih.gov/pmc/articles/PMC3521618/. https://doi.org/10.1136/jech.2009.096834.
52. Silverman JG, Decker MR, Gupta J, Dharmadhikari A, Seage III GR, Raj A. Syphilis and hepatitis B co-infection among HIV-infected, sex-trafficked women and girls, Nepal. Emerg Infect Dis [Internet]. 2008. [cited 2019 June 22];14(6):932–934. Available from: https://www.ncbi.nlm.nih.gov/pmc/articles/PMC2600282/. https://doi.org/10.3201/eid1406.080090.

53. Greenbaum JV, Dodd M, McCracken C. A short screening tool to identify victims of child sex trafficking in the health care setting. Pediatr Emerg Care [Internet]. 2018. [cited 2019 June 22];34(1):33–37. Available from: https://journals.lww.com/pec-online/fulltext/2018/01000/A_Short_Screening_Tool_to_Identify_Victims_of.8.aspx. https://doi.org/10.1097/PEC.0000000000000602.
54. Jenny C, Crawford-Jakubiak JE. The evaluation of children in the primary care setting when sexual abuse is suspected. Pediatrics [Internet]. 2013[cited 2019 May 05];132(2):e558–e567. Available from www.pediatrics.org/cgi/doi/10.1542/peds.2013-1741. https://doi.org/10.1542/peds.2013-1741.
55. Moore JL, Kaplan DM, Barron CE. Sex trafficking of minors. Pediatr Clin North Am [Internet]. 2017. [cited 2019 May 05];64(2):413–421. Available from https://doi.org/10.1016/j.pcl.2016.11.013.
56. Choi KR. Risk factors for domestic minor sex trafficking in the United States. J Forensic Nursing. 2015. [cited 2019 May 05];11(2):66–76. Available from: https://journals.lww.com/forensicnursing/Abstract/2015/04000/Risk_Factors_for_Domestic_Minor_Sex_Trafficking_in.2.aspx; https://doi.org/10.1097/JFN.0000000000000072.

Chapter 17
The Subspecialties

Kanani E. Titchen, Jack Garden, Shirley Louis, Natalia Vasquez-Canizares, and M. Susan Latuga

Introduction

In this chapter, experts in cardiology, adolescent medicine, neonatology, and rheumatology share their reflections about trafficked patients they have encountered. In addition, a survivor of human trafficking offers her experience working with neonatologists and social workers and emergency medicine workers – all of whom failed to see how she and her baby were being victimized.

Before these encounters, despite working with trafficked patients for years, we had never particularly thought of transplant recipients, rheumatology patients, or parents in the neonatal intensive care unit as being vulnerable to trafficking. But the truth is that people of all backgrounds are vulnerable to labor and sex trafficking, and those with chronic disabilities may be particularly vulnerable due to their

K. E. Titchen
Division of Adolescent and Young Adult Medicine, Department of Pediatrics, University of California San Diego and Rady Children's Hospital, San Diego, CA, USA

J. Garden
Department of Cardiology, Thomas Jefferson University Hospitals, Philadelphia, PA, USA

S. Louis · M. S. Latuga (✉)
Department of Pediatrics, Division of Neonatology, Children's Hospital at Montefiore, Albert Einstein College of Medicine, Bronx, NY, USA

N. Vasquez-Canizares
Department of Pediatrics, Division of Rheumatology, Children's Hospital at Montefiore, Albert Einstein College of Medicine, Bronx, NY, USA

K. E. Titchen, E. Miller (eds.), *Medical Perspectives on Human Trafficking in Adolescents*, https://doi.org/10.1007/978-3-030-43367-3_17

dependence on and submission to caregivers, social isolation, and desensitization to increased touching that may accompany intimate care or medical procedures, among other reasons [1, 2]. In turn, human trafficking can have a direct impact on health and the ability to manage chronic medical conditions [3–5].

It takes a team of medical, social work, mental health, legal, and anti-trafficking specialists to care for these patients [6]. Anti-trafficking education efforts must be expanded to include all medical subspecialties to identify and assist the many human trafficking victims and survivors who present for medical care each year.

Cardiology and Transplant Medicine

Case Presentation

As an adolescent medicine physician, you receive an inpatient consult for a patient who is an organ transplant recipient. "Jay" is 19 years old, currently living on the street or with friends, and has decided to stop taking his transplant rejection medications. He is hemodynamically unstable, and upon first glance when you enter the room and introduce yourself, Jay appears sick. He consented to hospitalization but is refusing all treatments except for comfort measures. The adolescent medicine service has been consulted in an effort to connect Jay to a medical home and help him understand the importance of adhering to his medication and treatment regimen. You notice in Jay's chart multiple treatments for a series of sexually transmitted infections (STIs) over the past several years, and when you walk closer to his bed, you meet a young man in a hospital gown with a name tattooed across his neck and an expression of annoyance on his face. When you speak with him, he tells you immediately and as a matter of fact that he wants to die. When you ask gently, "Why? Why do you want to die?," he refuses to answer. You move on. You ask about him, about his symptoms, about school and work, about relationships, about friends, and these topics seem to be safe for him: he answers you with reluctant, brief responses. And the point is that he *answers you.* You are connecting. You thank him for being open with you. You share with him that you see a lot of teens and young adults from a lot of different backgrounds and that many of them seek an "adopted family" for a place to belong. Jay makes eye contact now. The tattoo on his neck, the unstable housing, the series of STIs, and his loss of interest in life coupled with his refusal to take life-sustaining transplant medications raise red flags for human trafficking, so you shift the conversation slightly. You admit that some of your patients need to do various things to get by, to survive. You have his attention now. You ask him when the first time was that he *chose* to have sex. He pauses. "Chose?"

"Yes, chose." And you repeat the question.

"Oh, I guess around 14."

You continue softly, "You paused before you answered. Was there a time you didn't choose?"

He looks away and looks annoyed, "Yeah." The curtain comes down.

"Are you able to tell me about that?... If not, it's OK." No response.

You see that he has ended the interview, so you tell him that you could come back later if he wants. He doesn't answer. You offer that if he needs help, if he is in trouble, you know some people who might be able to help. He comes to life, meets your eyes, and says somewhat defiantly that he is already in "the (name withheld) program" for human trafficking victims and survivors. But now he is back on the street and not going to his program. He "fell back in" with his trafficker and after a recent spate of neglect and abuse, he had decided that life was not worth living.

You talk more about his hospitalization, about his desire to die, but his mind is made up. You realize you are out of your depth and understand that he already has a team in place – a social worker, a psychiatrist, a primary care physician, and one of the leading anti-human trafficking teams in the country, as well as his team of medical professionals including transplant medicine, surgery, anesthesiology, infectious disease specialists, and organ specialists.

He continues under the care of the organ transplant service, and the consult is closed.

We don't know what became of Jay, and a number of aspects of Jay's case are concerning: upon admission to the hospital, Jay's name in the electronic medical record was not de-identified to "John Doe," so he was very much searchable and susceptible to contact (and threats) by his trafficker. Although social workers and mental health professionals were involved in Jay's hospitalization, it remains unknown how much Jay had permitted his non-medical support system from "the program" to be involved in his medical recovery. At the time of Jay's hospitalization, there was no International Classification of Diseases (ICD) code for "victim of human trafficking," and the consulting physician had not been notified about a human trafficking situation: as a result, the consultant spent time assessing for human trafficking that might have been better spent establishing trust with Jay, answering *Jay's* questions, ascertaining Jay's short-term and long-term goals and needs, coordinating care with Jay and his team, and/or exploring motivational interviewing techniques to better understand Jay's reluctance to take his medication. (The ICD-10 code T74.51 now can be used to document "adult forced sexual exploitation, confirmed." See Table 17.1). In addition, the medical team and consulting physician could have better informed Jay about the need for such personal questions, what Jay's hospitalization and outpatient follow-up might look like, and what Jay's medical team might be able to do to help him. Candor and transparency about the possibilities and limitations of care provision are essential when working with all adolescent patients - and especially with trafficked youth.

Heart Disease and Human Trafficking

Heart disease is associated with multiple defined predisposing circumstances or "risk factors." These are a constantly evolving combination of genetic and environmental influences that contribute to cardiac disease, such as family history of cardiovascular ailment, hypertension, hyperlipidemia, diabetes, obesity, tobacco use, alcohol abuse, substance abuse, stress, diet, and lack of exercise, among others. Individuals whose life circumstances are characterized by one or more of these features are at augmented hazard of heart disease.

Human trafficking, for the purposes of labor and sexual exploitation, is increasingly recognized as a malignant and pervasive phenomenon. Definite epidemiologic understanding of its numerical incidence has been incomplete. This is a reflection of fundamental societal and institutional handicaps in acknowledging and appreciating its very existence and frequency, much less in identifying populations at risk.

A medical conversation of what is known about victims of human trafficking and its extrapolation to the current cardiovascular care paradigm is illustrative in defining opportunities for recognition and therapy. Trafficking victims engage in onerous physical labor, repeated high-risk sexual behavior, or both. These life circumstances

Table 17.1 ICD-10 codes for human trafficking

ICD-10 codes for human trafficking	
T74.51	Adult forced sexual exploitation, confirmed
T74.52	Child sexual exploitation, confirmed
T74.61	Adult forced labor exploitation, confirmed
T74.62	Child forced labor exploitation, confirmed
T76,51	Adult forced sexual exploitation, suspected
T76.52	Child sexual exploitation, suspected
T76.61	Adult forced labor exploitation, suspected
T76.62	Child forced labor exploitation, suspected

have well-understood healthcare ramifications and, therefore, intersections with the healthcare system either as acute or chronic conditions. As a result, the nexus of this shadowed population and cardiac care providers is likely vastly underappreciated.

The daily life experiences of those subjected to human trafficking are ill-defined and difficult to accurately characterize, even as survivors are stepping forward to educate others about their experiences of trafficking and with respect to the healthcare they have received. Victims of trafficking live in a shadow world of coercion and exploitation, sometimes with reduced access to consistent healthcare [3, 7]. When there is opportunity for medical interaction, it generally is carefully monitored to assure minimum information is revealed as to where and how they live, what they do, and who they are [3]. Because of their focus on short-term economic gain, traffickers may see little value in or perceived benefit to comprehensive diagnoses or therapy for their victims beyond the bare minimum.

Alcohol, Tobacco, and Illicit Substances and Cardiovascular Health

Within this callous, utilitarian environment, various features of trafficked persons have emerged. They may be poorly nourished, profoundly overworked, and physically and emotionally abused [3]. Compared to their non-trafficked peers, among child sexual exploitation (CSE) youth there is a high incidence of tobacco use, as well as alcohol and substance abuse [8].

Tobacco usage is one of the earliest detected and most powerful risk factors in heart disease. Smoking cigarettes has been associated with roughly 1 out of 5 deaths from cardiovascular disease and increases risk 2–4 times that of nonsmokers. In the United States, although cigarette and cigar use among adolescents has decreased 1–3% since 2011, electronic cigarette ("e-cigarette") use in the past 30 days among high school students increased from 1.5% in 2011 to 20.8% in 2018 [9]. Nicotine increases blood pressure and viscosity or thickness of blood that can predispose to narrowing of arteries, arterial injury, and clotting within these damaged vessels. Tobacco smoke, primarily or via second-hand exposure, contains high levels of carbon monoxide, which reduces the capacity of blood to carry oxygen and deliver this critical nutrient to all organs resulting in functional compromise.

Legal, inexpensive, and readily available, alcohol also is deeply embedded in our civilization as a cultural touchstone. Nearly all individual or communal life events mournful or celebratory are entwined with an alcoholic thread. This is no different in the world of human trafficking: among 365 CSE youth in Los Angeles, over half reported alcohol use [8]. The medical impact of our cultural embrace of alcohol is enormous and indisputable. Multiple assessments have demonstrated that behind only smoking and obesity, alcohol consumption is the third leading cause of preventable death in the United States [10]. In the context of cardiovascular disease, alcohol is a direct toxic substance, injuring often beyond repair cardiac myocytes and Purkinje fibers and the cardiac conduction system. Acute alcohol excess increases blood pressure, decreases the force of the heart's contractility, and can induce irregular heart rhythms [11]. Any of these physiologic responses, individually, can presage morbid and mortal events and even more ominously when in combination. While low levels of consumption of certain alcoholic variants have been associated with beneficial cardiac outcomes, the risk-to-benefit ratio of drinking appears higher in younger individuals who have a greater frequency of excessive and/or binge drinking and adverse consequences of acute intoxication [10].

While alcohol is a legally sanctioned intoxicant for adults, extralegal substances such as cocaine, crack cocaine, amphetamines, and opioids also threaten cardiovascular health. A study of 237 New York City CSE adolescents found that 26% reported cocaine use, while 14% used heroin [12]. Cocaine is a direct vasoconstrictor, inducing blood vessels to narrow in caliber, leading to a hazardous elevation in blood pressure, increasing shear forces of blood, leaving open the possibility of injury to the intima (surface layer) of that vessel, clotting, and obstruction. These pharmacologic agents also can prompt spasm of the muscular band of tissue within the vessel. The combined effect of vascular hypertension and vasospasm can be devastating. Abrupt diminution of vascular perfusion, in effect starves the heart muscle cells of required oxygen, may result in chest pain, myocardial ischemia, and muscle death (and thereby myocardial infarction, stroke, arrhythmia, and sudden cardiac death). Chest pain, an extraordinarily common symptom, is the single most frequent prompt for emergency services [13]. Other acute pathologic manifestations of cocaine ingestion include myocarditis, cardiomyopathy, and catastrophic great vessel pathology, i.e., dissection or rupture.

If the mode of ingestion of illicit substances is intravenous (IV) and characterized by poor or absent hygienic consideration with sharing of syringes and/or their repeated use without sterilization, there is a substantial incidence of transmission of infectious diseases. These most commonly include hepatitis B and C and the human immunodeficiency virus (HIV). Among sex trafficking victims, there is pervasive compelled high-risk sexual exposure with its attendant hazards of unwanted pregnancy and sexually transmitted infections including HIV [14–16]. A shared consequence of poorly sterilized syringes and inattention to basic sterile technical consideration is an elevated incidence of injection-related bacterial infection. The skin is heavily colonized with bacteria, and poor hygiene often introduces pathogens into the skin, subcutaneous tissue, and bloodstream. The resulting pathology includes cellulitis, abscesses, and compartment symptoms that can be life-threatening and exact cardiovascular consequences. Such patients may be seen by dermatologists, orthopedists, infectious disease specialists, as well as cardiologists.

Trafficked persons are disproportionately vulnerable to homelessness and substance use, and thus they are also vulnerable to infection of cardiac valvular structures or infectious endocarditis in which bacteria, disseminated through the bloodstream, settle on the heart valves and propagate [17, 18]. Valvular infection is destructive, undermining the integrity of the valve and thereby compromising cardiac function. Furthermore, portions of the infectious mass can detach and embolize, often with mortal consequence. Intravenous drug use has a particular predilection for involvement of the tricuspid valve of the right heart and septic pulmonary embolic infections. (See Chaps. 11, 12 and 13 for more on substance use, unstable housing, IV drug use, and human trafficking.)

HIV, Malnutrition, and Cardiac Disease

HIV, whether acquired through IV drug use or as a reflection of high-risk sexual encounters, also is associated with independent discrete cardiac pathology. As stated above, cardiomyopathy has been attributed to an inflammatory involvement of cardiac muscle or myocarditis. While this may result in degradation of systolic function, there is a proposed secondary manifestation that can impair diastolic function. The diastolic component is postulated to be mediated by an autoimmune mechanism. The net result can be clinical congestive heart failure [19].

Malnutrition and a harsh physical and emotional environment have been associated with an increased prevalence of cardiac disease [19–21]. Trafficked victims may be poorly nourished and live in harsh physical conditions [3]. Insufficient intake of calories and proteins on a longstanding basis results in a loss of skeletal and myocardial muscle mass. As cardiac muscular mass diminishes, correspondingly so does the ability to generate the contractile reserve to maintain adequate cardiac output and meet the body's demands for perfusion with blood and oxygen. As in a cascade of dominoes, the resultant stress and secondary functional impairment of other vital organ systems function as a negative feedback loop, further contributing to the heart's inability to function [21]. (See Chap. 10 for more on disordered eating and human trafficking.)

Severe, coerced physical and sexual abuse in childhood has been associated in longitudinal studies with incremental hazard of myocardial infarction and stroke relative to the general population. This propensity remains even when conventional cardiovascular risk factors have been taken into account implying a discrete causal relation [22].

Individuals whose lives are characterized by oppressive environments with limited access to basic standards of hygiene and nutrition are vulnerable to transmission of infectious diseases that may convey primary or secondary cardiovascular manifestations [23]. These pathologic entities include mycobacterial disease (tuberculosis or atypical mycobacterium), ovum and parasitical infection, and enteric, pulmonary, or cerebrovascular pathogens either viral, bacterial, or fungal. In one study of 106 survivors of sex trafficking, 68% reported cardiopulmonary difficulty [24]. The superimposition of prevalent and frequent high-risk sexual activity widens the range and severity of these pathologic entities disproportionate to the general population.

The harshness of living circumstances of those victimized by human trafficking can delay or prevent recognition of underlying medical conditions. A tragic consequence of this diagnostic and therapeutic barrier is the development and progression of otherwise preventable cardiovascular ailment. Diabetes mellitus, hypertension, hyperlipidemias, genetic predisposition to blood clotting, and arrhythmia are profound accelerants of cardiac pathology in the most propitious of care environments. Organ failure may necessitate transplantation, the sequelae of which may be difficult to manage, as demonstrated by the human trafficking victim-survivor described at the beginning of this chapter.

Conclusions

Formulating a diagnosis is essential for providing care that can improve the quality of life and ensure its very continuance. However well-educated and cognizant cardiologists must also always be aware of the limitations of our training and capacity. While empowered to suspect that a patient we are caring for may be ensnared in the immensely complex universe of human trafficking, we must also appreciate our limitations in attempting to directly intervene. Systemic healthcare protocols need to be constructed on a national and international basis involving government, social service, law enforcement, and medical and mental healthcare resources for individual healthcare professionals to relay specific concerns regarding individual patients. There is still much work, funding, and energy required in establishing these care matrices. Each clinician must always recall the vow that in the course of attempting to heal we must first do no harm.

Cardiology is by definition not a frontline nor primary discipline and inhabits a consultative niche in modern-day medicine. Nevertheless, whether it be in the emergency department, a hospital consultation, or outpatient clinic or office encounter, we frequently, perhaps daily, encounter patients in this cohort. The great tragedy is that while our clinical acumen and diagnostic and therapeutic tools have taken enormous strides forward, our collective awareness of very existence of trafficked persons has lagged far behind. This failure of the medical community, and in this consideration, cardiac care providers, is a reflection of a fundamental and pervasive failure of education of the existence of this issue and population. One cannot diagnose or detect what one does not know or consider. Cardiovascular specialists require education to appreciate the magnitude of the problem of human trafficking, the distinguishing characteristics socially and demographically of the population at risk, and the pathologic entities to which trafficking predisposes.

Neonatology

Case Presentation

Amy is a 24-year-old woman who has just given birth to a baby girl at 29 weeks gestation due to preterm labor. She has a remote history of assault. You are the neonatologist caring for Amy's daughter in the neonatal intensive care unit (NICU).

For the first few weeks, Amy's daughter requires continuous positive airway pressure (CPAP) and is slowly started on feedings with breast milk. You update Amy at the bedside to discuss her respiratory status and feeding and inquire about pumping. On day of life 22, on one of your 24-hour shifts, Amy is accompanied by a woman you have never met. Amy introduces her as a friend. Amy appears to be exhausted. Concerned, you remark that she appears tired and ask her how she is doing. She apologizes and explains that she has been "working hard and has been picking up extra shifts at work." Although you have details about Amy's daughter's most recent radiograph, you don't want to share any medical information in front of Amy's friend. You decide to return to update Amy. However, by the time you finish rounds, Amy and her friend have left.

Amy's baby continues to progress. When Amy's baby turns 1 month old, she is weaned from CPAP to nasal cannula. She is tolerating nasogastric tube feedings into her stomach and is starting to take small volumes of milk by mouth. When you meet with Amy, she appears progressively fatigued. She has lost weight, appears malnourished, and wears disheveled clothing. Amy is now always accompanied by a friend, either male or female. Notably, it is rarely the same friend. None of the men appear to be the father of her infant. She has minimal conversation or physical contact with those accompanying her. Concerned, you again ask, "Is everything ok?" Amy explains that despite having medical insurance, aspects of her daughter's care have not been fully covered. The extra work shifts have been helping her to manage those expenses.

The change in Amy's appearance and demeanor is also a concern shared by other members of the NICU team. Nursing and ancillary staff express their worries about Amy and are suspicious of her friends. Her friends display no concern for Amy or her baby. Instead, they watch Amy while she spends time with her infant.

You assume Amy is not telling the truth and propose an explanation for the change in her appearance. The weight loss, fatigue, disheveled clothing, and suspicious characters make you concerned about substance use. The rest of the NICU team has the same worry. Coincidentally, a well-dressed man who previously has accompanied Amy to the NICU expresses his concern to the healthcare team that Amy is "unfit" to take her of her baby. He feels Amy should not be allowed to take her daughter home. Given his composure and appearance compared to Amy's, social workers question Amy about his allegations. No one interrogates this man.

Amy's Reality

In reality, the change in Amy's physical appearance was a direct result of physical, emotional, and mental distress precipitated by human trafficking. Amy initially sought work as a server at a local strip club. This business served as a gateway into human trafficking. During her time at the strip club, she was offered a more lucrative position stripping, and needing the income, she agreed. After a short time, Amy was held captive by her "employers," violently raped, beaten, psychologically tormented, and coerced into sex trafficking. Her perpetrators used Amy's financial needs and the medical debt associated with her daughter's hospitalization in the NICU to trap her. Her story reveals a resounding theme among a majority of trafficked persons and fits the definition of human trafficking: the use of a person for "compelled labor or commercial sex acts through the use of force, fraud, or coercion" [25].

Fearing for her life as well as that of her infant, Amy kept these horrors to herself. Her turmoil manifested as physical signs: weight loss, increasing fatigue, dehydration, and unkempt appearance. Despite knowing Amy as a devoted active participant in her infant's care, the healthcare team interrogated her regarding the changes in her appearance. Based on the accusations of this man, a stranger to the NICU, the healthcare team questioned Amy regarding her ability to care for her infant. This experience revictimized her and deepened her mistrust of the medical system. Ultimately, the NICU staff acknowledged Amy's unwavering commitment to her daughter from day one. Her daughter was rightfully discharged to her mother's care.

Ironically, it is within the medical framework that Amy would ultimately find empathy and justice. She rarely received routine medical care for injuries sustained during her work. Instead, she visited the emergency department (ED), typically accompanied by one of her captors. During one of these visits, an ED physician was able to interview her alone. He showed patience and compassion, enough that Amy expressed that she "was made to feel like a human again." *Although she never told the ED physician what a profound effect he had had on her life*, Amy later stated that this brief momentary interaction served as the turning point to her eventual dissociation from "the life" of human trafficking. Feeling human and valued as an individual led Amy eventually to seek legal help and the social services she needed.

NICU Staff and Human Trafficking

Healthcare professionals (HCPs) in the NICU have a unique relationship with families. Infants remain in the hospital for weeks to months, allowing HCPs to observe interactions over time. In addition, parents often visit with their extended social network, including family and friends. This continuity of care allows HCPs to develop a bond with the families, which in cases like these is integral to the infant's and family's safety and well-being.

Risk Factors

Risk factors for human trafficking include youth, a prior history of abuse, low socioeconomic status, marginalized ethnic minorities, and migrant worker status [26–32]. Changes in appearance, e.g., a mother who was previously well appearing but now comes in untidy, wearing revealing clothing, stressed and anxious, could be a warning sign. This mother may no longer make eye contact or may be accompanied by an individual who is one of her traffickers. Traffickers may employ seasoned victims (termed "bottom girls") to monitor their newer victims. By doing so, bottom girls curry favor with the trafficker, may get a day or night off, or may receive special gifts from the trafficker. Traffickers may pit their victims against each other and prevent bonding among victims. Bottom girls may appear controlling, dominate the conversation, insist on being present for all communications, and not allow the mother to speak.

The NICU as a Safe Space

Family meetings should provide a safe space for those suspected of being trafficked. In addition to discussing the care and progress of their child, as healthcare professionals, we should offer support and encouragement during these sessions. Ideally, those suspected of being trafficked will leave knowing the healthcare team is partnering with them and not against them. As in all cases of human trafficking, HCPs should avoid the rescue mentality and forced disclosure. Instead, HCPs should focus on emotional support and validation. In summary, the longitudinal relationships NICU staff have with infants, their families, and social support networks offer a unique opportunity to identify potential victims of human trafficking.

Rheumatology

Case Presentation

"Ruby" is a 15-year-old girl with juvenile dermatomyositis (JDM) who is here for routine follow-up with you, the pediatric rheumatology subspecialist. Ruby had been diagnosed with JDM at age 4 after presenting with proximal muscle weakness and skin rash. According to Ruby, after being initially treated with oral prednisone, hydroxychloroquine, and methotrexate, she had achieved clinical remission and had been off immunosuppressive medications for 5 years.

Background

You first met Ruby a year ago when she presented with a JDM exacerbation for which you initiated daily prednisone, hydroxychloroquine, and weekly methotrexate. At that time, you discussed with her and her mother the benefits and risks associated with these treatments, including possible infection, hepatotoxicity, and teratogenicity. You counseled Ruby privately on safe sexual practices, contraception, and abstaining from alcohol consumption. You followed Ruby's clinical course weekly for the first month, monthly for the next 6 months, and every 3 months thereafter.

Signs of Trouble

Early in the relapse of her disease at age 14, Ruby reported symptoms of depression and self-cutting after ending a relationship with her boyfriend. She had started smoking cigarettes and marijuana, and her grades in school had declined. She had started to receive mental health support for suicidal ideation.

You treated Ruby for persistent JDM disease activity with monthly high-dose intravenous methylprednisolone pulses and intravenous immunoglobulin (IVIG) infusions, along with minor adjustments to the previously prescribed immunosuppressive regimen. Signs of exogenous Cushing's syndrome on physical exam from systemic steroid use were consistent with good adherence to her medications.

However, Ruby's JDM clinical management was persistently complicated by continued psychosocial stressors and high-risk sexual behavior such as frequent unprotected sexual activity with repeated use of Plan B, "occasional" alcohol drinking, and daily smoking.

Because you recognized Ruby's continued high-risk behavior and contraception counseling due to risk of pregnancy and teratogenicity while on treatment with methotrexate, you referred Ruby to adolescent medicine.

Psychosocial Complications and Partnership with Adolescent Medicine

Today, 15 years old, Ruby reports being "out of school." She now has a pierced tongue and has started sleeping at "a friend's house." Ruby has not followed up with her referral to adolescent medicine, and she again reports having frequent unprotected sex, smoking marijuana on a daily basis, and that recently she had been found drunk in school.

Because of these behaviors that are increasing her risk for poor health, you decided to stop methotrexate despite the possibility of disease flare and an increased risk of cumulative steroid burden. Ruby continues treatment with hydroxychloroquine and prednisone, which you slowly taper over the following year until reaching a lower daily dose.

Juvenile Dermatomyositis

Juvenile dermatomyositis (JDM) is a multisystemic autoimmune disease primarily characterized by vasculopathy and perivascular inflammation of the skin capillary vessels and those of the striated muscles [33]. Onset is especially common from 4 to 9 years of age with a peak age of 5.5 years for boys and 6 and 13 years for girls. About 25% of children can be diagnosed before age 4, and the female-to-male ratio ranges from 1.5:1 to as high as 2.7:1 [33]. The main clinical manifestations include a pathognomonic rash (the heliotrope rash or Gottron papules over the extensor surfaces of the finger joints, elbows, knees, or ankles) and proximal muscle weakness [34]. Atypical manifestations may include the amyopathic form of the disease that predominantly has skin manifestations without weakness, a distal more than a proximal muscle weakness, or a more extensive muscle involvement without skin manifestations [33]. These signs should lead the physician to suspect an alternative diagnosis such as polymyositis or a neuromuscular disorder and should always be confirmed with a muscle biopsy [35].

Prompt recognition of presenting signs and symptoms and rapid implementation of immunosuppressive therapy are essential to reduce morbidity and mortality from JDM and to improve prognosis. Some of the factors that can adversely influence outcome include delay in diagnosis and institution of therapy and inconsistent or nonadherence to medical therapy, as demonstrated by Ruby's case above [33]. Delayed or inadequate corticosteroid (CS) treatment seems to be one of the most important predictors of poor outcome and a chronic illness course [36]. A major social stressor such as human trafficking will have significant consequences on treatment success and disease progression if this situation goes unnoticed and unaddressed by the medical team.

Close follow-up of patients with JDM is essential to adequately monitor for complications that could arise from both the disease and the immunosuppressive medications used to treat it, and a multidisciplinary approach is important for managing JDM successfully. Treatment should be aimed to suppress the immunoinflammatory response, preserve muscle strength and joint range of motion, prevent complications, and maintain general health, normal growth, and development [33]. Chronic corticosteroid (CS) use may lead to adverse effects including Cushing's syndrome and growth retardation – both of which can be especially challenging for adolescents who may be more focused on external appearance – as well as osteopenia and osteoporosis with risk of fractures, avascular necrosis, and increased cardiovascular risk [33, 37]. The use of steroid-sparing agents early in the disease course along with an adequate compliance is crucial to prevent these complications and improve disease outcome [38]. Patients need to be properly counseled on the risk of adrenal crisis with abrupt CS discontinuation, as this can be life-threatening. Other immunosuppressive agents, mainly methotrexate, can cause liver toxicity and are teratogenic, producing deleterious effects to the fetus and mother. Because the immune system is suppressed by the use of CS and other immunosuppressive medications to control the excessive immunomodulatory response in JDM, the risk for infections is increased. Adolescents and females of reproductive age need to be counseled on safe sexual practices to prevent sexually transmitted infection (STI) and pregnancy and should be strongly encouraged to use effective contraceptive methods such as long-acting reversible contraceptives (LARC). Alcohol consumption is strictly prohibited due to the risk of hepatotoxicity [37].

Case Continuation and Resolution

At age 16, Ruby was diagnosed with genital herpes infection in the emergency department. Testing for HIV, chlamydia, and gonorrhea are negative. She was treated with acyclovir and again referred to adolescent medicine.

During her first visit with adolescent medicine, Ruby disclosed intermittent use of condoms with five male sexual partners over the previous 2 years. She continued to smoke marijuana on a weekly basis and reported a strained relationship with her mother regarding curfew. Ruby was counseled on safe sexual practices, and she refused hormonal contraception, stating that she preferred to use condoms and Plan B. The adolescent medicine specialist respected Ruby's choices and scheduled her for 3-month follow-up to revisit her contraceptive choices and risk of STI. Ruby did not show for this follow-up appointment.

At age 17, Ruby returned to the rheumatology clinic for concerns of disease flare and myalgias. She had self-discontinued prednisone and was intermittently taking hydroxychloroquine. Laboratory work-up revealed elevated muscle enzymes and aldolase. Ruby reported binge-drinking alcohol with loss of consciousness on two occasions, as well as frequent physical activity, which were possible explanations for her laboratory abnormalities. Her physical exam was remarkable for normal muscle strength, absence of rash, and normal nailbed capillaries; in other words, there are no clinical signs of active disease. Because of her heavy alcohol consumption, Ruby was referred back to adolescent medicine.

Upon follow-up with adolescent medicine, she reported a new outbreak of genital herpes, three new sexual partners in the previous month, and increased marijuana use, declaring she had "nothing else to do." Ruby again declined hormonal contraception, choosing to rely on condom use and Plan B. Later, Ruby returned to her primary care physician with concerns for pregnancy.

Over the ensuing months, Ruby presented repeatedly to adolescent medicine with new outbreaks of genital herpes, and by the time she was 18 years old, Ruby reported ten lifetime male partners. She was no longer in school, was unemployed, and reported domestic physical abuse by her fiancé. On exam she was noted to have a new tattoo on the right postauricular area and an erythematous blister on her left index finger, reportedly from an accidental burn with a glue gun. Upon further questioning by the adolescent medicine physician,

Ruby disclosed exchanging sex for money to pay her rent. She was considering doing this again due to financial pressure.

Questions for Discussion

Is Ruby a victim of human trafficking? How does transactional or exchange sex compare to human trafficking? (See Sect. 4.1 for comparisons of transactional sex with sex trafficking.)

If Ruby is not a victim of human trafficking, what are her risk factors and red flags for human trafficking? (See Sect. 4.2 for more on risk factors for sex trafficking.)

What are the resilience factors in Ruby's life? (Refer to Chaps. 2 and 21 for information on adolescents and resilience.)

What concerning signs did this rheumatologist notice and act on? What more could have been done to help Ruby when she was a minor? What more could have been done to help Ruby once she turned 18? (See Chap. 18 for information on medicolegal aspects of human trafficking and mandatory reporting.)

What are the responsibilities of subspecialists in recognizing signs of human trafficking or risk factors for trafficking and assisting these patients?

Future Directions

Training is needed to help medical subspecialists understand their roles in identifying and providing trauma-sensitive care to patients who are victims and survivors of human trafficking.

In order to heighten awareness of human trafficking among medical subspecialists, case studies/series are needed from subspecialties including but not limited to orthopedic surgery, dermatology, nutrition, endocrinology, cardiology, pulmonology, rheumatology, gastroenterology, and others.

Information is needed regarding the percentage of survivors with chronic diseases such as diabetes and asthma who present to healthcare settings for acute-on-chronic conditions. What are suggestions for improving medication availability and adherence for this population?

Trauma-sensitive, efficient methodology is needed to bridge trafficked patients who present for acute-on-chronic disease care to mental health professionals, social workers, and primary care physicians for follow-up and for investigation into and treatment of underlying trauma.

References

1. Reid JA. Sex trafficking of girls with intellectual disabilities: an exploratory mixed methods study. Sex Abus. 2018;30(2):107–31.
2. Office for Victims of Crime Training and Technical Assistance Center [Internet]. Victims with Physical, Cognitive or Emotional Disabilities, from Human Trafficking Task Force e-Guide. Washington, D.C.:U.S. Department of Justice, Office for Victims of Crime (OVC) and Bureau of Justice Assistance (BJA); 2011 [updated 2019; cited 2019 Oct 2]. Available from: https://www.ovcttac.gov/taskforceguide/eguide/4-supporting-victims/45-victim-populations/victims-with-physical-cognitive-or-emotional-disabilities/.
3. ZimmermanC, YunK, ShvabI, WattsC, TrappolinL, TreppeteM, et al. The health risks and consequences of trafficking in women and adolescents: Findings from a European study. [Internet] London: London School of Hygiene & Tropical Medicine; 2003. Available from https://researchonline.lshtm.ac.uk/id/eprint/10786.
4. Zimmerman C, Hossain M, Yun K, Gajdadziev V, Guzun N, Tchomarova M, et al. The health of trafficked women: a survey of women entering post-trafficking services in Europe. Am J Public Health. 2008;98:55–9. https://doi.org/10.2105/AJPH.2006.108357.
5. Pocock NS, Kiss L, Oram S, Zimmerman C. Labour trafficking among men and boys in the Greater Mekong subregion: exploitation, violence, occupational health risks and injuries. PLoS One [Internet]. 2016;11(12):e0168500. https://doi.org/10.1371/journal.pone.0168500.
6. Titchen KE, Katz D, Martinez K, White K. Ovarian cystadenoma in a trafficked patient. Pediatrics. 2016;137(5):pii: e20152201. https://doi.org/10.1542/peds.2015-2201.
7. Zimmerman C, Hossain M, Watts C. Human trafficking and health: a conceptual model to inform policy, intervention and research. Soc Sci Med. 2011;73(2):327–35. https://doi.org/10.1016/j.socscimed.2011.05.028.
8. Cook MC, Barnert E, Ijadi-Maghsoodi R, Ports K, Bath E. Exploring mental health and substance use treatment needs of commercially sexually exploited youth participating in a specialty juvenile court. Behav Med. 2018;44(3):242–9. https://doi.org/10.1080/08964289.2018.1432552.
9. Gentzke AS, Creamer M, Cullen KA, Ambrose BK, Willis G, Jamal A, et al. *Vital signs:*tobacco product use among middle and high school students — United States, 2011–2018. MMWR Morb Mortal Wkly Rep. 2019;68:157–64. https://doi.org/10.15585/mmwr.mm6806e1.
10. O'Keefe JH, Bhatti SK, Bjwa A, DiNicolantonio JJ, Lavie CJ. Alcohol and cardiovascular health: the dose makes the poison…or the remedy. Mayo Clin Proc. 2014;89(3):382–93. https://doi.org/10.1016/j.mayocp.2013.11.005.
11. Klatsky AL. Alcohol and cardiovascular health. Integr Comp Biol. 2004;44(4):324–8. https://doi.org/10.1093/icb/44.4.324.
12. CurtisR, TerryK, DankM, DombrowskiK, KhanB. Commercial sexual exploitation of children in New York City, volume one: the CSEC population in New York City: size, characteristics, and needs. New York (NY): The John Jay College of Criminal Justice; 2008.p. 122. Report No.:1. Available from https://www.ncjrs.gov/pdffiles1/nij/grants/225083.pdf. Accessed 28 Sept 2019.
13. Maraj S, Figueredo VM, Morris DL. Cocaine and the heart. Clin cardiol. 2010;33(5):264–9. https://doi.org/10.1002/clc.20746.
14. Goldenberg SM, Silverman JG, Engstrom D. Exploring the context of trafficking and adolescent sex industry involvement in Tijuana, Mexico: consequences for HIV risk and prevention. Violence Against Women. 2015;21(4):478–99. https://doi.org/10.1177/1077801215569079.
15. Silverman JG, Raj A, Cheng D, Decker MR, Coleman S, Bridden C, et al. Sex trafficking and initiation-related violence, alcohol use, and HIV risk among HIV-infected female sex workers in Mumbai, India. J Infect Dis. 2011;204(Suppl 5):S1229–34. https://doi.org/10.1093/infdis/jir540.

16. Sarkar K, Bal B, Mukherjee R, Chakraborty S, Saha S. Ghosh Arundhuti, et al. sex-trafficking, violence, negotiating skill, and HIV infection in brothel-based sex workers of eastern India, adjoining Nepal, Bhutan, and Bangladesh. J Health Popul Nutr. 2009;26(2):223–31.
17. Sprang G, Cole J. Familial sex trafficking of minors: trafficking conditions, clinical presentation, and system involvement. J Fam Violence. 2018;33:185–95. https://doi.org/10.1007/s10896-018-9950-y.
18. ChonK.Human trafficking and opioid abuse. US Department of Health and Human Services Office on Trafficking in Persons Human trafficking and opioid abuse Published May 17, 2016. Available at http://www.acf.hhs.gov/blog/2016/05/human-trafficking-and-opioid-abuse. Accessed 28 Sept 2019.
19. Lumsden RH, Bloomfield GS. The causes of HIV-associated cardiomyopathy: a tale of two worlds. Biomed Res Int. 2016;2016:8196560.
20. Li MK, Beck MA, Shi Q, Harruff RC. Unexpected hazard of illegal immigration: outbreak of viral myocarditis exacerbated by confinement and deprivation in a shipboard cargo container. Am J Forensic Med Pathol. 2004;25(2):117–24.
21. Webb JG, Kless MC, Chan-Yan CC. Malnutrition and the heart. CMAJ. 1986;135(7):753–8.
22. Rich-Edwards JW, et al. Physical and sexual abuse in childhood as predictors of early-onset cardiovascular events in women. Circulation. 2012;126:920–7.
23. Macias-Konstantopoulos W, Ma Z. Physical health of human trafficking survivors: unmet essentials. In: Chisolm-Straker M, Stocklosa H, editors. Human trafficking is a public health issue: a paradigm expansion in the United States. Cham: Springer; 2017. p. 185–210.
24. Lederer LJ, Wetzel CA. The health consequences of sex trafficking and their implications for identifying victims in healthcare facilities. Ann Health Law. 2014;23(1):61–80.
25. Greenbaum J, Bodrick N, Committee on Child Abuse and Neglect, Section on International Child Health. Global human trafficking and child victimization. Pediatrics. 2017;140(6):pii:e20173138. https://doi.org/10.1542/peds.2017-3138.
26. WhitbeckL, LazoritzMW, CrawfordD, HautalaD. Administration for Children and Families: family and youth services bureau street outreach program, Data Collection Study Final Report.
27. Reid JA, Jones S. Exploited vulnerability: legal and psychological perspectives on child sex trafficking victims. Vict Offenders. 2011;6(2):207–31.
28. Clarke RJ, Clarke EA, Roe-Sepowitz D, Fey R. Age at entry into prostitution: relationship to drug use, race, suicide, education level, childhood abuse, and family experiences. J Hum Behav Soc Environ. 2012;22(3):270–89. https://doi.org/10.1080/10911359.2012.655583.
29. Definitions and methodology. In: Trafficking Persons Report, 2013. United States Department of State. 2013. [cited 2019 January 22] Available from: https://www.state.gov/j/tip/rls/tiprpt/2013/210543.htm.
30. Country Narratives: United States. In: Trafficking Persons Report, 2019. United States Department of State. 2019. p. 484–492. Available from: https://www.state.gov/wp-content/uploads/2019/06/2019-Trafficking-in-Persons-Report.pdf Accessed 28 September 2019.
31. ShermanFT,GraceLG. The system response to the commercial sexual exploitation of girls, juvenile justice: advancing research, policy, and practice, 337 (Francine T. Sherman & Francine H. Jacobs eds., 2011).
32. Clawson HJ, Dutch M, Solomon A, Goldblatt Grace L. Human trafficking into and within the United States: a review of the literature. Washington, D.C.: Office of the Assistant Secretary for planning and evaluation (ASPE), U.S. Department of Health and Human Services; 2009.
33. Rider LG, Lindsley CB, Miller FW. Juvenile dermatomyositis. In: Textbook of pediatric rheumatology. New York: Elsevier Health Sciences; 2015. p. 351–83.
34. Ramanan A, Feldman BM. Clinical features and outcomes of juvenile dermatomyositis and other childhood onset myositis syndromes. Rheum Dis Clin N Am. 2002;28(4):833–57.
35. Huber AM. Idiopathic inflammatory myopathies in childhood: current concepts. Pediatr Clin N Am. 2012;59(2):365–80.

36. Bowyer SL, et al. Childhood dermatomyositis: factors predicting functional outcome and development of dystrophic calcification. J Pediatr. 1983;103(6):882–8.
37. Becker ML, Lovell D, Leeder SJ. Pharmacology and drug therapy: nonbiologic therapies. In: Textbook of pediatric rheumatology. New York: Elsevier Health Sciences; 2015. p. 140–60.
38. Feldman BM, et al. Juvenile dermatomyositis and other idiopathic inflammatory myopathies of childhood. Lancet. 2008;371(9631):2201–12.

Chapter 18
Medicolegal Aspects and Mandatory Reporting

Shea Rhodes, Stephanie Mersch, and Jordan Greenbaum

Case Presentation

A young woman is brought into the emergency department presenting with severe abdominal pain and vaginal bleeding. You are a pediatrician working in the ED that night. The patient tells you her name is Josie, and she is 19 years old. She is accompanied by a woman who identifies herself as Josie's mother. Josie seems nervous, and glances at the other woman throughout your initial interaction. You think she seems much younger than 19. You notice that she smells strongly of marijuana, that her teeth are yellowing, and that her gums are very light. She appears to be underweight. The patient tells you abruptly that she "knows" she is not pregnant and that she knows this because she took a pregnancy prevention pill after unprotected sex a little over a month ago.

You advise the other woman that per hospital practice you need to speak alone with Josie and that the woman will need to return to the waiting room. She mutters under her breath and glares at you, but complies. You attempt to build rapport with Josie and engender a feeling of safety by asking her if she is warm enough, needs an extra blanket, would like some water or a snack. You tell her you would like to ask her some questions to find out more about her and about her symptoms in order to find out what may be causing the pain and to see if you can help. You tell her she is free to answer or not answer any of the questions, and you ask her if she is willing to talk to you. She says she is, and she responds to your questions by telling you the bleeding started two days ago, has gotten worse over time (changing tampons every few hours now), and the pelvic pain began last night. She speaks quietly, and she is evasive while answering your questions about reproductive history but does tell you she has had gonorrhea in the past, as well as a prior pregnancy with elective termination.

S. Rhodes (✉) · S. Mersch
Institute to Address Commercial Sexual Exploitation, Villanova, PA, USA

J. Greenbaum
Institute on Healthcare and Human Trafficking at the Stephanie V. Blank Center for Safe and Healthy Children, Children's Healthcare of Atlanta, Atlanta, GA, USA

International Centre for Missing and Exploited Children, Alexandria, VA, USA

K. E. Titchen, E. Miller (eds.), *Medical Perspectives on Human Trafficking in Adolescents*, https://doi.org/10.1007/978-3-030-43367-3_18

Approach to Care

When interacting with potentially trafficked/exploited patients, it is important to keep in mind some key concepts of the "trauma-informed approach" [1, 2]. With such an approach, the practitioner takes into account the impact of prior traumatic experiences in shaping a patient's views of self, the world, and other people and in influencing behaviors and attitudes. Trauma-informed care is victim centered (patient's desires and best interests are given the highest priority) and human rights based. There are five core values upon which a trauma-informed approach is built: (1) physical and psychological safety, (2) trustworthiness, (3) choice, (4) collaboration, and (5) empowerment [3]. The most important value of those five is safety, because without a sense of safety, patients will feel anxiety and stress which will add new trauma, amplify old trauma, and influence their reception of treatment. Therefore, care is taken to facilitate a sense of physical and psychological safety.

Privacy

Safety begins with separation of the patient from the person accompanying them in order to speak with the patient alone. An effective way to do this is to inform the companion that it is your practice's policy to interview patients alone, so you'll need them to step out for a few minutes and you'll be glad to come get them when you are finished. If this is not effective, you can remove the patient from the examination room by indicating they need to come with you for a procedure (x-ray, laboratory testing), then take the patient to a comfortable and private room to talk. It takes time to build rapport, but this is an essential first step in building trust and encouraging the patient to talk about their experiences and needs. Open-ended questions about nonthreatening topics (what the child likes to do; what apps he/she enjoys) can begin to build this rapport. Asking the child if she/he is hungry, thirsty, or cold also conveys concern and a desire to assist.

Building Trust

Two additional components of trauma-informed care are respect and transparency, key ways you can build trust with the patient. It is essential that you convey a sense of respect for the patient and all they have experienced. This can be done by encouraging them to voice their opinions (including their objections), actively listening to what they say, informing them of what you would like to do during the evaluation (before doing it), and obtaining their permission for every step of the process. Asking their opinion about the various steps and encouraging questions and feedback incorporate a strength-based approach and facilitate a sense of agency and control, as does offering the patient choices whenever possible.

Disclosing to Josie Your Mandate to Report

Questions about medical history transition to those about recent mental health symptoms. Josie reports episodic periods of sadness without suicidal ideation. She experiences occasional nightmares and insomnia. You begin asking open-ended questions about her social history, and eventually she reveals that she is actually only 14 years old, and that the woman outside is not her mother. You tell her you're glad she told you this and would like to find out more if she feels comfortable discussing it. However, since she is below the age of 18 years, you need to let her know something about privacy first. That is, while you want to respect her right to have information kept confidential and will make every effort to abide by that, there are two conditions under which you will need to speak with others about your conversation. Those conditions include if you are concerned that Josie is not safe or that Josie may harm someone else. Under those circumstances you would need to talk with other professionals in order to solicit their help, since safety is of the utmost importance. If this happens, you and Josie would discuss how you would go about notifying the other people. You ask if she has any questions about that and she says "no."

Confidentiality

Informing the patient of the limits of confidentiality before beginning a discussion of sensitive issues is important so that the child does not feel betrayed later, should you disclose the need to involve authorities in the case. While discussing the limits of confidentiality early in a discussion may inhibit the patient from disclosing potentially important information, it is critical to respect their rights to privacy and choice [6]. In many cases, if sufficient time is spent building rapport and trust, a patient will decide to discuss their situation despite knowledge of confidentiality limits [7].

Josie Opens Up

You thank Josie for her honesty and tell her that you are concerned that she did not feel comfortable revealing her age at first and that the woman outside is pretending to be someone else. You ask her if she is comfortable telling you why she said she is 19 years old, and why the woman pretended to be her mother. Josie hesitates and does not meet your eye. You allow some silence and do not rush to fill the gap.

You are sitting at eye level with Josie, with an open posture. Josie tells you the woman is a 'friend' she met while 'on the run.' She pauses and at length you ask an open-ended question, "Can you tell me a bit more about that? About your being on the run and meeting this woman?" Your voice is calm, nonjudgmental, and conveys interest. Josie tells you she ran away 3 months ago because she 'doesn't get along' with her mom, and she met this woman at a bus stop. The woman introduced her to her boyfriend and offered to let Josie stay with them for a while. You would like to know more about Josie's difficult relationship with her mother but do not interrupt the flow of Josie's story and decide to come back to this later. Instead, you nod, repeat back a bit of what Josie said (which conveys interest and the fact that you are listening.) "So she told you that you were welcome to stay with her and her boyfriend. Tell me about that..."

The Value of Open-Ended Questions and Silence

Open-ended questions (e.g., "Then what happened?") are a helpful way to elicit information and give the speaker control over the conversation. They will often lead to a narrative with important details that can inform your evaluation and recommendations for referrals. Leading questions (those which introduce new information not disclosed by the patient) and suggestive questions (those that imply a preferred response) should be avoided, as should any question that implies blame or judgment. Furthermore, it is common for the flow of the story to be scattered or nonlinear if the child has experienced trauma. Allow the child to tell the story in the order they wish to, and come back to parts you wish to elaborate on later. Do not rush to fill silences, for these may offer the child time to think and to offer sensitive and critical information.

Josie's Disclosure

Josie goes on to tell you that she stayed in an apartment with a few other girls, and that these girls seemed 'young'. They would disappear at night and come back early in the morning, and talk about making money and getting drugs. After a few days, Josie's friend told her about the 'stroll' and asked her if she wanted to make some money. You ask, "What is 'the stroll'?" She tells you this is X Street, where the 'players' are and where 'you do sex for money'. You follow up with another open-ended question, "So then what happened?" She says the woman's boyfriend convinced her to do it, telling her she'd make lots of money because she's so beautiful. Josie was scared, and when they got there she didn't want to get out of the car, but he punched her and made her get out. She had sex with three men that night, and as many men nearly every night since then. When she 'earns enough' the woman and boyfriend give her methamphetamine; sometimes she uses it to stay awake when she 'works'. She also uses marijuana nearly every day. She does this to 'make it easier to handle.' She wants to leave, but another girl tried to do this and the boyfriend beat her up. Josie doesn't want to get beaten up. She doesn't feel she can leave, and she is afraid of the woman and her boyfriend.

Handling a Disclosure

Josie is providing important information that allows you to assess risk of exploitation (she has actually disclosed that it is occurring), evaluate safety, and determine the possible need for after-care referrals, such as a formal assessment for substance abuse. Once Josie finishes her narrative, you may want to follow up with additional questions about injuries from this and other possible acts of violence, condom use, anogenital signs/symptoms, etc. These are important issues that will help you with your medical assessment. However, you would want to avoid irrelevant questions that will not provide you with useful information (e.g., "How much did you charge for each sex act?"), since these questions may elicit distress and anxiety and are inappropriate for the situation.

While Josie is describing what she has experienced, it is important for you to pay close attention to verbal and nonverbal cues that might signal traumatic stress and anxiety. You do not want to retraumatize her with your evaluation, if at all possible. Should you notice signs of distress (loss of eye contact, flat affect, nervousness, tears, fidgeting, etc.), it is important to take steps to alleviate the stress. This can be done by pausing, acknowledging the difficulty of what the patient has experienced, acknowledging her feelings, and emphasizing the strength it takes to talk about stressful experiences. You may want to offer her control by asking, "I can see this is very hard for you. Would you like to take a break or continue to tell me about it?"

Supporting Josie

You tell Josie that you are very glad she felt she could tell you about what is happening, that this takes a lot of courage. You acknowledge aloud that she has been through a great deal and is a very strong young woman. You tell her you are very concerned about her safety, and for this reason you are going to need to tell authorities about what is happening. You need police and child protective services to help offer assistance, to provide services you can't provide. She becomes upset about this. You ask her to talk about why she doesn't want anyone else to know. She tells you she is afraid of what the boyfriend will do, and afraid she'll be sent back to live with her mother. She doesn't want to live with her mother, but wants to go back to her former boyfriend, who is 24 years old. You reiterate your concern and your desire to help. You emphasize that it is important for her to tell the child protective services worker about her concerns and her desire not to return to her mother's care. Also it's important for her to tell police about her concern regarding the boyfriend's violence. You encourage her to voice her opinions, as these are critical for others to know. You ask her for her thoughts on how you and she should go about informing authorities. Does she want to tell the police and the protective services worker herself? Does she want you to call them? Or would she prefer for both of you to talk to them?

A Careful Balancing Act

While you cannot ignore your mandatory reporting requirements, you can allow Josie as much control over the situation as possible. Encouraging her to help you decide how to contact authorities, talking about other referral options, and seeking her opinion about those options (you will need to obtain her consent to make non-mandated victim service referrals, such as to an anti-trafficking nonprofit organization) help her to feel respected and be able to impact her situation.

Addressing the Chief Complaint

> You tell Josie that before you call anyone, you want to address the main issue: the cause of her pain and bleeding. You describe the general physical exam and the anogenital and speculum exams. You ask permission to do these exams. She agrees, albeit reluctantly. You assure her that you will explain all that you are doing during the exam and will stop if Josie becomes uncomfortable. With Josie's permission, you ask a nurse to assist during the exam. The nurse provides emotional support to Josie and monitors her for signs of distress. During the anogenital and speculum exams, you notice a hymenal laceration and two small vaginal contusions. All injuries are carefully documented in her chart. The injuries do not require treatment. There is no vaginal or cervical discharge; a small amount of bright red blood is in the vaginal vault. After completing the exam and allowing Josie to dress and get comfortable, you ask about the cause of the vaginal trauma. Josie tells you she was 'raped with a bottle' two days ago. There was pain during the event and a small amount of bleeding thereafter. Later that day, she began bleeding more heavily, as above.

Trauma-Informed Physical Exam

The trauma-informed approach extends to the physical exam and diagnostic evaluation [2]. It is important to explain all the steps of the process before beginning them and to obtain patient permission to proceed. This allows patient control and maintains transparency. Keep attuned to signs of distress during the exam, and take steps to minimize retraumatization. For example, a child who has had a gang rape digitally recorded and been threatened with posting the video online may become very agitated by the appearance of a camera for injury documentation. You would need to ask permission to use a camera and respect the patient's response. If she becomes upset during the anogenital exam (this is common), take breaks, explain each step, and acknowledge the strength it takes to undergo the exam. When you are contemplating STI, pregnancy, and/or drug testing, it is critical to obtain permission for these tests, after an explanation of what they entail.

In this case, Josie has obvious anogenital injuries, but in many cases the exam will be unremarkable, even with a history of multiple episodes of vaginal and/or anal intercourse [8, 9]. There are reasons for this: the adolescent hymen is able to distend to accommodate objects larger than its resting diameter without sustaining injury, as is the anus; and when injuries do occur, they typically heal within a few days to weeks, without scarring [10].

[See Chap. 16 Table 16.1, for information about the trauma-sensitive gynecologic exam.]

Evaluating and Examining Josie

You discuss your recommendations for further workup: urine testing for pregnancy and sexually transmitted infections; serum testing for HIV, syphilis, hepatitis B, and hepatitis C; and complete blood count to test for anemia. Because her last tetanus booster was greater than 5 years ago, you recommend tetanus booster vaccine for the dirty wound. You also recommend prophylaxis for gonorrhea, chlamydia and trichomonas. You discuss the pros and cons of HIV PEP. You ask Josie what she thinks about this course of action and if she has any questions. Josie agrees to the evaluation.

The point-of-care urine pregnancy test is positive. You ask Josie how she feels about the result and she simply says that she's 'not surprised' and that she doesn't want to talk about it. You discuss the need for a transvaginal ultrasound, and she agrees to the procedure. The ultrasound shows a sub-chorionic hemorrhage, and you recommend admission for observation. You tell Josie that this will help you to provide better care, and will also give Josie some time to think about things. You're glad to talk with her at any time, about the pregnancy or any other issues. Josie seems nervous and says she doesn't want to be admitted; she wants to leave. She asks when the other woman will be allowed to come in. You offer to contact her real mother, but she doesn't want her mother to know what is happening. She tells you she wants to go, will 'work things out with the woman and her boyfriend,' and will then go live with her 24-year-old ex-boyfriend.

Mandatory Reporting

Healthcare professionals are required to report suspected child abuse or neglect to any law enforcement official "authorized by law to receive such reports," and you do not need the individual's agreement in order to make this disclosure [11]. [See Chap. 3 section "Reporting" for nuances with adolescents]. State law may require more specific requirements as to whom clinicians must report and what information must be reported.

Adult abuse may be reported to law enforcement in specific circumstances, including: if the individual agrees; if the report is required by a different law; if expressly authorized by law, and based on the exercise of professional judgment, the report is necessary to prevent serious harm to the individual or others; or in certain other emergency situations [12]. In these cases, you may be required to give the individual notice of the report [12].

Healthcare professionals are required to report the amount of information that is the minimum necessary needed to accomplish the intended purpose of disclosure, unless more is required by a different law [13, 14]. Healthcare organizations typically have policies regarding what information this entails sharing. When it is reasonable, the clinician may rely upon the representation of the law enforcement official regarding what information is the minimum necessary for their lawful purpose [14].

Typically, a clinician should report when the clinician suspects or has reason to believe that a child has been abused or neglected [15]. Mandated reporters of child abuse are required to report the facts and circumstances that led them to believe the child is being abused or neglected [15]. Clinicians should ensure that they also are following the state reporting requirements and should contact their organizations' general counsel if they have questions.

According to the Polaris Project, one in seven endangered runaways who were reported to the National Center for Missing and Exploited Children was likely a sex trafficking victim, and of those, 88% were in the care of social services or foster care when they ran away [16]. According to the National Foster Youth Institute, 60% of all child sex trafficking victims have histories of child welfare involvement [17].

Josie should be referred to an attorney and to a social worker to help determine the best course of action for her. State laws vary regarding custody and emancipation, so Josie would need to be directed to someone who understands her state's requirements.

Whether or not the clinician is required to disclose Josie's pregnancy is a complicated question. The Health Insurance Portability and Accountability Act (HIPAA) defers to state and other laws to determine the rights of parents to access and control protected health information of their minor children. Parents, or a minor's other personal representatives, typically are allowed access to the child's protected health information. However, if the minor is subject to certain exceptions, this is no longer the case. For example, if the minor is emancipated, they are treated as a legal adult [18]. In some states, minors are considered emancipated for medical purposes when they are pregnant. Furthermore, when a clinician believes that "an individual, including an unemancipated minor, has been or may be subjected to domestic violence, abuse, or neglect by the personal representative, or that treating a person as an individual's personal representative could endanger the individual, the covered entity may choose not to treat that person as the individual's personal representative, if in the exercise of professional judgment, doing so would not be in the best interests of the individual" [13] [4]. If Josie's mother were involved in her trafficking situation, the clinician could choose not to treat her as Josie's personal representative because it would not be in Josie's best interest.

Josie's indication that she wishes to leave the hospital without being admitted and without further medical care raises the issue of whether the healthcare professional faces legal implications if the patient leaves against medical advice (AMA). There is no perfect answer. The clinician has the option of calling Child Protective Services (CPS) to arrange for protective custody so that treatment can continue right away. The clinician also may choose to discharge Josie with a note in the medical record indicating "discharged AMA" and with detailed follow-up instructions, including possibly an instruction to return – although that doesn't seem promising in this scenario.

Above all, the decision to report the abuse depends on the medical determination as to the impact a delay in treatment would have on Josie's long-term well-being. An AMA discharge does not necessarily immunize a clinician from liability; however it does affirm the clinician's intent to provide further treatment [5]. Josie should be discouraged from leaving AMA and instead should be given information relative to the dangers and risks inherent. Likewise, the healthcare professional should reiterate that CPS will be informed due to mandated reporting requirements. All interactions should be clearly documented in the medical record, and a final attempt at referring Josie to legal counsel should be made.

There are several other reasons why a healthcare professional should refer Josie to legal representation. If Josie has any pending cases or convictions relating to her victimization, an attorney may be able to help her fight these through vacatur, expungement, and safe harbor laws: some states have "safe harbor" laws, which means that minors who have been prostituted will not be prosecuted for prostitution-related crimes. If Josie has already been convicted of prostitution-related crimes, an attorney may be able to help her through processes known as vacatur and expungement. Vacatur is when a conviction is set aside as if it never happened, while expungement is when convictions are removed from a person's record.

Each of these processes can help Josie move forward without the burden of a criminal record, and it is important to let Josie know that she has this opportunity.

Documentation

You are now documenting your evaluation of Josie. It is important to balance detail with the desire for confidentiality, knowing that authorities are likely to read your report. You want future medical professionals to have important health and safety information, but you also want to respect the child's privacy. When describing what the child told you, document as much of her responses verbatim as possible. Ideally you are not taking notes during your discussion with Josie, but to the extent that you can remember the wording of your questions and her comments, it is important to document this. Describe injuries carefully (written description of location, type of injury, approximate size, shape, color, etc.), and document the child's affect, general state of health, untreated medical conditions, and acute conditions. Remain objective in your documentation and do not write anything you are not prepared to say in court, under oath.

It is important for your institution to consider privacy issues for patients with a history of human trafficking. Policies and protocols already in place to protect highly sensitive information (e.g., mental health records) may also apply to cases of trafficking. Access to information regarding a patient's trafficking experiences should be limited to those who are working with the patient, and processes must be in place to restrict access by other medical staff and outside persons who lack legal rights to the record.

List of Resources Pertinent to the Chapter Topic

1. NHTRC – National Human Trafficking Hotline: https://humantraffickinghotline.org/
2. CSE Institute and ABA: https://www.americanbar.org/groups/domestic_violence/survivor-reentry-project/
3. Guttmacher Institute: https://www.guttmacher.org/
4. American Academy of Pediatrics Policy Statement – Child Abuse, Confidentiality, and the Health Insurance Portability and Accountability Act, 2010: https://pediatrics.aappublications.org/content/pediatrics/125/1/197.full.pdf
5. Shared Hope International: https://sharedhope.org/

References

1. Substance abuse and mental health services administration [Internet]. 2016. Trauma-informed approach and trauma-specific interventions. Available from: http://www.samhsa.gov/nctic/trauma-interventions.
2. Substance abuse and mental health services administration trauma and justice strategic initiative [Internet]. 2014. Concept of trauma and guidance for a trauma-informed approach; [1–27]. Available from: https://store.samhsa.gov/system/files/sma14-4884.pdf
3. Wilson C, Pence DM, Conradi L. Trauma-informed care. Encyclopedia of social work [Internet]. 2013 [cited 2019 May]. Available from: https://oxfordre.com/socialwork/view/10.1093/acrefore/9780199975839.001.0001/acrefore-9780199975839-e-1063. https://doi.org/10.1093/acrefore/9780199975839.013.1063.
4. Zimmerman C, Watts C. World Health Organization ethical and safety recommendations for interviewing trafficked women. 2003. Health policy unit, London School of Hygiene and Tropical Medicine. Available from: https://www.who.int/mip/2003/other_documents/en/Ethical_Safety-GWH.pdf.
5. Kaltiso SO, Greenbaum VJ, Agarwal M, McCracken C, Zimitrovich A, Harper E, Simon HK. Evaluation of a screening tool for child sex trafficking among patients with high-risk chief complaints in a pediatric emergency department. Soc Academic Emerg Medicine. 2018;25(11):1193–1203.
6. Adams JA, Harper K, Knudson S, Revilla J. Examination findings in legally confirmed child sexual abuse: it's normal to be normal. Pediatrics. 1994;94(3):310–7.
7. Smith TD, Raman SR, Madigan S, Waldman J, Shouldice M. Anogenital findings in 3569 pediatric examinations for sexual abuse/assault. J Pediatr Adolesc Gynecol. 2018;31:79–83.
8. McCann J, Miyamoto S, Boyle C, Rogers K. Healing of hymenal injuries in prepubertal and adolescent girls: a descriptive study. Pediatrics. 2007;119:e1094.
9. Uses and disclosures for which an authorization or opportunity to agree or object is not required, 45 C.F.R. § 164.512 (2016).
10. Uses and disclosures of protected health information: general rules, 45 C.F.R. § 164.502 (2013).
11. Other requirements relating to uses and disclosures of protected health information, 45 C.F.R. § 164.514(d) (2013).
12. U.S. Dept. of Health and Human Services. When does the privacy rule allow covered entities to disclose information to law enforcement [Internet]. Washington, D.C.: Office for Civil Rights; 2004 [updated 2013 July 26]. Available from: https://www.hhs.gov/hipaa/for-professionals/faq/505/what-does-the-privacy-rule-allow-covered-entities-to-disclose-to-law-enforcement-officials/index.html.

13. Child welfare information gateway [Internet]. Washington, DC: Department of Health and Human Services, Children's Bureau; 2016. Mandatory reporters of child abuse and neglect; [1–61]. Available from: https://www.childwelfare.gov/pubpdfs/manda.pdf.
14. Polaris Project. The facts [Internet]. 2016; [cited 2019 May]. Available from: https://polarisproject.org/human-trafficking/facts.
15. National Foster Youth Initiative. Sex trafficking: sex and human trafficking in the U.S. disproportionately affects foster youth [Internet]. [cited 2019 May]. Available from: https://www.nfyi.org/issues/sex-trafficking/.
16. Michon K. The ins and outs of minor emancipation – what it means and how it can be obtained [Internet]. Nolo; [cited 2019 October]. Available from: https://www.nolo.com/legal-encyclopedia/emancipation-of-minors-32237.html.
17. U.S. Dept. of Health and Human Services. Guidance: personal representatives [Internet]. Washington, D.C.: Office for Civil Rights; 2013. Available from: https://www.hhs.gov/hipaa/for-professionals/privacy/guidance/personal-representatives/index.html.
18. Alfandre D, Schumann JH. What is wrong with discharges against medical advice (and how to fix them). JAMA. 2013;310(22):2393–4.

Chapter 19
Survivor Insights

Christine Cesa, Marti MacGibbon, Erik Gray, Nat Paul, Suleman Masood, and Wendy Barnes

My Lived Experience

Christine Cesa, MA, Survivor Advocate

> Empathy is not connecting to an experience; empathy is connecting to the emotion that underpins an experience.
>
> –Brené Brown

For over half my life I was sex trafficked by people who should have protected and supported me. I never looked like an at-risk youth or like someone who would need help from the moment they walked in the emergency department or clinic. To be honest that was part of the problem: I looked like an ordinary girl. I had learned to not cause trouble, to not speak up, to fit in and deal with my pain. I often had a controlling person with me – however, they would have looked like a concerned friend or family member. To this day, I have trouble finding medical care in which the

C. Cesa (✉)
Office of Victims of Crime (Expert Consultant), Los Angeles, CA, USA

M. MacGibbon
Office for Victims of Crime (Expert Consultant), Sacramento, CA, USA

E. Gray
Innovations Human Trafficking Collaborative (Programs Director), Olympia, WA, USA

N. Paul
Bolivar, NY, USA

S. Masood
Subject Matter Expert, Falls Church, VA, USA

W. Barnes
Human Trafficking Response Program, Dignity Health, Seattle, WA, USA

K. E. Titchen, E. Miller (eds.), *Medical Perspectives on Human Trafficking in Adolescents*, https://doi.org/10.1007/978-3-030-43367-3_19

clinician understands that a survivor of human trafficking is a normal person and that human trafficking happens in our communities.

Language Matters

Marti MacGibbon, CADC-II, ACRPS

In the movement to end human trafficking, the participation of survivors is crucial and highly beneficial. Healthcare providers invite lived experience experts from diverse backgrounds to work with you in developing protocols and policies for your clinical setting. Be open to survivor voice. By "survivor voice," we mean survivor input: the actions, insights, and expertise of those with lived experience of human trafficking, including exiting the trafficking situation. Survivors are not victims who have been rescued: we are resilient, empowered stakeholders who use our expertise to open doors and keep them open so that others may walk out of exploitation and into autonomy. The collective voice of survivors should be reserved for legislative advocacy, petitions, and the like. Every survivor has a different experience, skills, and perspective, and our voices are unique. Our language matters. Too often, we survivors are lumped together into classifications or painted with broad strokes. Our individual voices and our language demonstrate the diversity and individuality of survivors' stories, skill sets, and beings.

Risk

Erik Gray

Inherited Trauma

Susceptibility to human trafficking began before I was born. Both of my parents grew up in abject poverty. My mother grew up in the Philippines and had to be sent away at a young age in order to feed the entire family. My father entered into the Texas foster care system after being homeless for several months around the age of 6 and experienced sexual abuse while in the foster care system.

Alcohol and Addiction

A majority of the time I spent with my father was when he was home, he was drinking. Whenever the ship would deploy, the sailors would drink copious amounts of alcohol. Whenever the ship returned, the sailors would drink copious amounts of alcohol. Ever since I can remember, I've regularly attended 30- to 40-person large navy parties, where alcohol was the primary focus. When I continued to be abused by men my father worked with, it was nothing new, and the chaotic environment encouraged poor decisions and no accountability. I started drinking alcohol around the age of 8. I was drinking regularly by 10 years old and started smoking cigarettes by 12. All of these were readily available to me.

Prejudice

Growing up in a navy family, I spent most of my time with predominantly Filipino, Islander, Hispanic, and/or Asian communities stationed overseas. I didn't live in a predominantly white community until I was 14 years old, which is when I started to be bullied. My first day of school, I ate lunch in the bathroom. Within my first month of school, I was placed into in-school suspension for the first time. Although I was popular and elected as student council secretary, the advisors were homophobic and later modified the results and announced a different winner of the election. Teachers, staff, and students frequently mocked my behavior, mannerisms, and their perceptions of my voice. There wasn't a single time I felt safe coming to school. All of this led to an environment where I felt increasingly unwelcome and unsafe. I would grow to need an inclusive and accepting environment and was pushed to find one elsewhere.

LGBTQ2IA+

I came out as bisexual when I was 14 years old, and this intensified the bullying. Growing up in a fairly conservative navy town, there weren't many accessible healthy role models or safe means of exploring this piece of my identity. While growing up, the only sex education taught referred to heterosexuality. Growing up in a homophobic Catholic community, there was no possibility of discussing the issue without substantial consequence. LGBTQ2IA+ issues were rarely brought up, and when they were it was never in a positive light. When my curiosity and need to explore my identity became more pressing, I pressed on.

I met a man named Brian on the Internet. He would groom me, make me feel loved, and make me feel really special. The first night I met Brian, he gave me methamphetamines. I continued to hang out with him, and he got me addicted to opiates, alcohol, and a variety of drugs. Shortly afterward, Brian began inviting other men over and trafficked me from the ages of 14–16. Brian's love for me and his claim to my body were nothing new to me: in retrospect, they remind me of my father.

I would continue in and out of the sex trade for 10 years. Eventually, I contracted HIV and was forced to trade sex for medications to survive AIDS.

Lack of Support Systems

Moving around constantly while growing up and being ousted out of my familial, spiritual, and community supports created an environment ripe for exploitation. Human trafficking is a crime that exploits our vulnerabilities. When I was younger, I expressed myself more androgynously. I would change into female clothing and hide in the newspaper box we never used near our mailbox at the top of the hill. While the people immediately around me rejected me for my gender expression and sexuality, the men online seemed to desire me even more. Brian showed me that my body was tradeable – that if I wanted something I couldn't otherwise have, all I needed to do was have sex and I could have nearly anything I wanted. He built up a dream of us driving range rovers and living in a house together. He made me feel loved and seen. He started "helping" me plan to get out of my non-accepting environment to live with him. When I didn't want to have sex, he would give me more drugs until I couldn't control my actions or body or was inebriated to a point where I couldn't verbalize or express non-consent.

I didn't have anybody with whom to express what I was going through. I didn't have the words to describe what I was going through at night. I didn't even have the words to describe what I was going through during the day with my sexuality and gender let alone the horrific sex acts I was being forced to do at night by this controlling man in his 30s when I was just 14. Whenever opportunities seemed to arise to talk about it, they were often swiftly shut down with a homophobic word or action that pushed me toward guilt and repentance.

Stand Alone

Erik Gray

I don't know how to escape it
I don't know how to breathe outside of it
I don't know how to exist outside of an existence built for me
I don't know how to feel special outside of exploitation
I don't know how to feel valued outside of sex
I don't know how to feel satiated outside of instant gratification
I don't know how to feel respected outside of violence and pain
I don't know how to feel understood outside of manipulation
I don't know how to feel validated outside of grief
I don't know how to feel normal outside of hate
I don't know how to feel calm outside of dead
–Dead Man Walking

Recovery, Resilience, and Trauma Resolution

Marti MacGibbon, CADC-II, ACRPS

Recovery is a dynamic, ongoing healing process involving a plan of action, emotional and spiritual renewal, self-discovery, and self-empowerment. Recovery is the creation of a new lifestyle; it includes the acquisition of self-protective behavioral skills and the development of tenacity and optimism in the face of challenges and adversity. Recovery taught me how to love myself, to forgive myself and others, and to embrace positive change. That's how I see it now, looking back over 24 years of continuous recovery from addiction. I'm one of the 23.5 million adults in the United States who reports long-term recovery from addiction to alcohol or other drugs.[1]

I'm also a survivor of human trafficking and complex posttraumatic stress disorder. Today I'm a nationally renowned humorous inspirational speaker and a national award-winning author. I hold five professional certifications in addiction treatment, advocate for victims and survivors of human trafficking, and advocate for people in recovery from addiction. I do not regret the nightmare experiences of my past. Thanks to cognitive reframing and the years I worked with a wonderful trauma therapist, I can look back and see the courage, strength, grace, humor, and generosity in my actions during the worst of times. Survivors are resilient, not only after exiting the trafficking but during the captivity phase. They arrive at your facility armed with tools for recovery: strength, innate and experiential knowledge, and courage.

> Service providers,
> be aware of the innate resiliency of all survivors, and of youth.
> Our brains are most plastic during adolescence,
> so young patients with substance use issues
> have a lot going for them in the healing process.
> Believe in your patients, and let them know you believe in them.
> Give them permission to be an integral part of their own healing.

My story, like every survivor's story, is unique to me, but shares common threads with all other survivors' stories, because the perpetrators use similar methods and target certain vulnerabilities – substance use issues, history of abuse and/or trauma, poverty, lack of shelter, mental health issues, disabilities, desperation. I was trafficked and sold to organized crime figures as an adult, but I was sexually abused and assaulted on multiple occasions at ages 15, 16, and 17. At one point, I was also commercially sexually exploited. Immediately after the first incident, when I was sexually assaulted and abused by a 26-year-old man who was a student teacher at my school, then sexually assaulted by his roommate, I used illicit drugs for the first time, in an attempt to manage the trauma. The age I first used is significant to my story – neuroscientists know that one big risk factor for addiction is the age you start using. We're most vulnerable to addiction in our teenage years, when the brain is most plastic, and adolescent substance use can affect emotional maturation.

As an adolescent, I used illicit substances – amphetamines, hallucinogens, cannabis – for a couple of years, then quit, became involved in some fringe Christian cults, and developed anorexia, all in an unconscious attempt to gain control over the chaos created by my trauma. At 17, I landed in the psychiatric ward, where I was misdiagnosed, overmedicated, and then confined in a room on a mattress with no sheets, clad only in one of those gowns that tie in the back and leave your body exposed. During the days I spent in chemical restraints, two male orderlies digitally raped me. I never reported any of the crimes committed against me. I believed I was ultimately responsible for everything that happened as I stumbled through crisis after crisis. Part of the biology of trauma and addiction is the shame and self-loathing that build up, accompanied by fear and a creeping sense of powerlessness that increase over time.

After escaping being trafficked as an adult, my trauma was so profound that I was unable to function in society for nearly 10 years. I used drugs intravenously, mostly methamphetamine, every day, except when I was in jail or on one occasion in the psychiatric ward on a 5150. Trapped in a cycle of trauma and addiction, I grappled with despair, rage, grief, and loss. My turning point, about a year before I turned my life around, came when I ended up in the ICU of a hospital. They found drugs in my bloodstream but didn't arrest me. I was so moved by their kindness and nonjudgmental treatment of me that I determined to get clean.

Be process-oriented, not results-oriented.
You never know how powerful a positive effect you can have on someone when you create a safe space within the healthcare setting.

I've considered the things that helped me to recover: in the little town where I lived, I found a healthcare clinic with a sliding scale; they had a licensed clinical social worker on staff, and she taught me mindfulness practices, cognitive behavioral therapy, and other skills. She helped me with trauma resolution via EMDR (Eye Movement Desensitization and Reprocessing) therapy. Female gynecologists treated me for healthcare issues resulting from being trafficked, and they were non-judgmental, kind, and empathetic. Because I lacked resources for formal rehab, I sought community resources and support groups to recover from addiction. I educated myself about the disease by studying books from my local library. Because I wasn't withdrawing from opioids or alcohol, the acute withdrawal didn't require a formal detox. Yes, it took many months to finally get a foothold. But I recovered, and I know thousands of people who have done the same, against long odds, just like me. Healthcare professionals have every reason to take heart from my story and to maintain optimism about patients.

1. Partnership for Drug-Free Kids, 2012 survey results https://drugfree.org/newsroom/news-item/survey-ten-percent-of-american-adults-report-being-in-recovery-from-substance-abuse-or-addiction/
2. The Neuroscience of Need: Understanding the Addicted Mind, from Stanford Medicine Archives SPECIAL REPORT Spring 2012 http://sm.stanford.edu/archive/stanmed/2012spring/article5.html

Intersectionality and Complex Systemic Oppression

Nat Paul, Survivor Advocate

Implicit and Explicit Bias and False Assumptions

For purposes of clarification on terminology, I use the following:

- *Victim*: Someone who is being actively trafficked in accordance with the legal definition as defined in the law.
- *Survivor*: Someone who is no longer being actively trafficked – these survivors can still be marginalized, oppressed, and vulnerable or in an exploitative situation that does not meet the definition of trafficking.
- *Potential Victim*: Someone who is in an oppressed status or stigmatized by society with core vulnerabilities to being trafficked or in a situation of exploitation that is not actively being trafficked.

These three terms represent merely a sliding scale of places through which an individual may or may not cycle in their life. With so much societal stigmatization around these terms, their use should not be forced upon anyone. A service should be acquired through checking a box on a form that they meet a legal definition without trying to force a person to own the term or definition used in legal/medical coding.

In order to fully respond to a potential victim of trafficking, one needs to constantly assess and weigh their own preconceived biases and assumptions as to what a victim looks like. Bias is as simple as the medical professional who refers to a "frequent flyer" in a psych ward admitted for suicide, the medical professional who doesn't look at self-harm and self-cutting through the lens of trauma and the patient's attempt to justify their emotional trauma with a physical pain they *can* comprehend. Bias is the medical professional's assessment that a "junkie" simply is not worth the time: instead they just patch the "junkie" and send them out the door. Bias involves marginalizing transgender street youth who are not in a place to legally transition by simply looking at the chart and constantly "dead-naming" them (calling them by their birth name rather than their chosen name) or assuming something from a text scribbled on a sheet of paper at intake. Bias is the assumption that labor trafficking is only happening in rural settings and mass farming locations without understanding that trafficking occurs in massage parlors, nail salons, hotel workers, garment industries, and even street-based markets of drug running. Bias is the police officer who brings into the emergency department a patient in handcuffs for drug charges without noting the potential force, fraud, or coercion that has victimized that patient and which legally qualifies as unidentified labor trafficking – buying into the sensational awareness campaigns that white girls are sex trafficked by black pimps. And this is the only representation you will find in an emergency department setting and in all forms of healthcare from HIV mobile testing units, to primary care facilities, to even a dentist's office.

Addressing the Hierarchy of Oppression

There are no "one-box-fits-all" victims of crimes, but there certainly is a "one-bias-negates-a-lot-of-identification" of victims. What we need is for medical professionals to provide comprehensive services while asking questions around *why* poorly stitched injuries/scars are present, asking *why* a poorly set healed bone happened, and noting gaps in medical history with clear awareness of physical trauma that should have been seen. Medical professionals need to address the challenging questions of *why* a black teenager is pregnant by a "boyfriend" in his 30s *who is always present with her*. Medical professionals need to ask about safety plans for addiction-related needs or suicidal ideation that may not be active. Medical professionals need to provide comprehensive services while addressing harm reduction approaches for a cutter, such as ensuring access to bandages and disinfectant to prevent infections. Medical professionals should address abscesses from narcotic injections or other complicated health issues *without bias* while keeping a door open for future dialog or engagement with services when the patient is ready/willing.

As illustrated in chapter "LGBTQIA+ Youth and Human Trafficking," the hierarchy of oppression in the United States leaves a homeless addicted transwoman of color without any programs or services: how do we improve our programs to meet the needs of a person that has no access to housing, employment, or services in the United States? If we overcome the systemic and pervasive biases that deny access to the most marginalized among us, then all other biases will fall away.

Prisoner of War

Suleman Masood, Survivor Advocate

I was 20 years old when I found myself in the ICU for the first time in my life. Initially, I didn't want to go, despite the lacerations, bruises, and wounds across my body. When most people think of a victim of human trafficking, they often imagine the fears associated with interacting with law enforcement. What many experts in the field fail to understand is that those same fears exist when a victim of human trafficking interacts with the healthcare system.

My victimization from human trafficking was not something that an expert in human trafficking would classify as "traditional." The manipulation and physical trauma I had experienced were that of a "prisoner of war." My trafficker created a fictitious world around me where he had made claims to work as a member of the

Department of Defense, US Air Force, and as the son of a high-profile member of the government in a Middle Eastern country.

Recruitment and Grooming

This individual had infected my family like a computer virus: every area in our home, neighborhood, and community brought us nightmares of him. In his quest to lure me, to "mentor" me, he spent countless hours with me and my family. Because of his status in both the United States and his home country, he was required to have security detail follow him wherever he went; the same was the case with those he considered "close" in his life. As a 16-year-old at the time, I thought it was fascinating to have black SUVs follow me to and from school: little did I know that these vehicles and their drivers would contribute to my trauma.

Transportation/Isolation

Shortly after completing high school and receiving a scholarship to attend UC Irvine, I was ecstatic to major in biology and start my journey toward becoming an oncologist. My mother was diagnosed with cancer, and after years of interning with a local doctor near my neighborhood, I was determined to fulfill my dream. My trafficker had other plans. Moving out of my parents' home to pursue my undergraduate degree was the ultimate moment of vulnerability in my life: I didn't know the area where I lived, I didn't have friends, and I certainly didn't have any money. (Hooray student loans!) My trafficker moved out to Santa Monica due to a change in his "work assignment," where he said he needed to monitor potential terrorist threats.

At this point a looming "debt" was beginning to blossom over my head, so I had incentive to accept my trafficker's offer to become "One of his Men." As such, I traveled to his many homes to move furniture, to do electrical work, and to paint all across cities in California. I was spending less of my time and energy in lecture halls studying and more time wanting to prove myself as one of my trafficker's men. While failing classes and being placed on academic probation, my trafficker was able to target my deepest vulnerability: my self-esteem. Growing up, I had never failed a class, and I had never been away from my family. I had worked hard and been successful in almost everything back in my hometown.

My trafficker called me various names: stupid, useless, a waste of an opportunity, etc. I was made to believe that I was not just a failed investment in my trafficker's eyes but, more importantly, my parents'. My trafficker launched a campaign to get me to drop out of school. Despite my trafficker making open threats throughout my relationship, the threats he was now making stuck with me. "I am going to give you two options, Suleman: either drop out of school to work for me, or I will put you in a body bag and drop you on the doorstep of your parent's house." The decision was pretty easy to make.

Exploitation

I started working around the clock: I worked 18 hours a day and delivered every single paycheck to my trafficker. If that wasn't enough, I was now experiencing both mental and physical trauma. All of the awards I had in school and sports he shredded in front of me, along with all of my personal documents that contained my name (social security, driver's license, etc.). The only active document I had that was sufficient for me to go out and work jobs was my passport. Unfortunately, I had no access to this because my trafficker would lock it in his safe. My personal identity was erased right in front of me. If that wasn't enough, I was beaten and starved daily. Some days I wasn't even allowed to go to work because I was beaten instead. My trafficker wanted the idea ingrained in me that he was no one to play with. There was no single day that was guaranteed for me during this experience.

Escape and Medical Care

When I found the courage to escape, I could only think of the love of my parents, who were under the impression I was studying at UC Irvine. (I found out later that my trafficker would have lengthy conversations with them to convince them that I did not love them and didn't want to have contact while I was out working.) I was able to talk my coworker into helping me escape. When I did, I was able to return to my parents. After so many beatings, I had one good eye, one good leg, and one ounce of hope left.

Throughout the night of my return, my parents pleaded for me to be admitted to an ICU. Both my stubbornness and fear of my trafficker's affiliation with the US government made me believe that I would be executed the minute my medical record became discoverable by my trafficker's men. I held off for two additional nights, and it finally took a very strong family friend to physically take me to the ICU. With lengthy and seemingly unnecessary questions from two nurses, I finally was able to see the physician. I began to tell my account of what had happened to me. The physician quickly notified the local sheriff's office.

The nurses spent time treating my lacerations – and leaving me physically exposed while I spoke with law enforcement about what had occurred. When these processes were completed, I had the chance to speak with the physician who did not waste time in telling me, "Listen, I am going to write this on your prescription as I say this to you: You need to go to therapy. I don't care where or how, but you need to. And you need to do this ASAP. If you don't, you will do this to someone else." This has stuck with me to this day and is why I vow to spend my life helping others to make sure the trauma I had experienced will never happen to anyone else.

Overlooked

Erik Gray

When I finally decided to try to leave Brian, I started to get sick from withdrawal. This felt a lot like what heartache looks like in the movies: lying in bed all day, nauseated and vomiting, eating lots of ice cream and junk food. I didn't know how to process it and felt that I must be in love. I didn't understand the impacts and effects of the chemical restraints Brian put on me. There were several incidents where I was trafficked for a night or a couple of days and never saw the trafficker again. Party and Play (PnP) is a common term and subculture within the gay community. This term refers to using methamphetamines and having sex, usually for hours or days at a time. Often used with methamphetamines is gamma-hydroxybutyrate (GHB, also known as "the date rape drug"). When combined, it's often called a "G-Tini" referencing methamphetamine or "T/Tina" and GHB.

I first ran away when I was 16 years old and then permanently when I was 17. I would become unstably housed, and PnP'ing would become a regular way for me to meet my basic needs and fuel my addiction. I would frequently trade sex for drugs and a place to stay, clearly indicating to my future traffickers that I was vulnerable and easily exploitable with nowhere to go. I couldn't go to my own closest friends without being thought of as being on a drug-addled rant. People from my street family to strangers I met off the Internet would traffic me to profit off my body, frequently drugging me, leaving me incapacitated and available for easy exploitation. Other times, my street family and Internet strangers and I would set up a fetish or kink scene based on "Bondage Domination Slave and Master" or "BDSM," and men would pay them without my knowledge or consent.

BDSM is a topic that is often overlooked when addressing trafficking. However, if we are to take a holistic psychosocial approach, it is a topic we have to cover. BDSM in and of itself does not make one vulnerable to human trafficking: however, BDSM can and does shape one's mind, perception of one's sexual self and others. Additionally, BDSM engages in power and control dynamics that are reinforced through orgasm and other physiologic processes and sensations. [See chapter "Human Trafficking in Adolescents and Young Adults with Co-existing Disordered Eating Behaviors" for more about power and control dynamics in human trafficking.] This creates a perfect accountability-free training ground for exploitation without informed, balanced, and empowering BDSM education. This can be particularly for submissive personality types. BDSM is also egregiously overlooked when addressing healing from human trafficking and is often stigmatized negatively. BDSM and human trafficking are not equivalent; however, they both exist in the same space.

Wakeup Sunshine

Erik Gray

There's something special about that time
I remember the first morning I woke up
And couldn't have thoughts
I felt like I'd been awake all night
I knew I was high
But like I couldn't think
If I could think I think I thought it was great
Because I could only feel my body
And I was really really high
So I thought maybe I was just really really high
And I don't know it was just different
But that's just it
I don't know
That moment that just disappeared out of my head
I'm really used to that moment
Getting plucked out
I'm really used to people messing with my head
So I can tell
When memories
Just go poof
Or zaPPppO!
It's annoying
And incredibly dehumanizing
I remember that moment like I remember drinking my first cup of coffee
Or riding my first bike
or figuring out that santa claus isn't real
and I remember with the intensity of
similar to that of getting déjà vu
it comes all at once
and you kind of want to declare it
DÉJÀ VU!!!
As if screaming it could make something happen
As if
Any agency existed at all
But today I remembered that moment
That moment when
I didn't remember what happened
It almost feels blissful
Remembering the not remembering
–Reality Check

Arriving at the ED: What Does Empathy Look Like?

Christine Cesa, MA, Survivor Advocate

When I walked into the emergency department, I often was met by a security guard and nurses in triage, and I was instructed where to sit. If someone was assertive, firm, or simply just having a tough shift and was aggressive with me, I would get afraid, my fight-or-flight response would kick in, and I would want to get out of a potentially dangerous situation. Sometimes I left. I would need to be told that I was safe, taken into a safe place to wait, and given empathic care, but often in a busy emergency department, that was not possible. Because of my level of experienced trauma and the fact that people in authority have sold, exploited, and taken advantage of me since I can remember, if someone was too harsh with me, I would totally shut down. Clinical staff should note that all trafficked persons are not always aggressive and belligerent: sometimes they are quiet and passive and will not speak for themselves.

Empathy, Kindness, and Dignity

If I had been seen by a clinician who was empathic, kind, and compassionate and treated me with dignity, it would have made all the difference. When I was being trafficked, many of the clinicians were connected to the person who exploited me, so it was impossible to trust them. It is still hard and deeply painful some days to be seen by clinicians.

One time, I was in terrible pain from what I thought might be a cyst on my ovary. There were days that I was doubled over in pain. I couldn't walk at times, and I wouldn't eat because the pain was too severe. I was working part time at a church when two women working there saw the level of pain I was in and asked me if I was OK. My response to these women was, "I'm OK." That is kind of my go-to line a lot of the time: that I am OK or fine. Eventually they both said, "You are not OK."

Here is the truth: I was in *immense* pain! In my mind due to my past of being sex trafficked as a minor, I was worried that I had many sexually transmitted infections and maybe something horrible had happened to me. I was also terrified of the actual exam and that maybe I would need some type of surgery. Just the thought of laying on a table and having a physician conduct a pelvic examination was terrifying.

Eventually, I went to a doctor at a county facility. The examination was traumatic. I still was having flashbacks and would emotionally shut down due to the trauma I had endured. The first thing I had to do was undress and lie on a table. I understand that this is necessary for the clinical exam. However, this is what happened to me my entire childhood: people wanted me to undress and lay me somewhere. I told the physician I had a lot of trauma. I told the physician I needed something to help me, that this was going to be really hard for me and I was in a lot of pain. She told me that they were an OB/GYN office and they "didn't help people that way." I said, "OK." When she began examining me, I started crying, and when she touched the area that was in pain, I screamed and jumped. She realized I wasn't drug seeking and helped me.

I don't want to have to explain human trafficking to you or feel like I've traumatized you when I am not feeling well. It is necessary that clinicians understand that a majority of my issues are related to my trauma from human trafficking and that I am not making them up. Any time I even remotely mention human trafficking, clinicians are so horrified that human trafficking exists that they can't imagine that someone they meet would be a survivor.

I don't want to be thought of as a prostitute, an addict, or someone who made horrible life choices. Those things do not describe me. I am sometimes nervous to disclose that I am a survivor of human trafficking. Will it impact the medical treatment I receive? Did she think negatively because of my background as a survivor of trafficking?

Recently, a clinician heard I was a survivor of trafficking and said, "Congratulations." I felt nauseous. Surviving human trafficking is not the same as surviving cancer. I was sold for sex and left to die, beaten and tortured, that doesn't feel like something to congratulate. Instead, congratulate who I am today. Congratulate the fact that I graduated from college and have a master's degree. Celebrate special milestones with me. Walk alongside me. We are all learning and growing, and let's honor and care for one another.

HIPAA and ICD-10 – My Privacy Matters

Christine Cesa, MA, Survivor Advocate

When a person has endured human trafficking, it should be *their* information to share. If clinicians do not make patients feel safe, honored, and treated with dignity, then patients will not share the reality of what is going on in their lives. Human trafficking has long-lasting health implications, and in my experience the longer a person has been victimized, the more serious the health implications will be.

In healthcare, the Health Insurance Portability and Accountability Act (HIPAA) is taken very seriously. However, are there parts of HIPAA which become gray? For example, do patients have to consent for a social work consult? Are we always operating in the best interests of the patient? Let's consider the new ICD-10 codes: are they helpful or hurtful? On the one hand, we may identify an individual who has been trafficked or who is at risk. They help clinical staff to identify and keep records on the number of cases of human trafficking patients. If a patient is identified as being a victim/survivor of trafficking and coded with the ICD-10 codes, they could be provided extra care consideration and provision. If the ICD-10 coding only lasted for a finite number of years and was then removed from the medical record, this could be helpful so that the individual would not continually have to explain his/her/their past, family history, or other related questions every time they needed care. If they could have the same nurse or healthcare professional who understood the history, it could be helpful. Perhaps then trafficked patients would stay for care and would not leave against medical advice.

However, let's consider that person 7 years later: they've gotten on their feet and have a new place to live, new job, and new friends. One ordinary day, they go to the clinic for routine care. Perhaps the clinical staff start asking safety questions when they see in the chart that the patient has experienced human trafficking. All well meaning, but perhaps the survivor doesn't wish to keep reliving this past and is simply seeking medical care for an unrelated cause. The experience of severe trauma should not mean that a patient is bound to vouch for his or her safety time and time again.

Value Survivor Leaders as Members of the Team

Christine Cesa, MA, Survivor Advocate

It can be overwhelming for clinicians to assess patients at risk for violence, especially human trafficking. Emergency medicine staff have expressed to me that they have many things to assess in triage, and now we are tasking the staff to assess at-risk patients for human trafficking.

Employing a survivor leader/advocate as part of the staff is important for a number of reasons. First, having a survivor advocate to provide training is critical for staff understanding of human trafficking as a public health issue. Survivor advocates have unique insights and perspectives that others likely will not be able to offer.

Second, having a survivor advocate on site to whom staff can turn with questions is critical to staff understanding of the complex dynamics around human trafficking, such as coercion, manipulation, complex trauma, and lack of options for survivors. The assistance of survivor advocates can help staff to feel empowered to identify patients and to know that trafficked patients will be provided the care and assistance that they need.

Third, survivor advocates are critical for the emergency response. Many survivors of human trafficking have experienced so much trauma and often are still being victimized when they arrive in the emergency department. They may be shut down, or they may respond to "outside" help from social workers and medical staff in a combative manner. The survivor may have been controlled, exploited, or recently arrested: therefore, security personnel, although well meaning, often can be triggering to the survivor. To some, the gender of the medical professional can be a barrier, no matter how empathic, kind, and knowledgeable that medical professional may be. Survivor advocates create a safe space for the survivor to know that they are not alone and that there is someone who has experienced human trafficking and now is able to provide assistance. The patient finds in the survivor advocate someone who is actively listening and who truly understands what they have been through, not because they read it in a book or took a class but because the survivor advocate has walked the same path, the same journey, and made her/his/their way out on the other side; and in so doing the patient understands that this is possible for them too. This is critical for patient success, healing, and restoration.

One patient recently said to me, "I can't believe someone is here who understands. I want to be an advocate too someday. Thank you for helping me."

Survivor advocates are as critical to the emergency response team as other clinical staff. If we value the response to our human trafficking patients and their care, we must value the experience and empathy that survivor advocate employees bring to our hospitals and clinics.

A Survivor Leader's Recommendations

Suleman Masood, Survivor Advocate

Safe Space

A medical professional's practice and intentions will never be sufficient unless they are able to create a safe space. Throughout my victimization, my trafficker made an effort to concentrate my injuries in areas covered by clothes. Because I had to be physically exposed in order to be treated, I was surprised that law enforcement was permitted to speak with me in the exam room and would have preferred to be dressed in a separate space for this line of questioning. Creating a safe space is key for a patient to disclose.

Withhold Judgment

No matter what the patient may look like the night they are admitted, it is imperative that no judgment is passed. While receiving an invoice during my discharge, a receptionist made comments to suggest that I was in a street fight or was a gang member because of my gender and age. Patients don't plan to come in looking like hell: in fact, their poor physical condition often is the very cause for admission.

Communicate

If an individual is victimized in one county and decides to move to another, it is crucial for the assigned victim advocate and the county representative of the new location to communicate with each other. When a victim moves away from the county they were victimized in, a lack of communication between a county representative and victim advocate may arise where one assumes the other will follow up and vice versa. This almost always leads to a delay in health insurance and benefits needed for a survivor to move on with their lives and start over.

Expedited Referrals

We need a common referral form for both doctors and medical social workers to help identify the risk factors of both sex and labor trafficking and to serve as an expedited referral that can be made to a partnering agency for trauma victims. This would greatly expedite the process and enhance the level of care for a patient. When healthcare professionals expedite care for patients, they become the driving force for their healing. My personal trauma (both physical and mental) has taught me sheer willpower, and I attribute my resilience to those who took the time to care for my well-being and ask the necessary questions to enhance my level of care.

We as professionals owe it to those at risk to reduce our naiveté and seek the knowledge necessary in keeping up with current crimes that affect families, such as human trafficking.

I Am a Survivor

Wendy Barnes, Author, *And Life Continues: Sex Trafficking and My Journey to Freedom*

> December 1998. Portland, Oregon
>
> I am so tired of living like this. Greg is evil, he is mean, but what can I do? He's the father of my kids. I don't have any money or anywhere to go. I'm pregnant. How can I bring another child into this world when this is the way I am living? Greg is right. I'm a horrible mother. Soon I will bring yet another child into this messed up life that I am living. (Excerpt from *And Life Continues: Sex Trafficking and My Journey to Freedom* by Wendy Barnes)

My name is Wendy Barnes and I am a survivor of sex trafficking. I was trafficked for 13 years from Seattle, Washington, to Southern California by my first boyfriend, a young man nearly my own age whom I met in high school when I was 15. He is the father of my three beautiful children, all born while I was being trafficked. In addition to the healthcare I received during my pregnancies, I had multiple encounters with healthcare professionals for other reasons while being trafficked.

Any time I visited a healthcare facility, I would have looked to the outside observer like an average person. There was nothing about my appearance that would have given anyone a clue that anything was wrong. In fact, all of Greg's "girls" worked very hard to not be noticed by anyone. If we had visible signs of injuries, our trafficker typically did not permit us to seek medical care; on the rare occasion he did, we were always careful to hide bruises or injuries from others, or we made up what we thought were "credible" stories to explain away the evidence.

Why Didn't I Reach Out for Help?

The intense brainwashing tactics our trafficker used to keep us in line and obedient also convinced us that we were worthless and that nobody would ever care about us except for him. These beliefs were beaten into us so deeply that we became what he made us to be. I believed I was worthless, that I was pathetic, and that nobody would ever love me but him.

What I remember most vividly from my many visits to the emergency department (ED) was how busy and overworked the nurses were. I saw the frustration in their eyes, heard the hurried tones in their voices, and I felt bad for them. I didn't want to add any more work to their already full plates. "Human trafficking" was not a common term while I was being trafficked from 1986 to 1999; but people did talk about domestic violence, and I knew I was a victim of that. I believed while I was trafficked that if anyone found out that I was a victim of domestic violence and that I had children in my home, then the police and child protective services (CPS) would be called; and I would have to be ready to leave Greg immediately, at that instant, to start a new life. I'm not certain how I came to believe that; it may have come from my trafficker directly or from listening to other people around me. I just knew that if I wasn't ready to leave my abuser, at the very moment someone found out about the abuse, then my children would be taken from me.

I remember being asked if I was a victim of domestic violence, and I always said, "NO." I could only imagine what would have happened if I had ever said yes: the nurse would have to call the police and CPS (whether she wanted to or not), drama would erupt, and there would be many people in the examining room, all talking *about* me but never *to* me. The nurse would now have even more on her plate because of me, and I would feel guilty about that.

In "the life" (slang for sex trafficking), we were always blamed by our trafficker for anything that did not go right. We learned early on that if we took responsibility for whatever was "wrong" and profusely apologized, sometimes the consequence from Greg wouldn't be as bad. Over time, we learned to take responsibility for anything that ever went wrong. We learned that anything that went wrong was always our fault, and because of that we always yearned to be "good." To me, being good meant that I did not cause anyone any trouble: *Don't be noticed, be invisible*.

Even so, when I visited a healthcare facility, I always hoped that one of the nurses would notice enough to talk with me in private. I always secretly wished that one of the nurses would look at me and say, "I want to know if you are truly OK. I want you to come back here in one week and check in with me. Ask for me specifically and I will come out to see you. I want to know that you are OK." Of course, I would not have shown up – the "rules" were too ingrained in me. But I wanted someone or anyone to know that I was not OK.

It would not be unreasonable for someone who has not been trafficked or abused to wonder why I didn't just tell the nurses what was going on. Surely that was a safe place to reveal my secrets, right? It may be difficult to understand what "reality" looks like to an abuse victim. The reality is I wasn't allowed to say "I'm not OK," even though I desperately needed to feel that I existed in the mind of another human being even if I wasn't present. I needed someone to *know* that I was not OK, but I couldn't *tell* them. In my childlike view of the world, just knowing that someone in the world knew that I was not OK would have made me feel less alone in the world.

During most of my trafficking experience, we moved around a lot. There were two times that I lived at the same location for more than a year, and it was during one of those times, in 1999, that a nurse practitioner perhaps unknowingly made a difference that would ultimately change my life.

I was 29 years old, pregnant with my third child, and living near 136th and Division in Portland, Oregon. Because we had lived in the same place for over a year, I was able to see the same nurse practitioner for my entire pregnancy. As had long been my practice, I had made sure never to go to the doctor if I had visible signs of injuries, and I had become very skilled at presenting as a "Single Mother of Two."

Near the end of my pregnancy, I was visiting the nurse practitioner once a week. I don't know what she had seen over the previous months that would make her think something was wrong; maybe she just had a gut feeling. At the end of my appointment one day, she helped me sit up on the exam table. As always, I stared down at the ground or maybe out the window. I heard her say, "Wendy," and I responded, "Yeah." I glanced her way but did not make eye contact. She waited.... I was so uncomfortable. *Why isn't she talking? Maybe she is trying to show me something?* I finally allowed myself to look directly at her.

Only then did she ask, in a very soft, calming voice, "Wendy, if something were wrong, would you tell me?"

This was such a strange question! As I quickly racked my brain for the appropriate answer to give her – an answer that would not make Greg angry with me – I also thought about how much I liked this lady. I didn't want to lie to her because I respected her. I wanted to tell her the truth but knew that was not an option. I knew that, as a nurse, she was a mandated reporter, and I mistakenly thought that if I told her the truth, she would have to call the police or social services even though I was no longer a minor. I looked down at my hands and spoke softly. "No."

Another pause of uncomfortable silence, and I looked up at her again. I could see that she knew something was wrong, but she had no proof. She couldn't call CPS or the police on me simply because I replied "No" to her question, or could she?

She continued, her voice still soft, "If there was help, if I can find you help, would you accept that help?"

I stiffened as the image of "help" flashed through my mind: the police barging through the door of our apartment with their guns drawn, Greg grabbing the kids and using them as hostages. Everyone screaming and yelling, the kids crying – and in the end, the kids and I would be outside in the cold rain with no place to go. That was my vision of "help."

I relaxed as much as I could and very politely told her that no, I did not want her help. Very kindly she replied, "If you ever change your mind, know that you can come back here, and I will find you help."

I wish I could have felt what you might be feeling now as you read this. Relieved? Safe? Tempted to let her help me? But I could not feel anything, not in that instant. My training to be on guard 24 hours a day, 7 days a week, 365 days a year was stronger than her kindness at that moment. Instinctively I knew I had to keep my guard up to protect Greg, to protect myself and my kids. I was so afraid of saying or doing something "wrong" that I could not process what was happening. I didn't realize at that moment that my nurse practitioner had planted a seed, a seed that would soon take root.

I would typically walk to and from my obstetric (OB) appointments because we lived only about a mile away, and I treasured that time for a bit of peace and quiet. On my walk home, these were my thoughts, the conversation I had with myself that day:

> That sure did feel like she cared about me.
> But Greg always said nobody would ever care about me but him.
> Seemingly out of nowhere, another voice broke into the conversation in my mind:
> But what if Greg is lying?
> What else could he be lying to you about?
> What if Greg doesn't really love you?

That last thought was too much for me to bear. If Greg didn't love me, then I thought that would make me unlovable. That thought was so painful that I remember, even today, how I aggressively pushed it out of my mind. I was afraid of that reality, that Greg had been lying to me this entire time, that this was just a game to him and that he didn't really love me, that he didn't love any of us. I was determined never to let that thought enter my consciousness again.

What happened next was even more powerful. What happened next was a shift in my soul. The words I am about to use are not words that were said; they reflect something that happened within me, to me. It was a realization.

> When was the last time I had felt safe enough, without fear of retribution, to say the word 'No' to an adult?
> When had anyone ever respected my 'No?'

The nurse practitioner's seed had taken root in my soul. When I got home from my appointment, I had a strength within me that I had never felt before. I had so much strength that when I got home, I moved out of the bedroom I shared with Greg and into the bedroom with my two children. I informed the other "girls" and Greg that this is where my kids and I would be and that even though I know that I'm not allowed to go anywhere or do anything without his permission, I was taking a stand and removing myself from this chaos and will stay in my room with my kids for the rest of my life. Perhaps that sounds childlike to you. It was the most adult I had ever felt. It took all the strength I could muster. I had put my foot down. I was emotionally removing myself from the monster.

Even though the nurse had planted the seed and the seed had taken root, it took time for the new plant to sprout and for a flower to blossom. How much time? Two weeks later I gave birth to my third child, and 2 weeks after that, the "help" that had flashed through my mind when the nurse was talking to me came true. A SWAT team came to our door. At first, I envisioned this would lead to freedom from this life. That vision quickly soured as my hands were placed behind my back and my wrists were enclosed with handcuffs.

The girls and women who were under Greg's control at that time ranged from 14 to 36 years old. I was 29. Because I had three children with Greg and had been with him the longest and he had placed most of the cars and apartments he used in my name, the police assumed that I was just as responsible for the trafficking as he was. I was too afraid to talk to the police, to tell them my story; silence in police presence was one of the many rules Greg demanded, and I complied without hesitation. Otherwise, the consequences were unthinkable. I always did what Greg told me to do: "Put your eyes to the ground and don't say a word." Within a short time, I was pleading guilty to two counts of promoting prostitution. The judge sentenced me to 2 years in prison. It was there, in prison, that the nurse's seed had a chance to bloom.

I have shared this story with audiences across the United States for the past 10 years. It took that long for it to occur to me, "I should find her and tell her what she did for me." It was an arduous process, but I was finally able to contact the clinic and request my records so I could find that nurse practitioner and tell her how much I appreciated what she had done to make me feel safe enough to say no. I wanted to tell her how she had planted that seed of dignity that had changed my life. After a few weeks, I got a letter in the mail from the clinic, informing me that they destroy records after 10 years. They had no idea which nurse practitioner had helped me so long ago.

I wish to this day that I knew who she was. I want her to know that her kindness was not ignored or brushed aside. Instead, I honor that kind and gentle nurse practitioner with this message. "Thank you for seeing me. Thank you for speaking softly so I would feel comfortable. Thank you for creating an environment that made me feel safe. It was your words, your kindness that was the seed that took root, sprouted, and has grown into a beautiful flower that thrives in the bouquet of flowers I am today."

Now, I am the Coordinator of Dignity Health's Human Trafficking (HT) Response Program. Dignity Health is one of the largest healthcare systems in the country and the largest hospital provider in California. In 2014, Dignity Health launched their HT Response Program to assist in the identification of HT victims/survivors and provision of trauma-informed care and services. In my role I share my expertise and experiences to help healthcare professionals understand the often complex dynamics of sex and labor trafficking and the importance for trauma-informed intervention strategies, like the PEARR Tool.

Dignity Health partnered with HEAL Trafficking and Pacific Survivor Center to develop this tool, the "PEARR Tool," which guides healthcare professionals on how to provide trauma-informed victim assistance in healthcare settings. PEARR stands for Provide privacy, Educate, Ask, Respect and Respond. Respecting a patient's decision to disclose or deny victimization or accept or reject services is key to a trauma-informed approach. To learn more about the PEARR Tool, please visit dignityhealth.org/human-trafficking-response. And, to all the nurses, nurse practitioners, doctors, and medical staff who have ever taken the time to plant a hopeful seed for others like me: “Thank you.”

Afterword

The contributors to this chapter include award-winning authors, speakers, and patient advocates who contract with medical and nonprofit organizations, governmental bodies, and training programs to advise on policy, evidence- and experience-based content, and a sustainable approach to educating professionals about human trafficking and ending human trafficking. We are deeply grateful for their contributions to this textbook. If you wish to hire a Survivor Consultant, please contact the individuals directly through their webpages or listed organizations, or contact the National Survivor Network: www.nationalsurvivornetwork.org/consultantspeakers-bureau/.

Chapter 20
Educating Our Students

Sara Schreiber, Micaela Cayton Garrido, and Michelle Lyman

Case Presentation

You are a pediatric intern called down to the Emergency Department (ED) for an admission. Your patient Carmen, an 18-year-old woman, sits on a stretcher in the ED hallway, waiting with her uncle for you to admit her to the hospital. Carmen's chief complaint is "I cannot move my hands." She presents for full thickness burns on the palmar and dorsal surfaces of both hands as well as over her forearms.

Carmen states that she was using cooking oil as part of her job as a line cook at her uncle's fast food restaurant where she works. The burns occurred five days ago when hot cooking oil overflowed onto her arms. She has been treating herself by wrapping cloth around her hands and forearms.

The cloth has been sticking to her skin which is red and edematous, and because it is painful, she has avoided removing the cloth over the last two days. Carmen states she previously has experienced burns due to her work, but this time the burns are more severe and interfere with her work.

The emergency medicine physician estimates that burns cover 7% of Carmen's total body surface area. Complete blood count indicates a mild leukocytosis, while a CRP is within normal limits and there are no electrolyte abnormalities. Carmen's vital signs have remained normal and stable, with the exception of mild tachycardia.

Carmen appears exhausted, and the burns cause extreme pain with the slightest movement. The burns ooze a green discharge, and you note limited range of motion due to swelling. Carmen says the pain has progressively worsened over the last three days. When you

S. Schreiber (✉)
SBH Health System, Bronx, NY, USA

M. C. Garrido
Legal Aid Society of Metropolitan Family Services, Chicago, IL, USA

M. Lyman
University of North Carolina Hospitals, Chapel Hill, NC, USA

K. E. Titchen, E. Miller (eds.), *Medical Perspectives on Human Trafficking in Adolescents*, https://doi.org/10.1007/978-3-030-43367-3_20

ask why Carmen has not been able to seek medical care sooner, her uncle answers for her, saying that they were unable to afford insurance and cannot afford a hospital stay. Now that the pain has prevented full movement, it is interfering with her work and her ability to earn her room and board.

The uncle says he was Carmen's legal guardian until she turned 18 earlier this year. He answers all of the questions on her behalf while Carmen sits quietly on the stretcher and avoids eye contact. When you ask the uncle to leave the room, he insists that anything you have to say to Carmen you can say to him – he has raised her for several years and they have no secrets. The uncle is forceful, and Carmen appears even more uncomfortable as you explain that standard best-practice medical care necessitates that you have private time alone with your patient. Carmen's uncle refuses to leave. You postpone this conversation about privacy, stating that with signs of infection and the possibility for dehydration, Carmen needs to be admitted for rehydration and antibiotics.

Once Carmen is wheeled away from her uncle to complete registration and to be brought to her room upstairs, there is a palpable sense of relief; she is visibly more relaxed and talks more freely. However, Carmen also volunteers that she is worried about missing work and wants to get back as soon as she can. She cannot remember the last time she visited a doctor.

You recognize the opportunity for a private and confidential conversation and begin a HEEADSS (Home & Environment, Education & Employment, Activities, Drugs, Sexuality, and Suicide/Depression) psychosocial assessment where Carmen shares that she has neither graduated nor attended school for the last five years. She spends most of her time working for her uncle who says he needs the extra help to make enough money to pay for her food and lodging. Carmen started living with her uncle at age thirteen when her mother was incarcerated for drug possession.

When you asked about a history of violence or abuse, Carmen avoids eye contact and states, "Life with my mom was tough. She would often take off for days at a time and I know she'd be using." Carmen initially thought that living with her uncle would be a relief because she was hoping for a more consistent adult in her life and an escape from the chaos of men who rotated in and out of her mother's life.

Now, she lives with her uncle and relies on him for her sole source of transportation. Carmen's wages go straight to her uncle purportedly to pay for expenses, and she is not able to participate in any activities outside of her work.

When asked about work, Carmen tells you about the fast food restaurant and the other workers there, "There's a couple of guys who use cocaine to take the edge off of the night shift. I don't touch the stuff, not after seeing what it did to my mom. Sometimes they'll bring in booze and I have a few drinks."

Carmen tells you that she has a couple of coworkers who are in their 30s and 40s who she says "are creepers," and you notice that she becomes visibly uncomfortable and squirms in her hospital bed as she talks about them. You tell Carmen that part of your job is to make sure that she is safe, and you ask Carmen if anyone at work has made her feel unsafe. Carmen looks around nervously and tells you "No, I feel safe at work."

Carmen's uncle has found his way back into the patient room. Carmen instantly becomes stiff in her bed and refuses to look up. Your interview with her is concluded as the uncle angrily makes calls in the room, speaking with someone on the other line.

On the morning after Carmen's admission, her uncle is waiting for the medical team. He is insistent that his niece be released immediately. Carmen does not speak and is sitting stiffly on the bed dressed in her street clothes. The uncle expresses that they cannot afford another night in the hospital, and Carmen will be signing herself out against medical advice. He refuses to discuss the situation with the medical team and simply repeats that they are leaving, and he knows the consequences.

How to Teach the Case

When using case-based learning to teach health professional learners, there are several steps to help guide the individual or group to the key elements of the case. The first is to establish the objectives of the case: what should the learners take away or accomplish after finishing the case? Establishing key definitions, such as the definition for human trafficking in this scenario, will be at the forefront of the review. The second step is for learners to identify systematically the components of the history taking and physical exam that led to their conclusions about the case: what about the case suggests human trafficking? Learners may synthesize their existing knowledge with new definitions and theory. Learning need not be limited to arriving at the final diagnosis and identification of human trafficking, but instead incorporate trauma-sensitive approaches to care and discussions of systems-level changes as well as advocacy on behalf of patients.

Carmen's story is based on an amalgamation of human trafficking survivors seen in healthcare settings and highlights common patterns of physical injury and mental health concerns associated with human trafficking. These health concerns negatively impact victims' and survivors' ability to rebuild their lives and increase the likelihood that survivors will need healthcare well after their exit from human trafficking. Thus, human trafficking education for health professional students is critical to ensure successful patient interaction and possible intervention. Although there are many lessons to be learned from Carmen's story, not all of which can be contained in a single chapter, the following elements are essential to a trauma-sensitive human trafficking curriculum. These lessons are not exclusive to a specific profession but can be applied broadly to nearly all members of the healthcare team.

This chapter considers all parts of the case review as a method to teach learners about human trafficking. Figure 20.1 shows the progression through the case, from accessing Carmen's chief complaint to taking a more detailed history, performing a physical exam, and finally applying all of the knowledge to form a differential diagnosis and plan of action. However, as Fig. 20.1 illustrates, there are multifactorial elements that influence all parts of the encounter from the history the patient provides to the differential diagnoses that learners may consider. Finally, the chapter reviews other forms of human trafficking medical education, comparing the goals of those different modalities.

Chief Complaint

For many patients, there may be several health concerns that would warrant assessment and treatment by a health professional. However, there may be one specific health concern that brought the patient into the healthcare setting specifically, and they are seeking a solution to that one problem or concern. With persons who have been or

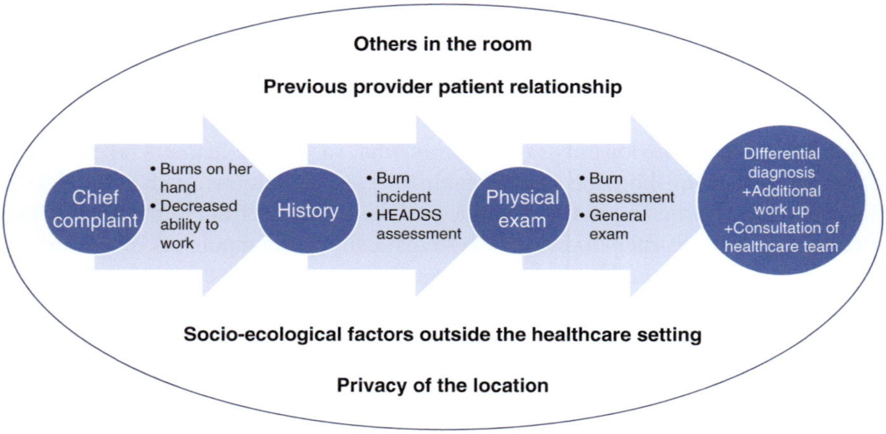

Fig. 20.1 Steps for case review with Carmen's case as an example

are being trafficked, there are many obstacles that may interfere with their access to care. When they do have access to care, it may also be under close supervision.

Carmen presents with burns that have been untreated for several days. Her main concern is treatment for the burns that would impact her ability to work.

History Taking

In addition to investigating the immediate medical reasons and chief complaint that brought her to medical attention, it is important to address the multifaceted socio-ecological clues of Carmen's trafficking. [For more about the social ecological framework of human trafficking, see Chap. 1, Table 1.] Her case demonstrates the critical role of the healthcare setting in a survivor's life: notably, it provides an opportunity to identify human trafficking and ask Carmen about her living and working situation. History taking represents the opportunity for the clinician to identify trafficking and offer assistance [1].

Through respecting patient autonomy and using a trauma-informed approach, clinicians enable a safe space for medical and psychosocial care (which may or may not include disclosure) and the potential for follow-through intervention and assistance [2].

Trauma-Informed Care

A trauma-sensitive healthcare environment maximizes patient-centered interaction at every level of care. Practitioners are aware of the possibility of trauma in a patient's physical symptoms, emotional responses, and interactions with practitioners and other hospital staff [3]. Practitioners recognize that trauma can affect a patient's decision-making process, and they create a *trauma-sensitive* environment to foster a safe physical, emotional, and psychological space for patients [4]. Trauma-informed healthcare professionals practice compassion and understanding of patients who may come across as being "difficult" or presenting with seemingly negative coping skills and do not force patients to disclose to connect them to services and supports [3, 5].

To be clear, the goal is *not* disclosure; rather the goals are to address the immediate needs of the patient, build trust, and communicate an open-door policy so patients are aware that ongoing medical and psychosocial support without judgment or invasive questioning is available [2].

Creating a Safe Space for the Patient

When healthcare professionals suspect that a patient is a possible human trafficking survivor, they must account for additional safety considerations. The first step is making sure the patient is alone or separated from their companion to enable a more in-depth conversation. As in Carmen's case, traffickers often seek to control a patient's interactions with others, including in the hospital setting [6]. A companion who answers on behalf of the patient or who insists on being present at all times raises a red flag [2]. If a healthcare professional senses an unhealthy power dynamic between the patient and their companion, it is best practice to separate the patient, even if momentarily, to enable a more in-depth assessment [2]. A healthcare professional may be able to achieve separation naturally during the exam but also might need to use other more creative techniques, such as asking the patient's companion to fill out paperwork in a separate area [7].

When alone, in addition to posing open-ended, nonjudgmental questions, clinicians should seek to discuss the patient's situation using patient-centered, motivational interviewing-style questions. This helps build trust and enables more openness from the patient [5]. The medical safe haven at Dignity Health in Sacramento, California, created and piloted the use of the PEARR (Provide Privacy, Educate, Ask Questions, Respect and Respond) tool to help guide clinicians through addressing the potential for trafficking with patients [8] (see Chap. 21, Fig. 21.1). Not only does it reinforce the privacy required to ask sensitive questions, but it also provides survivor-informed, patient-centered questions for patients. The U.S. Department of Health and Human Services has also created a screening tool guided by survivor leaders and subject matter experts (HHS) [9]. Both the PEARR and the HHS tool provide informed questions and steps for screening for trafficking; however neither has formal validation in part because of their innovative nature and the lack of research that exists about human trafficking and long-term outcomes.

Mandatory Reporting

For healthcare professionals, when human trafficking concerns arise, mandatory reporting requirements may need consideration [1]. It is important to be familiar with reporting requirements under state laws. This may create a conundrum: how might healthcare staff build trust with a patient if the law mandates reporting? Learners may consider how and when in the interview that they would address the issue of mandatory reporting with their patient. They should be encouraged to consider the effects on the patient-provider relationship of reporting human trafficking without the adolescent patient's consent. In the chapter scenario, Carmen is 18 years old, but if she were 17, how would that change the interaction and kind of questions that must be asked? [See Chap. 18 for information on mandatory reporting.]

Patient Autonomy

Patient-centered care places emphasis on the patient's sense of agency and choice among all the options available to them. Conversely, medical paternalism strips away a patient's autonomy and sense of agency and may place victims of human trafficking at increased risk for retribution from their traffickers [10]. For example, if a health professional decides on behalf of a patient when and how that patient should leave the trafficking situation, this could create conditions that put the patient at risk for harm by their trafficker(s). In addition to putting the patient at risk for interpersonal violence, medical paternalism may destroy the trust built with the patient. Additionally, medical paternalism may mimic the dynamics of power and control a survivor has with their trafficker, as can happen during the physical exam, possibly triggering memories of past traumatic events or causing revictimization.

It is of utmost importance for clinicians to avoid medical paternalism [10]. For health professional learners, it is important to dissect and discuss the emotions and tension that arise while assisting patients like Carmen and seeking to respect their autonomy. In Carmen's case, you suspect that her living situation is unsafe, but because she is legally an adult, she is free to decide when and with whom she leaves the hospital, even against medical advice. A clinician's job includes communicating to the patient what is medically necessary, guiding decision-making by providing relevant information, and being empathic and compassionate even if the adult patient chooses a course contrary to their own best interest [10].

Physical Exam

Patient autonomy also plays a large role in the physical exam. Trafficking often strips individuals of their agency over their own bodies. Invasions into their space and physical contact with healthcare professionals can cause retraumatization. Thus, creating a safe space for trauma-informed physical examinations is paramount. This necessitates the employment of trauma-informed techniques in both the preparation of the physical space and the treatment of the patient during the examination itself. Ideally the exam would take place in a quiet or calm location with respect for the patient's privacy through the use of curtains/blinds. The patient should be provided a support person if the patient desires this, and the clinician should ask permission to conduct the exam before touching the patient. A trauma-informed examination demystifies the process for the patient, uses terminology that the patient understands, and mirrors the patient's words when appropriate. This includes an explanation of the exam, how long the process could take, reasons why the examination is necessary, and that the exam can be stopped at any time [9]. [See Chap. 16 for detailed information on the trauma-informed gynecologic exam.]

Differential Diagnosis

In Carmen's situation in the case study, in addition to needing a primary and secondary burn assessment to gauge hydration status and extent of skin damage, you must consider the effects of delayed treatment and increased risk of infection [11]. The discharge, leukocytosis, and edema around the burn are supporting evidence of a potential infection that developed in the 3 days since her burn. You will need to consider potential sequelae including sepsis, need for skin graft, and potential loss of function to her limb with a consult to the plastic surgery or orthopedics team to assess her hand for possible surgical intervention.

It is important to also consider the potential mental health challenges affecting Carmen. Individuals who have been trafficked are at increased risk for developing posttraumatic stress disorder (PTSD), complex type. While complex PTSD is not an official diagnosis under the Diagnostic and Statistical Manual of Mental Disorders, 5th Edition: DSM-5 diagnosis, studies of women and children who have been abused or exposed to prolonged interpersonal violence often exhibit symptoms that are not captured within the PTSD diagnostic criteria [12].

A patient with PTSD may present with emotional dysregulation, hyperarousal, depressed mood, anxiety, and avoidance symptoms, to name a few. Although someone can develop PTSD from one isolated traumatic event, complex PTSD stems from exposure to ongoing, interpersonal traumatic stress. A patient with complex trauma might appear with pervasive personality disturbance, particularly borderline personality features (e.g., impaired affect modulation, self-destructive and impulsive behavior, identity disturbance, impaired relationships), persistent somatization, depression, and recurrent dissociative symptoms [13]. [See Chap. 9 for detailed information about the psychological effects of human trafficking.]

In Carmen's case, the limited history you were able to gather makes a diagnosis of PTSD difficult. During your interview with Carmen, she mentioned substance use. Trafficked persons may develop substance use disorder as a result of trafficking, either as a result of manipulation by their trafficker [14] or as a means of coping with the trauma of trafficking. While Carmen does not currently use substances, several of her coworkers – who may also be trafficked – do use substances to perform at work and cope. [See Chap. 13 for more information on human trafficking and substance use.]

Clues/Clinical Red Flags

In addition to the specificities of Carmen's case, several other socioecological indicators constitute push and pull factors and red flags for human trafficking.

Understanding Push and Pull Factors of Trafficking

To better understand and empathize with patients, it is crucial for healthcare providers to be aware of the factors that *push* individuals into being trafficked and the factors that *pull* individuals into being trafficked (see Table 20.1), which can be understood using a socioecological model [17–19]. Now, take a look at Carmen's push and pull factors (see Table 20.2).

When to Include Trafficking in the Differential Diagnosis: Identifying Red Flags

It is important to recognize red flags that may indicate your patient is a victim of human trafficking. Red flags may appear through patient interaction, timeline of symptoms, immediate presentation, history of trauma, and access to resources (see Table 20.3). Next, take a look at Carmen's red flags (see Table 20.4).

Table 20.1 Trafficking push and pull factors [15, 16]

	Push	Pull
Societal	Lack of awareness of sex and labor trafficking Sexualization of children Lack of resources	Demand for cheap labor
Community	Peer pressure Societal norms Social isolation Gang involvement Under-resourced schools, neighborhoods, and communities	Promise of fame and luxury Promise of better socioeconomic opportunities or life conditions
Relationship	Family conflict, disruption, or dysfunction	Seeking marriage or a relationship
Individual	History of adverse childhood experiences especially sexual or physical abuse Homelessness or runaway LGBT Foster care Juvenile/criminal justice system history Stigma and discrimination Substance use/abuse Low IQ Physical disability Earlier pubertal maturation	Seeking a better life than before Drug and alcohol dependency

Table 20.2 Carmen's push and pull factors [15, 16]

	Push	Pull
Societal	Lack of resources and awareness Carmen got "lost in the system"	Demand for cheap labor
Community	Seeming lack of support when Carmen was living with her mom and when her mother was incarcerated Rarely sees doctors, lack of exposure to help	Pressure to make money since Carmen was on her own
Relationship	Lack of other family support	Uncle is only caregiver Carmen feels indebted to her uncle and feels the need to make money for him
Individual	Early history of abuse and neglect Carmen has not attended school for 5 years	Seeking place to live due to maternal incarceration Seeking more stable, less chaotic life than with mom

Table 20.3 Trafficking red flags [20]

Labor	Recent immigration history (especially if lack of access to immigration documentation) Work-related (typically preventable) injuries Sweatshops, commercial agricultural work, domestic care, construction sites, restaurant, custodial work Prohibited from leaving work site Current working circumstances are not what an individual had been promised
Sex	Trades sex for food, shelter, money, drugs, other necessities Has a trafficker or pimp or "daddy" or "boyfriend" Sexually transmitted diseases Signs of rape or sexual abuse Inappropriately dressed for the weather
Both	Bruising, broken bones, other indications of medically under or untreated problems Not paid directly, owes a large debt and unable to pay it off Posttraumatic stress or other psychiatric disorders Unfamiliarity with city or town, claims of just visiting Fearful, anxious, depressed, submissive, tense, or nervous/paranoid Heavy security and surveillance at place of work/living Critical illnesses that are uncontrolled like diabetes, heart disease, asthma, cancer Malnourished, poor personal hygiene Not in possession of travel documentation or valid identification documents Apparent intimidation by person accompanying the person Signs of substance use/addiction Use of a "translator" during history Does not drive or travel alone Lives and works in the same place, works excessively long/unusual hours Tattoos or physical branding

Table 20.4 Carmen's red flags

Patient interaction	Limited answers in the presence of trafficker/uncle Carmen does not clearly identify as being trafficked
Familial trafficking patterns	Earlier history of abuse and neglect, push factor toward trafficking
Barriers to patient communication	Having uncle/trafficker in the room Uncle/trafficker unwilling to leave patient alone at first Uncle/trafficker abruptly ending care
Limited access to resources	Does not have access to her paycheck Limited mobility dependent on her uncle/trafficker

Research suggests that the interaction with Carmen or someone like her in your clinical practice is highly probable. One study of 173 foreign-born and US-born trafficking survivors who were trafficked in the USA for sex or labor demonstrated that 73% of all respondents wanted to see a healthcare provider while in their trafficking situation. Sixty-eight percent of all respondents reported that they were successful in seeing a healthcare provider while being trafficked and primarily visited emergency or urgent care practitioners, primary care providers, dentists, and obstetrician gynecologists [21]. Data show that healthcare professionals see trafficked patients in a variety of fields; thus, healthcare professional students need comprehensive curricula on human trafficking. [See Chap. 17 for more on trafficking and medical subspecialties.]

Action Steps: Safety Planning and Establishing Follow-Up

A nuanced discussion on documenting trafficking and creating a safety plan involves the following steps:

Healthcare staff must consider the unique needs of the patient. To practice using the case scenario, consider Carmen's safety planning needs not just with her uncle but with her coworkers as well [19].

Next, refer to the stages of change model (Fig. 20.2) as a guide to determine safety planning methods and strategies. The stages of change model rely on a motivational interviewing technique to help healthcare staff determine how best they can support a survivor seeking services [21]. It is important to listen closely to the language the patient is using to determine at which stage of change the patient is functioning. A practitioner should be familiar with what "change talk" (e.g., "I want to get out of this situation") vs. "sustain talk" (e.g., "I have nowhere to live"; "It's not so bad"; "I'm living my best life") sounds like. A patient using "change talk" is likely in a *preparation* or even *action* stage of change, while a patient using "sustain talk" is likely still in the *precontemplation* stage of change and requires using motivational interviewing skills in order to help bring the patient into a contemplation stage of change. Remember that it is always impor-

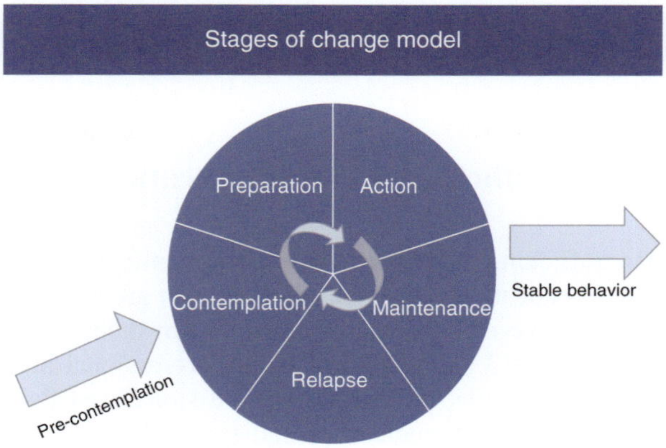

Fig. 20.2 Stages of change model [21]. (Adapted from Prochaska and DiClemente's Transtheoretical Model of Behavior Change)

tant to focus on building a trusting relationship through maintaining a nonjudgmental stance since the end result is increased motivation to change [22].

Trafficking survivors often have needs that extend beyond medical care, including housing, legal troubles, food insecurity, and more [5]. The wide breadth of services a trafficking survivor may require, highlights the need for a team-based approach and for protocols that make connections to resources seamless [2].

Safety planning must account for the following:

1. Awareness of who has access to patient's medical records and how notes are written in the electronic medical record (EMR) [22, 23]
2. Awareness of how to employ International Classification of Diseases, Tenth Revision, Clinical Modification (ICD-10) codes for human trafficking and ensuring that all medical personnel are trained in understanding these codes
3. Awareness of the party responsible for the patient's payment (the trafficker, insurance company, etc.) [22, 23]

In the chapter scenario, Carmen is at the age of majority, but her uncle has acted as her guardian for many years. He attempted to prevent her admission to the hospital, and he may be financially responsible for her hospital stay. Because of his extensive control in her life, he may have forced her to sign Health Insurance Portability and Accountability Act (HIPAA) forms and permissions allowing him to view her medical records. Direct documentation in open medical records should be carefully considered and any hospital-wide protocol for patient safety and confidentiality followed [23].

Scheduling follow-up appointments is an important method for building rapport and helps address the long-term medical issues that result from human trafficking (e.g., PTSD, chronic pain, etc.). Provide a prescription-style written follow-up appointment for the patient to show the patient's trafficker as proof of need for medical follow-up [24]. [Refer to Chap. 19 Survivor Insights for more on the importance of provider-patient trust.]

Existing Human Trafficking Medical Education

Currently, human trafficking medical education is not uniform nor universal. There is a broad variety of educational materials and an even greater number of institutions that use none of the existing materials to inform their providers of human trafficking [25, 26]. A 2013 summation of health professional human trafficking education revealed 27 programs for healthcare professionals (HCPs) [27]. There are many curricula across different medical specialties and disciplines for nurses [28], physicians [29], dentists [30], midwives [31], and mental health counselors [32].

Across training and education resources, modalities range from international guidelines [33] to workshop presentations [34]. Amidst the various training initiatives, there is a call for standardization among training programs; core competencies in HCP education could ensure consistent improved care of trafficked patients [35]. Several professional organizations have issued statements of support regarding collective human trafficking training within their professions, including the American Nurses Association (2010) [36, 37], American College of Obstetricians and Gynecologists (2011) [38], Institute of Medicine (2013) [39], American Medical Women's Association (2014) [40], American Academy of Pediatricians (2014) [41], Association of American Family Physicians (2015) [42], and the American Medical Association (2015) [43]. Currently, there is not a single leading professional group that oversees the content of human trafficking curricula, and the lack of standardization suggests the potential for discrepancies in care.

Training Objectives and Desired Outcomes

Medical educators outline common goals of educational interventions in a stepwise approach, with HCP participation and learning as the foundation for altering clinical behavior and improving quality of care for human trafficking survivors [27]. Because the power dynamic of human trafficking relies on the trafficker's manipulation and withholding of resources [36], improving the health of survivors requires HCP training with a human rights-based framework centered on providing the trafficked person with resources that enable them to make decisions in their best interest [35, 44].

Reviews of existing trafficking curricula emphasize the need for education centered on gender-sensitive, trauma-informed care (TIC) and material that is evidence based and survivor informed [35]. A 2015 qualitative study of mental health professionals highlighted the need for TIC: providers identified the effects of trauma as frequent barriers to care. In a study of 130 trafficking survivors, mental health professionals struggled with lack of patient engagement and difficulties assessing patients' history due to the sequelae of trauma [45]. Without training, clinicians may not be skilled at assisting patients through their trauma, which can impede effective and sensitive delivery of essential healthcare.

Curricular Assessment

Methods to assess an educational intervention's effectiveness include data collection preceding and following the intervention to measure knowledge acquisition [46]. The Health and Human Services Department's SOAR program (Stop, Observe, Ask, Respond to human trafficking) utilized this method when testing its pilot program with 180 HCPs [27]. Another assessment method is the use of self-survey after training related to the care of trafficked persons [47]. Some surveys employ clinical vignettes of real trafficking cases to assess objectively whether HCPs can identify trafficking in healthcare settings [45]. While surveys of self-reported changes in confidence reveal learner attitudes, clinical vignette assessments offer more objective results.

Researchers may also collect evidence of behavior changes associated with training. One 2015 study tracked HCPs who had received trafficking training versus those who had not. They found that those with training more often self-reported that after encountering a victim of sex trafficking, they had called the National Human Trafficking Hotline or referred the patient to human trafficking services [48]. Despite these few studies, there remains a dearth of direct curricular evaluation and assessment: only 20% of all programs participate in the evaluation of learner clinical performance [35], while other researchers note that none of the existing programs have withstood critical review [24]. In summary, a critical assessment and evaluation of human trafficking training programs are clearly needed to guide the implementation of effective training for healthcare professionals and to create the systems-level changes necessary for care of these patients.

The Future of Training Programs

The effectiveness and success of current programs inform the design of future trafficking trainings. Standardization across trafficking education is a primary objective, as researchers suggest that current resources are too diverse to assure consistent TIC (23, 31–32, 40). Reviews focus on the need for training to expand to more HCPs with the inclusion of those early in health professional training – such as medical, nursing, social work, and dental students – to ensure broad coverage across all healthcare specialties [49]. In addition, critical components of human trafficking for both sex and labor should be informed by content experts, educators, and survivors. One such study used a two-round Delphi method to obtain consensus among

30 professionals with expertise on the subject matter of human trafficking about the critical components to shape a framework for HT education and emphasized measurable content [50]. In a follow-up study using similar methodology, survivors of human trafficking shared expertise based on their lived experiences to inform criteria for HT education approaches and emphasized, by contrast, more "holistic" content emphasizing trauma-informed care and a strengths-based approach [51].

An alternative approach to standardized education has been the systematic analysis of training content. Researchers, including HT survivors, categorize components of current training based on essential elements to provide improved standards of care for HT victims [35, 49, 52]. This content may be used to create a standard model of training across a broad range of healthcare professions at the beginning of healthcare training.

References

1. Chisolm-Straker M, Baldwin S, Gaïgbé-Togbé B, Ndukwe N, Johnson PN, Richardson LD. Health care and human trafficking: we are seeing the unseen. J Health Care Poor Underserved. 2016;27:1220–33.
2. Shandro J, Chisolm-Straker M, Duber HC, Findlay SL, Munoz J, Schmitz G, et al. Human trafficking: a guide to identification and approach for the emergency physician. Ann Emerg Med. 2016;68:501–508.e1.
3. Macias-Konstantopoulos W. Human trafficking: the role of medicine in interrupting the cycle of abuse and violence. Ann Intern Med. 2016;165:582–8.
4. National Association of School Psychologists. Creating trauma-sensitive schools: supportive policies and practices for learning. Bethesda: National Association of School Psychologists; 2015.
5. Alpert EJ, Ahn R, Albright E, Purcell G, Burke TF, Macias-Konstantopoulos WL. Guidebook on identification, assessment, and response in the health care setting. Boston: Massachusetts General Hospital, Massachusetts Medical Society; 2014.
6. Baldwin SB, Eisenman DP, Sayles JN, Ryan G, Chuang KS. Identification of human trafficking victims in health care settings. Health Hum Rights. 2011;13:E36–49.
7. Raymond JG, Hughes DM. Sex trafficking of women in the United States: International and Domestic Trends. PsycEXTRA Dataset; 2001. https://doi.org/10.1037/e624522007-001.
8. Dignity Health. Using the PEARR tool [Internet]. [cited 2019 Oct 4]. Available from: https://www.dignityhealth.org/hello-humankindness/human-trafficking/victim-centered-and-trauma-informed/using-the-pearr-tool.
9. Office on Trafficking in Persons. Toolkit and guide: adult human trafficking screening [Internet]. [cited 2019 Oct 4]. Available from: https://www.acf.hhs.gov/otip/resource/nhhtacadultscreening.
10. Macias-Konstantopoulos WL. Caring for the trafficked patient: ethical challenges and recommendations for health care professionals. AMA J Ethics. 2017;19:80–90.
11. Burn Management [Internet]. World Health Organization; 2007. Available from: https://www.who.int/surgery/publications/Burns_management.pdf.
12. van der Kolk BA, Roth S, Pelcovitz D, Sunday S, Spinazzola J. Disorders of extreme stress: the empirical foundation of a complex adaptation to trauma. J Trauma Stress. 2005;18:389–99.
13. Taylor S, Asmundson GJG, Carleton RN. Simple versus complex PTSD: a cluster analytic investigation. J Anxiety Disord. 2006;20:459–72.

14. Polaris Project. The victims & traffickers [Internet]. [cited 2019 Oct 4]. Available from: https://polarisproject.org/victims-traffickers.
15. Ronda-Pérez E, Moen BE. Labour trafficking: challenges and opportunities from an occupational health perspective. PLoS Med. 2017;14:e1002440.
16. Lederer LJ, Wetzel CA. The health consequences of sex trafficking and their implications for identifying victims in healthcare facilities. Ann Health L. 2014;23:61.
17. Substance Abuse and Mental Health Services Administration. SAMHSA's concept of trauma and guidance for a trauma-informed approach [Internet]. Rockville, MD: Substance Abuse and Mental Health Services Administration; 2014. Report No.: HHS Publication No. (SMA) 14–4884. Available from: https://store.samhsa.gov/system/files/sma14-4884.pdf.
18. American College of Obstetricians and Gynecologists. Committee opinion: effective patient-physician communication [Internet]. 2014. Available from: http://www.acog.org/Clinical-Guidance-and-Publications/Committee-Opinions/Committee-on-Health-Care-for-Underserved-Women/Effective-Patient-Physician-Communication.
19. National Research Council. Victim and support services. Confronting commercial sexual exploitation and sex trafficking of minors in the United States. Washington, D.C.: National Academies Press; 2013.
20. Office on Trafficking in Persons. 10 ways you can help end trafficking [Internet]. [cited 2019 Oct 4]. Available from: https://www.acf.hhs.gov/otip/about/ways-endtrafficking.
21. Administration for Children and Families, National Human Trafficking Training and Technical Assistance Center. Adult human trafficking screening tool and guide [Internet]. 2018 [cited 2019 Jun 10]. Available from: https://www.acf.hhs.gov/otip/resource/nhhtacadultscreening.
22. Naar-King S, Suarez M. Motivational interviewing with adolescents and young adults. intrinsicchange.com; 2011.
23. Hemmings S, Jakobowitz S, Abas M, Bick D, Howard LM, Stanley N, et al. Responding to the health needs of survivors of human trafficking: a systematic review. BMC Health Serv Res. 2016;16:320.
24. Ottisova L, Smith P, Shetty H, Stahl D, Downs J, Oram S. Psychological consequences of child trafficking: an historical cohort study of trafficked children in contact with secondary mental health services. PLoS One. 2018;13:e0192321.
25. National Human Trafficking Hotline. Using the stages of change model [Internet]. 2012 [cited 2019 Oct 4]. Available from: https://humantraffickinghotline.org/resources/using-stages-change-model.
26. Berlinger N, Zacharias RL. Resources for teaching and learning about immigrant health care in health professions education. AMA J Ethics. 2019;21:E50–7.
27. Powell C, Dickins K, Stoklosa H. Training US health care professionals on human trafficking: where do we go from here? Med Educ Online. 2017;22:1267980.
28. Cole H. Human trafficking: implications for the role of the advanced practice forensic nurse. J Am Psychiatr Nurses Assoc. 2009;14:462–70.
29. Tracy EE, Konstantopoulos WM. Human trafficking: a call for heightened awareness and advocacy by obstetrician-gynecologists. Obstet Gynecol. 2012;119:1045–7.
30. O'Callaghan MG. Human trafficking and the dental professional. J Am Dent Assoc. 2012;143:498–504.
31. Dovydaitis T. Human trafficking: the role of the health care provider. J Midwifery Womens Health. 2010;55:462–7.
32. Coverdale J, Beresin EV, Louie AK, Balon R, Roberts LW. Human trafficking and psychiatric education: a call to action. Acad Psychiatry. 2016;40:119–23.
33. World Health Organization. Understanding and addressing violence against women [Internet]. Available from: https://apps.who.int/iris/bitstream/handle/10665/77394/WHO_RHR_12.42_eng.pdf;jsessionid=80525E002E239B82E6628B6C657155B6?sequence=1.

34. Office on Trafficking in Persons. SOAR to health and wellness training [Internet]. [cited 2019 Oct 4]. Available from: https://www.acf.hhs.gov/otip/training/soar-to-health-and-wellness-training.
35. Stoklosa H, Grace AM, Littenberg N. Medical education on human trafficking. AMA J Ethics. 2015;17:914–21.
36. Baldwin SB, Fehrenbacher AE, Eisenman DP. Psychological coercion in human trafficking: an application of Biderman's framework. Qual Health Res. 2015;25:1171–81.
37. American Nurses Association. Position Statement: the nurse's role in ethics and human rights: protecting and promoting individual worth, dignity, and human rights in practice settings. Silver Spring, MD; 2010.
38. American College of Obstetrics and Gynecology. Committee Opinion No. 507: Human Trafficking. 2011;118(3):767–70.
39. Institute of Medicine, National Research Council. Confronting commercial sexual exploitation and sex trafficking of minors in the United States. Washington, D.C: National Academies Press; 2013.
40. American Medical Women's Association. Position paper on the sex trafficking of women and girls in the United States. Washington, D.C.; 2014.
41. American Academy of Pediatrics. Annual Leadership Forum attendees vote on Top 10 resolutions [Internet]. 2014. Retrieved from: http://www.aappublications.org/content/early/2014/03/20/aapnews.20140320-1.
42. American Academy of Family Physicians. Summary of actions: 2015 national conference of constituency leaders, resolution 2006. 2015. Retrieved from http://www.aafp.org/dam/AAFP/documents/events/alf_ncsc/business/Org%20and%20Fin_2016.pdf.
43. American Medical Association. Physicians response to victims of human trafficking [Internet]. 2015. 65-66 Retrieved from https://policysearch.amaassn.org/policyfinder/detail/H-65.966?uri=%2FAMADoc%2FHOD.xml-0-5095.xml.
44. Schwarz C, Unruh E, Cronin K, Evans-Simpson S, Britton H, Ramaswamy M. Human trafficking identification and service provision in the medical and social service sectors. Health Hum Rights. 2016;18:181–92.
45. Domoney J, Howard LM, Abas M, Broadbent M, Oram S. Mental health service responses to human trafficking: a qualitative study of professionals' experiences of providing care. BMC Psychiatry. 2015;15:289.
46. Grace AM, Lippert S, Collins K, Pineda N, Tolani A, Walker R, et al. Educating health care professionals on human trafficking. Pediatr Emerg Care. 2014;30:856–61.
47. Ross C, Dimitrova S, Howard LM, Dewey M, Zimmerman C, Oram S. Human trafficking and health: a cross-sectional survey of NHS professionals' contact with victims of human trafficking. BMJ Open. 2015;5:e008682.
48. Beck ME, Lineer MM, Melzer-Lange M, Simpson P, Nugent M, Rabbitt A. Medical providers' understanding of sex trafficking and their experience with at-risk patients. Pediatrics. 2015;135:e895–902.
49. Ahn R, Alpert EJ, Purcell G, Konstantopoulos WM, McGahan A, Cafferty E, et al. Human trafficking: review of educational resources for health professionals. Am J Prev Med. 2013;44:283–9.
50. Stoklosa H, Miller CL, Duke G, Chisolm-Straker M. A framework for the development of healthcare provider education programs on human trafficking part one: experts. J Hum Traffick. 2019:1–22.
51. Chisolm-Straker M, Miller CL, Duke G, Stoklosa H. A framework for the development of healthcare provider education programs on human trafficking part two: survivors. J Hum Traffick. 2019:1–15.
52. Bohnert CA, Calhoun AW, Mittel OF. Taking up the mantle of human trafficking education: who should be responsible? AMA J Ethics. 2017;19:35–42.

Chapter 21
Building Resilience and Fostering Prevention

Mary Steigerwald, Wendy Barnes, and Amy Williamson

Introduction

According to the Federal Trafficking Victims Protection Act of 2000, with reauthorization in 2017, sex trafficking is defined as "a commercial sex act that is induced by force, fraud, or coercion, or in which the person induced to perform such an act has not attained 18 years of age" [1]. As a major health issue, it affects individuals, families, communities, and societies around the world [2]. Trafficked persons experience injuries, infections, untreated chronic disease, and mental health problems. Although health-care professionals come into contact with victims and survivors of sex trafficking, few recognize them, resulting in potentially significant health consequences for this vulnerable population [3].

The role of the health-care professional goes far beyond screening and medical care. Clinicians, educators, advocates, researchers, and health-care providers are uniquely positioned to engage in broader preventive efforts that target populations across the risk continuum, as well as to guide and help build resilience within survivors [4–6].

M. Steigerwald (✉)
Departments of Women, Children and Psychiatry, Dignity Health, Phoenix, AZ, USA

W. Barnes
Human Trafficking Response Program, Dignity Health, Seattle, WA, USA

A. Williamson
University of Arizona, Dignity Health Medical Group and Phoenix Children's Hospital, Department of Obstetrics and Gynecology and Pediatric and Adolescent Gynecology, Phoenix, AZ, USA

K. E. Titchen, E. Miller (eds.), *Medical Perspectives on Human Trafficking in Adolescents*, https://doi.org/10.1007/978-3-030-43367-3_21

Building Resilience

Colloquially, resilience is the process of adapting well in the face of adversity, trauma, tragedy, threats, or significant sources of stress. Resilience has been defined as "the capacity to recover from difficulties" or "bouncing back." While most people generally adapt well over time to life-changing situations and stressful conditions, it is resilience that enables one to do so. Resilience is an ongoing process that requires time and effort and ultimately allows trafficked persons to overcome their struggles. For survivors of sex trafficking, recovering from trauma and building resilience may require months, years, and even decades of intensive medical and psychiatric care [7]. Resilience does not mean that a person is exempt from difficulty or distress. Emotional pain and sadness are common in people who have suffered major adversity or trauma in their lives. In fact, the road to resilience is likely to involve considerable emotional distress. Although the research on resilience can guide the development of treatment, resilience rates among survivors of child sexual abuse range between 10% and 53% [4].

Resilience has been studied for many decades with varying definitions, yet a consensus on an operational definition does not exist. Discrepancies also exist in conceptualizations of resilience as a personal trait versus a dynamic process [4]. There is also a growing consensus to consider resilience as a two-dimensional concept that comprises the person's life circumstances and ability to positively adapt. Some researchers believe that resilience must include positive adaptation in a number of areas of life, while others believe that positive adaptation in only one area linked to the adversity under consideration is sufficient. The majority of studies define resilience or adaptive functioning as the absence of psychological symptoms, thereby focusing on relative resilience [4].

As we search for answers about resilience among survivors of sex trafficking, it may be helpful to better understand the dynamic nature of resilience and the contributing factors of recovery.

Commercially sexually exploited (CSE) youth are at high risk for mental health problems, including depression, posttraumatic stress disorder (PTSD), and substance use given their exposure to violence and trauma, as well as difficult and dangerous living situations [6]. Established protective factors associated with resilience following child sexual abuse (CSA) have shown to strengthen the survivors' belief in their future and ability to cope with adverse effects. Strong evidence suggest individual factors such as education, interpersonal and emotional competence, control beliefs, active coping, optimism, family social support, social attachment, and external attribution of blame all aim at attaining positive mental health [4]. Research suggests education to be one of the best established protective factors on an individual level [4]. Educational engagement, plans, motivation, and positive attitude toward learning contributed to resilience in both adolescents and adults. Attachment to family or peers was additionally found to be protective for girls and women [4].

Throughout this chapter, we explore the personal journey of Wendy, a survivor of sex trafficking beginning at the age of 17, and examine what inspired coping, healing, and resilience throughout her life. Her personal experience provides insight into research findings of the protective factors that were most beneficial through her healing process.

> For almost thirteen years I lived with my trafficker, and as many as ten other girls and women who were also under his control. The relationships we formed in this horrible environment were intense, close, and bonded. I've always said that the bond created by shared torture and pain is stronger than the bond of love. We were beaten, we cried, and we had to make enough money so 'we' wouldn't get into trouble. Six of us lived together in this environment for more than five years, during which we shared a connection that was deeper than most people can imagine, a connection built on our shared experience of torture and abuse: abuse that involved drugs and what we thought to be 'love'.
>
> After many years of rebuilding myself and my life, I was able to articulate the reasons we stayed, and was able to describe the painful and difficult journey of integrating into the 'real world,' as I like to call it. Over the years, I have missed my 'friends,' the other girls who cried with me, suffered with me. We comforted each other for so long that we will always be a part of each other. I hope they are also doing well, although I know that they were probably experiencing the same dilemmas and life challenges that I was. Over the two decades, since I escaped the trafficking situation, I have spoken to most of them from time to time. Sadly, the one thing that remains constant is that I am truly the only one that has really made it out. The girls who shared my horror continue to struggle with drug addiction, are in and out of jail, continue to engage in bad relationships, and overall, are not doing well at all.
>
> People ask me what made the difference for me, why was I able to create a life worth living and the others weren't? The simple answer is: My Mother's Couch – the tangible symbol of her undying acceptance and love for me. I could always come home and she would always love me no matter what. That has been my go-to answer to the question, but, honestly, the real reason would fill a book.
>
> —Wendy

Foster Healing

A published peer review of intervention programs for CSEC and adolescents and the programs' effectiveness to foster healing within this population found that despite differences in approach or delivery, most programs appear to foster healing, with very few reporting negative outcomes to some degree [8]. It is important to note that many intervention programs had limited outcome data and did not contain validated measures. However, the findings did highlight the critical role clinicians play in the identification and support of this vulnerable population in order to promote evidence-informed, holistic health in a nonjudgmental care environment. A key tactic for how frontline practitioners approach this topic may include universal education about violence and routine screening of children and adolescents for commercial sexual exploitation rather than relying on the assumptions of who may be affected by this type of abuse [8].

My ‘rescue’ came in the form of a two-year prison sentence. While in prison, I went through a year-long drug and alcohol treatment program, which tragically is no longer in existence at this prison. I think of that time as my needed ‘time out’ from life. I don’t recall any substantial emotional growth during that time, but I did receive many compliments from the counselors in the program. They told me they saw something promising within me and that the only way I would ever end up back in prison again was if I did not learn to ask for help when I needed it. These compliments from people I respected planted a seed, but as we know, seeds need water and light.

—Wendy

Although several approaches have been recognized for the treatment of sexual abuse in children and adolescents, no specific evidence-based treatments have been identified for victims/survivors of child sex trafficking or CSE youth. The most studied treatment for youth with PTSD is cognitive behavioral therapy (CBT). CBT has effectively treated trauma in young adults, including exposure to community violence and sexual trauma. CBT focuses on the interconnectedness of thoughts, behaviors, emotions, and physiologic responses. CBT was delivered to sexually exploited girls in the Democratic Republic of the Congo during a randomized controlled trial [9]. The outcomes demonstrated a reduction in trauma symptoms, decreased anxiety and depression, and improved prosocial behavior. This treatment was delivered in a group setting by trained facilitators, without a mental health background, who adapted the treatment for the girls’ culture. The study suggested part of the success and positive outcomes included the support of peers who had experienced similar trauma. It is believed that CBT can be culturally adapted for commercially sexually exploited and sex trafficked youth in the United States. There are other potential evidenced-based modalities that could be adapted for sex trafficked youth, including multisystemic therapy (MST), a model originally designed to treat antisocial behavior. MST utilizes a natural approach to treatment and engages multiple systems to facilitate care of the patient, including the patient, friends, family, school, and other advocates [6]. Dialectical behavior therapy (DBT), which has been used to treat victims of domestic violence and childhood sexual abuse, may also be beneficial to prevent self-harm and maladaptive coping mechanism. The cornerstone of DBT involves learning skills of distress tolerance, mindfulness, and emotional regulation [6]. DBT usually includes one weekly individual session of psychodynamically oriented therapy provided by a therapist with extensive specialty training. Psychodynamic therapy encourages exploration and discussion of the full range of a patient’s emotions. Psychodynamic therapists work to identify and explore recurring themes and patterns in patients’ thoughts, feelings, self-concept, relationships, and life experiences with a goal to help patients free themselves from the bonds of past experience in order to live more fully in the present [10]. [See Chap. 9 for more on psychology, psychiatry and human trafficking.]

Often youth become involved in sexual exploitation before getting a high school diploma and learning life skills. Several successful interventions identify the need for a holistic approach to treatment beyond medical and mental health treatment, including supportive services, education, life skills, and job training [6]. It is important for providers to practice a multidisciplinary, team-based holistic approach and incorporate social service agencies that can offer financial, social, legal, and immigration support, as well as support basic daily needs.

> When I was released from prison, I still held the beliefs my trafficker had instilled in me: 'I am nothing. No one else will ever care about me. I am stupid and dumb and I will never make it in the world without him.' My job was to change that script. Although it seemed overwhelming, I was determined to do it. I don't know why I ultimately succeeded where others cannot. I honestly do not feel that there is anything within me genetically, or otherwise, that would have written the genuine script for my life.
>
> Thirty days after my release from prison I was accepted into a two-year transitional living program for women within the criminal justice system with an open case with Child Protective Services (CPS). Some of the women had their children with them in the program and others, like me, did not. The court had permanently removed all three of my children from my care and permanently severed my rights, even though the court saw something in me that inspired them to give me a chance. In this program, there were three on-site counselors who worked Monday through Friday, 8 a.m. to 5 p.m. Each counselor's approach was very different from the others, and each had valuable impact on my ability to learn how to live. One counselor was abrupt; no excuses allowed. You follow the rules no matter what! Another counselor was the complete opposite, frequently asking about my feelings and always available when I needed someone to talk to. The third counselor was more of a case manager, making sure I went to appointments on time and handled any household or living issues that arose. All three of the counselors influenced my development and I needed all three disciplines. The program taught us how to go shopping, how to clean our house, how to talk with people, how to make it to appointments on time, and how to dress appropriately.
>
> There were many rules! Not only the program rules but also the rules that governed my four-year parole and probation. Although there were so many rules, I also understood that these rules would help keep me safe. The more I understood the 'why' behind a rule, the more apt I was to follow it without opposition. My first parole officer was not like the typical parole officer; he actually saw me as a person. Just as the counselors had, he saw something within me that made him believe in me. He believed that I would be successful in changing my life. I couldn't understand what he saw; I only know he was nice and I respected him. I was not as confident as he was about my changes, but I didn't want to be the one to prove him wrong to his fellow parole officers, so I grasped onto his belief that I would be successful and I used that as my motivation to keep moving forward.
>
> I somehow found myself enrolling in community college nineteen days after I was released from prison. This was not something that I had planned. At that point, I had no plan for what I was going to do. All I knew at the time was that no one would ever hire me without an education and that I needed to do something to keep parole officers and correction counselors happy. When they appeared happy, then I felt I was doing something right. And if I did enough thing right, maybe this would lead me on the road to success.
>
> —Wendy

Despite the many challenges, physical health needs, psychosocial adversities, and mental health complexities, many commercially sexually exploited youth like Wendy have successfully exited sex trafficking and developed resilience. Multiple lines of research have identified a common set of factors that predisposed children to positive outcomes in the face of significant adversity, including the availability of at least one stable, caring, and supportive relationship between a child and the important adult(s) in his or her life. Although these relationships usually begin in the family, they can also include others such as neighbors, teachers, social workers, or coaches, among others [11].

Fostering Prevention

Monica was 16 years old. Her mother was working two jobs and Monica was in charge of watching her 14-year old brother at night. She started a new school, where she met a man who was older, 35, and was very attentive and interested in her. Her 14-year-old brother noticed that every night at midnight, a taxi would pick her up. Her brother took a photo of the taxi that picked her up and sent the photo to a VICE detective. She was being trafficked and the police were able to stop her victimization and arrest the trafficker thanks to her younger brother.

—as shared by Dominique Roe-Sepowitz

Monica's story highlights the fact that any adolescent can be trafficked and anyone, even a 14-year-old younger brother, can help prevent it. Preventive strategies are key in addressing this issue. The prevention of sex trafficking must be addressed on multiple levels. Prevention strategies include everything from government programs and legislation intended to deter trafficking to educational programs that alert communities, families, and health-care providers to be aware of the problems and the dangers. Linking survivors to critical medical and psychological care, legal assistance, and appropriate social service support will provide them with protection and support needed for healing and empowerment [7].

This section is intended to highlight some of the successful prevention strategies that are currently in place throughout communities in the United States. Prevention must also address revictimization. Adolescents who have been trafficked are much more likely to be victimized again. They may require specialized care that is designed to address the trauma that they have experienced.

It is also important to highlight laws in place, both nationally and internationally, as they provide a framework to structure prevention strategies.

International Legal Efforts

Under the auspices of the United Nations (UN), an international governmental body authored the Global Compact for Safe, Orderly and Regular Migration in 2018. One of the objectives detailed in this document is to "prevent, combat and eradicate trafficking in persons in the context of international migration." This document supports an earlier UN document, the Protocol to Prevent, Suppress and Punish Trafficking in Persons, Especially Women and Children, also known as the Trafficking Protocol or UN TIP Protocol; it is one of the three Palermo Protocols and was adapted by the UN in the year 2000. Law enforcement and other authorities are encouraged to work together by exchanging information that allowed the successful prosecution of perpetrators. The UN's recognition of human trafficking as a major human rights issue and the development of the Global Compact and the Trafficking Protocol provide all countries and governments a legal framework to develop laws to protect human rights. Furthermore, the documents state that victims of trafficking should receive appropriate housing, counseling and information, medical and psychological assistance, and employment and educational opportunities [12, 13] (see Chap. 3 for more about human rights and trafficking of adolescents).

National Legal Efforts

In the United States, the Trafficking Victims Protection Act (TVPA) was initially authorized in 2000 and was the first federal law to address human trafficking. This law has been reauthorized and is now known as the Trafficking Victims Protection Reauthorization Act of 2017 (TVPRA). The law focuses on prevention, protection, and prosecution. Most importantly it defines trafficking survivors as victims, not criminals [6].

Two additional federal acts are now in place to aid and improve victim services. The first is the Justice for Victims of Trafficking Act (JVTA) of 2015, S. 178 (114th), which seeks to improve the response to trafficking in the United States. An Advisory Council on Human Trafficking was created and required the formation of a victim's fund to provide grants for prevention programs and mandate additional training requirements for first responders. In particular, the JVTA amended the Runaway and Homeless Youth Act (RHYA) to include adolescents who are trafficked in the list of individuals who are eligible for services under the RHYA.

The Preventing Sex Trafficking and Strengthening Families Act of 2014 is designed to reduce the incidence of sex trafficking among children involved in the foster care system. Individual states are charged to develop procedures and policies to screen and identify service needs for children in the foster care system. States are also *encouraged* to adopt procedures and policies in regard to protecting *all* youth under age 26 at risk for trafficking regardless of their involvement in foster care. State welfare agencies are required to report the number of children involved in sex trafficking under their care to the U.S. Department of Health and Human Services, which then reports these data to Congress. A key purpose for collecting and reporting these data is to provide services for adolescents who have been trafficked and to develop protocols for locating missing and runaway children through the National Center for Missing and Exploited Children [14].

Education

Educating law enforcement, first responders, health-care professionals, teachers, parents, communities, and youth about the dangers of sex trafficking may go a long way to preventing human trafficking in the first place. The end of this chapter contains some key educational programs and resources (see Chap. 20 for more on education and human trafficking).

Health-Care Provider Tools and Education

Education programs and tools have been created to assist health-care providers. It is well known that sex trafficked victims and survivors present to both emergency rooms and primary care physician offices with medical issues. Most often victims of sex trafficking are not identified even when seeking medical care. In an effort to build provider knowledge, programs such as Physicians Against the Trafficking of Humans (PATH), Human Trafficking 101, and the Provide Privacy, Educate, Ask, Respect, and Respond (PEARR) Tool were developed by health-care organizations. See Fig. 21.1 and Table 21.1 at the end of this chapter for the PEARR Tool and a list of references.

Missed Opportunity

> I met my trafficker, Greg, when I was fifteen and in high school. He was a year older than me and was charming and popular. He took the time to make me feel special; something that was missing in my life from my parents and other adults. I was completely smitten, and it didn't take much for him to convince me that we would live 'happily ever after together.' That was truly all I had ever wanted: someone to love me forever. By the time I was sixteen, I was pregnant with his baby. At this point, I saw him as my boyfriend and future husband. Looking back now, I can see that I was experiencing the 'grooming stage'; slow, methodical and intentional manipulation of a person to a point where they can be victimized.
>
> When I realized I was pregnant, I visited a local OB/GYN. I was extremely frightened, but I knew from my upbringing that my feelings did not matter. I took to heart the adage that 'children are to be seen and not heard,' so I kept quiet and did not volunteer any information to the medical staff. I answered their questions and listened carefully to everything the doctor and nurse told me. By that time, Greg had been emotionally abusive several times; but at the time, the only information I had about domestic violence was what I had learned from watching The Burning Bed (1984) with Farrah Fawcett. Since the slight emotional abuse I was experiencing from my 'boyfriend' was not depicted in the movie, I thought that the things Greg said to me were 'normal' and that the only reason he was mean sometimes was because I had caused a problem and it was my fault.
>
> The pregnancy-related visits to the medical clinic would have been the perfect opportunity for the nurse or doctor to provide me with education on domestic violence and sex trafficking. I likely presented with some of the signs of an abused person. Privacy was not an issue; my mother, not Greg, typically took me to my appointments, and she rarely went into the exam room with me. The nurse and physician had many opportunities to discuss domestic violence and sex trafficking with me and to share brochures that included resources and a vision of what success would look like to a person in my position.
>
> When I was six months pregnant, I got a phone call from the nurse, who explained that one of my lab tests had come back positive for gonorrhea. I was shocked, I felt dirty and disgusting. I was completely embarrassed and was silently trying to figure out how to get up the nerve to ask the nurse how I got the disease. After a few moments, her voice brought me back to the present. "Wendy, Wendy? Are you still there?"
>
> Thoughts were racing through my head. I couldn't possibly have gotten gonorrhea from the father of my baby! I assumed that I must have contracted gonorrhea from a one-time sex encounter I had before I knew Greg. I must have had it this entire time! But then why wouldn't it have been detected at the beginning of my pregnancy? I asked the nurse if I had

PEARR Tool

Trauma-Informed Approach to Victim Assistance in Health Care Settings

In partnership with HEAL Trafficking and Pacific Survivor Center, Dignity Health developed this tool, the "PEARR Tool", to guide physicians, social workers, nurses, and other health care professionals on how to provide **trauma-informed assistance** to patients who are at high risk of abuse, neglect, or violence. The PEARR Tool is based on a **universal education approach**, which focuses on educating patients about abuse, neglect, or violence prior to, or in lieu of, screening patients with questions.

The goal is to have an informative and normalizing, yet developmentally- and culturally-appropriate, conversation with patients in order to create a context for them to share their own experiences.

A double asterisk ** indicates points at which this conversation may end. Refer to the double asterisk ** at the bottom of this page for additional steps. The patient's immediate needs (e.g., emergency medical care) should be addressed before use of this tool.

P – Provide Privacy

1. Discuss sensitive topics **alone** and in **safe, private setting** (ideally private room with closed doors). If companion refuses to be separated, then this may be an indicator of abuse, neglect, or violence.** Strategies to speak with patient alone: State requirement for private exam or need for patient to be seen alone for radiology, urine test, etc.

   Note: Companions are not appropriate interpreters, regardless of communication abilities. If patient indicates preference to use companion as interpreter, see your facility's policies for further guidance.**

   Note: Explain **limits of confidentiality** (i.e., mandated reporting requirements) before beginning any sensitive discussion; however, do not discourage person from disclosing victimization. Patient should feel in control of all disclosures. Mandated reporting includes requirements to report concerns of abuse, neglect, or violence to internal staff and/or to external agencies.

E – Educate

2. Educate patient in manner that is **nonjudgmental** and **normalizes** sharing of information. Example: "I educate all of my patients about [fill in the blank] because violence is so common in our society, and violence has a big impact on our health, safety, and well-being." **Use a brochure or safety card** to review information about abuse, neglect, or violence, and offer brochure/card to patient. [Ideally, this brochure/card will include information about resources (e.g., local service providers, national hotlines)]. Example: "Here are some brochures to take with you in case this is ever an issue for you, **or someone you know.**" If patient declines materials, then respect patient's decision.**

A – Ask

3. Allow time for discussion with patient. Example: "Is there anything you'd like to share with me? Do you feel like anyone is hurting your health, safety, or well-being?"** If available and when appropriate, use **evidence-based tools** to screen patient for abuse, neglect, or violence.**

   Note: All women of reproductive age should be intermittently screened for intimate partner violence (USPSTF Grade B).

4. If there are indicators of victimization, **ASK** about concerns. Example: "I've noticed [insert risk factor/indicator] and I'm concerned for your health, safety, and well-being. You don't have to share details with me, but I'd like to connect you with resources if you're in need of assistance. Would you like to speak with [insert advocate/service provider]? If not, you can let me know anytime."**

   Note: **Limit questions** to only those needed to determine patient's safety, to connect patient with resources (e.g., trained victim advocates), and to guide your work (e.g., perform medical exam).

   USPSTF = US Preventive Services Task Force

R R – Respect and Respond

5. If patient denies victimization or declines assistance, then **respect patient's wishes.** If you have **concerns about patient's safety**, offer hotline card or other information about resources that can assist in event of emergency (e.g., local shelter, crisis hotline).** Otherwise, if patient accepts/requests assistance with accessing services, then **provide personal introduction** to local victim advocate/service provider; or, **arrange private setting** for patient to call hotline:

   National Domestic Violence Hotline, 1-800-799-SAFE (7233);
   National Sexual Assault Hotline, 1-800-656-HOPE (4673);
   National Human Trafficking Hotline, 1-888-373-7888 **

** Report **safety concerns** to appropriate staff/departments (e.g., nurse supervisor, security). Also, **REPORT** risk factors/indicators as required or permitted by law/regulation, and continue **trauma-informed** health services. Whenever possible, **schedule follow-up appointment** to continue building rapport and to monitor patient's safety/well-being.

PEARR Tool – Risk Factors, Indicators, and Resources

Child Abuse and Neglect

Risk factors include (not limited to): Concerns of domestic violence (DV) in home; parents/guardians exhibiting mental health or substance use disorders; parents/guardians who are overly stressed; parents/guardians involved in criminal activity; presence of non-biological, transient caregivers in home.

Potential indicators of victimization include (not limited to): Slower-than-normal development, failure to thrive, unusual interaction with parent, signs of mental health disorders [e.g., depression, post-traumatic stress disorder (PTSD), self-harm], sudden difficulty in school, medical or physical neglect, sudden changes in behavior, new or unusual fears/anxiety, unexplained injuries (e.g., bruises, fractures, burns – especially in protected areas of child's body), injuries in pre-mobile infants, sexually transmitted infections (STIs).

For additional information, *see Child Welfare Information Gateway: www.childwelfare.gov*

Abuse/Neglect of Vulnerable Adults (e.g., elder and dependent adults)

Risk factors include (not limited to): Concerns of mental health or substance use disorder with caregiver, caregiver exhibits hostile behavior, lack of preparation/training for caregiver, caregiver assumed responsibilities at early age, caregiver exposed to abuse as child.

Potential indicators of victimization include (not limited to): Disappearing from contact; signs of bruising or welts on the skin; burns, cuts, lacerations, puncture wounds, sprains, fractures, dislocations, internal injuries or vomiting; wearing torn, stained, bloody clothing; appearing disheveled, in soiled clothing; appearing hungry, malnourished.

For additional information, *see National Association of Adult Protective Services (NAPSA): napsa-now.org; Centers for Disease Control and Prevention (CDC): cdc.gov/violenceprevention/elderabuse/index.html*

Domestic Violence/Intimate Partner Violence (IPV)

DV/IPV can affect anyone of any age, gender, race, or sexual orientation. **Risk factors** include (not limited to): Low self-esteem, low income, low academic achievement, young age, aggressive/delinquent behavior as youth, heavy alcohol/drug use, depression, suicide attempts, isolation, anger, and hostility.

Potential indicators of victimization include (not limited to): Injuries that result from abuse or assault, e.g., signs of strangulation, bruises, burns, broken bones; psychological conditions such as anxiety, depression, sleep disturbances; sexual and reproductive health issues, e.g., STIs, unintended pregnancy.

For additional information, *see National DV Hotline: thehotline.org; CDC: cdc.gov/violenceprevention/intimatepartnerviolence/index.html*

Sexual Violence

Sexual violence crosses all age, economic, cultural, gender, sexual, racial, and social lines. Some statistics from Rape Abuse & Incest National Network (RAINN): More than 300,000 persons are victimized annually; ages 12-34 are the highest risk years. Female college students (ages 18-24) are three times more likely than women in general to experience sexual violence. One in 33 American men have experienced an attempted or completed rape. And, 21% of transgender, genderqueer, noncomforming (TGQN) college students have been sexually assaulted.

Potential indicators of victimization include (not limited to): STIs, pregnancy, depression, PTSD.

For additional information, *see RAINN: rainn.org; CDC: cdc.gov/violenceprevention/sexualviolence/index.html*

Human Trafficking (e.g., labor and sex trafficking)

Although human trafficking crosses all age, economic, cultural, gender, sexual orientation, racial, and social lines, traffickers often target persons in situations of vulnerability. **Risk factors** include (not limited to): Running away or homelessness (particularly for youth), history of interpersonal abuse or violence, involvement in commercial sex industry, minority/immigrant status.

Potential indicators of victimization include (not limited to): Accompanied by controlling companion; inconsistent history; medical or physical neglect; and submissive, fearful, hypervigilant, or uncooperative behavior.

For additional information, *see National HT Hotline: humantraffickinghotline.org*

As defined by the Substance Abuse and Mental Health Services Administration (SAMHSA), **a trauma-informed approach** includes an understanding of trauma and an awareness of the impact it can have across settings, services, and populations. This includes understanding how trauma can impact patients, families, communities, and the professionals attempting to assist them.

SAMHSA describes the guiding principles of a trauma-informed approach as follows: safety; trustworthiness and transparency; peer support and mutual self-help; collaboration and mutuality; empowerment, voice, and choice; and consideration of cultural, historical, and gender issues.

To learn more, *please see SAMHSA's Concept of Trauma and Guidance for a Trauma-Informed Approach: https://store.samhsa.gov/system/files/sma14-4884.pdf*

For more information, visit dignityhealth.org/human-trafficking-response

Dignity Health. Pacific Survivor Center. HEAL

Fig. 21.1 PEARR Tool: trauma-informed approach to victim assistance in health-care settings

PEARR Tool – **Contact List of Resources and Reporting Agencies**

Local, Regional, and State Resources/Agencies

County Child Welfare Agency:

County Welfare Agency for Vulnerable Adults:

Sexual Assault Response Team (SART) Center or Child Advocacy Center (CAC):

Local Law Enforcement Agency:

Local FBI Office:

Local DV/IPV Shelter – Program:

Local Runaway/Homeless Shelter:

Local Immigrant/Refugee Organization:

Local LGBTQ Resource/Program:

National Agencies, Advocates, Service Providers

National Human Trafficking Hotline: 1-888-373-7888 (888-3737-888)

National Domestic Violence Hotline: 1-800-799-SAFE (7233)

National Sexual Assault Hotline: 1-800-656-HOPE (4673)

National Teen Dating Abuse Hotline: 1-866-331-9474

National Runaway Safeline for Runaway and Homeless Youth: 1-800-RUNAWAY (786-2929)

StrongHearts Native Helpline: 1-844-7NATIVE (762-8483)

National Suicide Prevention Lifeline: 1-800-273-8255

Notes

The PEARR Tool was developed by Dignity Health, in partnership with HEAL Trafficking and Pacific Survivor Center, with support from Dignity Health Foundation.

Dignity Health. PACIFIC SURVIVOR CENTER HEAL

Fig. 21.1 (continued)

been tested at the beginning of my pregnancy, and she confirmed I did not have gonorrhea when I was first pregnant.

Then I asked how would I have gotten it? I didn't have sex with anyone but Greg. I don't understand how I could have this now, but not when I was first pregnant. The nurse remained silent, perhaps waiting for the reality to hit me—the reality that the only way I could have contracted gonorrhea was from Greg. Once it dawned on me, I still needed confirmation from her.

Wait…, if I didn't have it when I first started seeing you, and I haven't had sex with anyone else besides Greg, then that would mean that Greg had sex with someone else and transferred gonorrhea to me – is that right? The nurse confirmed that if I had not had sex with anyone else, then it was transferred to me through Greg. The reality that Greg had been cheating on me was a hard pill to swallow. I automatically felt that it was my fault, that I must not be good enough for him. The nurse was quiet, giving me time to process this difficult news. After a few moments, she asked me if I was okay. I played it off like I was okay, even though I was not. I asked her how I could get rid of the disease and if my baby was okay. The nurse explained that the baby was fine and that she would order a prescription for both of us that would eliminate the infection.

I took the pills as prescribed, as did Greg. Looking back, it seems like another golden opportunity for the medical staff to ask me about abuse, but I don't remember the doctor or nurse ever asking me about it or addressing the issue again.

—Wendy

Nurses and physicians have a unique opportunity to prevent or intervene in human trafficking by educating and listening to their patients. The circumstances under which a 16-year-old girl gets pregnant may be suspect [15]. Victims of human

Table 21.1 Resources for preventing human trafficking

Prevention of trafficking resources		
Resources	Description	Website
Polaris	Polaris is an organization dedicated to helping trafficking survivors, accumulating public databases on human trafficking, turning this knowledge into action plans, and involving law enforcement and businesses to prevent human trafficking. In 2007, Polaris developed the National Human Trafficking Hotline and the BeFree (233733) text. This 24/7 toll-free hotline can provide support, make referrals for anti-trafficking services, and accept tips. During 2017 the hotline received over 26,000 calls.	https://humantraffickinghotline.org/mission
TRUST	Training and Resources United to Stop Trafficking (TRUST) is an agency that was formed to coordinate anti-trafficking efforts in Arizona. TRUST encourages communication between service providers, law enforcement, media, health-care providers, and the legal system. This organization provides centralized resources for education including research papers, documentaries, and news articles. They also provide local training programs designed to raise awareness and promote best practices for support services related to the issue of commercial sexual exploitation of children (CSEC).	trustaz.org/about-trust.html
Prevention Project	There are multiple programs that are designed to be used to educate teachers and provide programs in schools. One very successful program is the Prevention Project. The program was designed by the Richmond Justice Initiative, a nonprofit organization. This program has been implemented in eight states within the United States, and according to their 2017–2018 impact statement reports, they have reached over 9000 students. The mission of the Prevention Project is to eradicate human trafficking. The program educates children and adolescents about the dangers of trafficking and teaches young people character building and leadership skills so that young people will not be vulnerable to the manipulation of the traffickers. One goal includes empowering students to become leaders, so in turn, the students become part of the solution. In one survey, 86% of the students who completed the program reported they would know how to help, if presented with a trafficking situation [9, 10].	https://www.prevention-project.org

(continued)

Table 21.1 (continued)

Prevention of trafficking resources		
Resources	Description	Website
Project Concern International	Project Concern International (PCI) has a program aimed at preventing and raising awareness surrounding human trafficking. One aspect of their program involves empowerment and prevention. PCI developed after-school programs, such as Girls Only! designed for adolescents ages 8 to 12. These classes involve frank discussions regarding real-life situations and threats, with a goal to teach adolescents how to make positive life choices and avoid manipulation from sex traffickers.	https://www.pciglobal.org/us-initiatives/#localpartners
PROTECT	Prevention Organized To Educate Children on Trafficking (PROTECT) is a program based in California. In January 2018, public schools in California were required to educate students on sex trafficking as part of health education. This education was mandated through the California State Human Trafficking Prevention Education and Training Act (AB 1227). PROTECT focuses on training educators and students, as well as training the key county stakeholders in California. PROTECT is currently offered in nine counties within California, as well as Nevada and Utah.	https://protectnow.org
The Ugly Truth Campaign	The Ugly Truth Campaign is founded on the premise that communities need to understand both the social and economic pressures that drive people into the sex trade and the suffering that the victims of trafficking endure. If trafficking goes unrecognized, the communities will lack the outrage and determination to eliminate the billion-dollar sex trade industry. This campaign challenges the glamorization and myths of the sex trade.	http://www.uglytruth.org/the-campaign
CEASE	Centre to End All Sexual Exploitation (CEASE), a Canadian program, has a Sex Trade Offender Program (STOP), which offers a post-court diversion program. CEASE works under the premise that without demand, there would be no sex trafficking industry. This has also been known as "john school." The program is intended for those who have been charged with trying to purchase sex services for the first time. These programs can also be required as part of probation. The program is a daylong course where the participants hear from survivors, parents, and community members about the negative impact of purchasing sex.	http://www.ceasenow.org

(continued)

Table 21.1 (continued)

Prevention of trafficking resources		
Resources	Description	Website
PATH	Physicians Against the Trafficking of Humans (PATH) is an organization that was founded by the American Medical Women's Association (AMWA) in 2012. PATH has developed programs and videos that are meant to educate health-care providers on trafficking. Their website is a resource for health-care providers, including a toolkit, screening tools, and educational materials. AMWA-PATH developed a free four-hour continuing medical education (CME) accredited training program entitled Learn to Identify and Fight Trafficking (LIFT), which provides critical information for health-care providers.	https://www.amwa-doc.org/our-work/initiatives/human-trafficking https://www.doc-path.org
Additional information and resources		
National Human Trafficking Hotline	1-888-373-7888	
PEARR Tool	PEARR stands for Provide Privacy, Educate, Ask, Respect, and Respond. The PEARR Tool provides a trauma-informed approach to victim assistance in a health-care setting. This tool is helpful in educating hospital staff on ways to provide patient education and to offer assistance in a trauma-informed, compassionate manner. This tool was developed by Dignity Health in partnership with HEAL Trafficking and Pacific Survivor Center (Fig. 21.1).	Figure 21.1

trafficking may present for medical attention under a variety of circumstances, such as following an acute sexual assault, or for treatment of a physical injury, overdose (intentional or unintentional), for an acute medical or psychiatric condition, or management of a pregnancy [16]. Every high-risk patient should be educated on various types of violence, including sex trafficking and intimate partner violence. The PEARR Tool (Fig. 21.1) can help make this education a routine part of the examination.

> In my case, I was not trafficked until after my baby was born. I was so dependent emotionally on my boyfriend–trafficker, looking back I honestly can't say that education would have prevented my sex trafficking. However, my first encounter with being trafficked was so traumatizing that I do believe that if I had been given the knowledge of what was really happening to me, I might very well have reached out for help instead of staying in that situation for over a decade.
>
> —Wendy

Business Partnering

Involving local businesses in prevention is key as well. The surrounding community benefits when businesses commit to preventing sex trafficking: if victims do not have safe employment alternatives to trafficking, they will be more likely to return to the life [17]. Therefore, identifying businesses that are willing to employ victims/survivors of sex trafficking in a safe environment may help prevent reentry into "the life" (a term often used to describe the subculture of sex trafficking).

Hotels have joined forces with Polaris to help combat human trafficking. Businesses are training victims for careers in the hospitality industry and creating charity programs to aid victims in need of emergency shelter [18].

Streetlight USA

Streetlight USA is a therapeutic group home that provides residential, trauma-informed care for adolescents that have been commercially sexually exploited. Streetlight began in 2008 and to date has served over 1000 girls. This facility provides emergency housing and crisis planning as well as a long-term home through the age of 18. Teens receive support and faith-based counseling and mentoring and education at an on-campus school [19].

Fostering Prevention Requires Community Support

The prevention of sex trafficking in adolescents is an overwhelming topic that requires input from multiple members of society. We need the help of politicians, attorneys, health-care professionals, social workers, educators, parents, and business leaders in order to form an organized, coordinated approach to the problem. Together, we can prevent youth from becoming involved in the sex trade and can help those who are already involved to leave the life and lead healthy and fulfilling lives.

References

1. United States Department of State. Trafficking in persons report [Internet]. U.S. Department of State; 2019. Available from: https://www.state.gov/wp-content/uploads/2019/01/282798.pdf.
2. Greenbaum VJ, Dodd M, McCracken C. A short screening tool to identify victims of child sex trafficking in the health care setting. Pediatr Emerg Care. 2018;34:33–7.
3. Barnes W. In: SDJ F, editor. And life continues: sex trafficking and my journey to freedom: CreateSpace Independent Publishing Platform; 2015.

4. Domhardt M, Münzer A, Fegert JM, Goldbeck L. Resilience in survivors of child sexual abuse: a systematic review of the literature. Trauma Violence Abuse. 2015;16:476–93.
5. Greenbaum VJ, Titchen K, Walker-Descartes I, Feifer A, Rood CJ, Fong H-F. Multi-level prevention of human trafficking: the role of health care professionals. Prev Med. 2018;114:164–7.
6. Ijadi-Maghsoodi R, Cook M, Barnert ES, Gaboian S, Bath E. Understanding and responding to the needs of commercially sexually exploited youth: recommendations for the mental health provider. Child Adolesc Psychiatr Clin N Am. 2016;25:107–22.
7. Stoklosa H, Grace AM, Littenberg N. Medical education on human trafficking. AMA J Ethics. 2015;17:914–21.
8. Moynihan M, Pitcher C, Saewyc E. Interventions that Foster healing among sexually exploited children and adolescents: a systematic review. J Child Sex Abus. 2018;27:403–23.
9. O'Callaghan P, McMullen J, Shannon C, Rafferty H, Black A. A randomized controlled trial of trauma-focused cognitive behavioral therapy for sexually exploited, war-affected Congolese girls. J Am Acad Child Adolesc Psychiatry. 2013;52:359–69.
10. Shedler J. The efficacy of psychodynamic psychotherapy. Am Psychol. 2010;65:98–109.
11. National Scientific Council on the Developing Child. Supportive Relationships and Active Skill-Building Strengthen the Foundations of Resilience: Working Paper No. 13. [Internet]. Center on the Developing Child: Harvard University. 2015 [cited 2019 Sep 30]. Available from: https://developingchild.harvard.edu/resources/supportive-relationships-and-active-skill-building-strengthen-the-foundations-of-resilience/.
12. United Nations Convention against Transnational Organized Crime and the protocols thereto. Palermo, Italy: United Nations Office on Drugs and Crime; 2000.
13. The General Assembly. Modalities for the Intergovernmental Conference to Adopt the Global Compact for Safe, Orderly and Regular Migration [Internet]. United Nations; 2018 Jan. Available from: https://undocs.org/A/Res/72/244.
14. Preventing Sex Trafficking and Strengthening Families Act of 2014 (H.R. 4980). 2014.
15. Reid JA. Entrapment and enmeshment schemes used by sex traffickers. Sex Abus. 2016;28:491–511.
16. Greenbaum VJ. Commercial sexual exploitation and sex trafficking of children in the United States. Curr Probl Pediatr Adolesc Health Care. 2014;44:245–69.
17. National Research Council. Confronting commercial sexual exploitation' ' and sex trafficking of minors in the United States. 2013.
18. Polaris Project. Hotel companies step up to fight human trafficking [Internet]. Polaris. 2019 [cited 2019 Sep 30]. Available from: https://polarisproject.org/blog/2019/01/16/hotel-companies-step-fight-human-trafficking
19. StreetLightUSA [Internet]. 2019 [cited 2019 Sep 30]. Available from: https://www.streetlightusa.org/programs.

Index

K. E. Titchen, E. Miller (eds.), *Medical Perspectives on Human Trafficking in Adolescents*, https://doi.org/10.1007/978-3-030-43367-3